I'm Too Young to Get Old

I'm Too Young to Get Old

Health Care for Women After Forty

JUDITH REICHMAN, M.D.

TIMES 𝔗 BOOKS

RANDOM HOUSE

Library of Congress Cataloging-in-Publication Data
Reichman, Judith.
    I'm too young to get old : health care for women after forty / Judith
Reichman.—1st ed.
      p.   cm.
    Includes bibliographical references and index.
    ISBN 0-8129-2417-7
    1. Middle-aged women—Health and hygiene.   2. Middle-aged women—
Diseases.   3. Menopause.   I. Title.
RA778.R4225   1996
613'.04244—dc20   95-34614

Manufactured in the United States of America

9 8 7 6 5 4 3 2

First Edition

I'm dividing my dedication—like the book—into four parts:

PART I is dedicated to my daughters, Ronit and Anat, whose love has made me feel that my own fertility and pregnancies were the most important events of my life.

PART II is dedicated to my patients, who have taught me more about our hormonal transitions than all the textbooks and articles written by the "experts."

I dedicate PART III to Henri Galina-Rosin, an admired friend who devoted much of her life to advancing women's causes. She died a year ago after a valiant fight against ovarian cancer. Henri, I miss you and I'm devastated that we did not (as yet) have the medical ability to save you.

Finally, I wish to dedicate PART IV to my husband, Gil Cates, whose love and caring have helped me appreciate our maturing psyche and, yes, sex, hormones, and rock and roll . . .

Thank you.

Acknowledgments

I want to thank my patients, who shared their symptoms, concerns, choices, compassion, and intelligence with me. They were the driving force behind this book.

I am very grateful to my literary agents, Maureen and Eric Lasher, who encouraged me to write this book and to broaden its scope. When they suggested that I collaborate with a professional writer, I replied, "I can write my own book; I went to Barnard!" So thank you, Barnard College, for making me (and many other women) feel we can express ourselves.

I want to thank my editor, Betsy Rapoport, and copy editor, Patricia Romanowski, for preventing this book from becoming a thousand-page tome that no one would have wanted to read.

I owe a debt of gratitude to the staff at Cedars-Sinai Medical Center Library, who helped me obtain the articles and medical literature I needed to complete this book.

Thank you, Debbie Craig, for typing and retyping and correctly punctuating so much of what I wrote.

I wish to thank the physicians who were willing to read and offer suggestions on specific chapters: Jim Brenner, M.D., Ron Leuchter, M.D., Mark Surrey, M.D., and Robert Swezey, M.D.

I imposed on my close friendship with a number of women whose opinions I value. My thanks go to Lynne Wasserman, Marcia Brandwynne, and Francis Rothschild for reading the book and telling me when it became too complicated or too wordy.

Thank you to my office staff, who had to cope with my late hours during the last eighteen months.

Lastly, I want to thank my family, who accepted and supported my disappearance into our den—to write "the book." I know I closed the door (and agree this was unfriendly), but it was temporary and now I'm back. We'll just have to stay young—so we can make up for those lost hours. I missed you.

Contents

PART III
Health Concerns After 40:
We Are More Than Our Reproductive Organs

PART IV
Protecting Our Future Health

PROLOGUE
Woman Care: An Uphill Medical Struggle

For many years, I was simply too busy to pay attention to my age. If anything, I tried to appear older. Being young was an added insult to being a woman and did nothing to impress my medical school professors or convince my patients that I was a "real doctor." Residency became a blur of work, study, night calls, being a wife, and motherhood. Despite my understandably drawn appearance, I was still told by my mentors that I looked "too young" to counsel women on their care or to convince them that I was capable of performing their surgery.

During this time, I was trained to regard women's health only as it related to their reproductive function: birth control, fertility, pregnancy, and delivery. Once women no longer needed this type of care, they became surgical candidates, and I was taught the art of hysterectomy and pelvic surgery. We ignored other aspects of midlife woman care, as did the general medical establishment. Research projects involving tens of thousands of patients were scientifically conducted to learn about heart disease, high blood pressure, diabetes, lung cancer, colon cancer, nutrition, exercise, and new medications. The studies were performed almost exclusively on men, since it was felt that women, with their pesky hormones, had too many variables to yield clear results!

I've spent the last twenty years treating women and, of course, getting older. In the midst of giving my patients birth control, helping them get pregnant, delivering their babies, treating their infections, performing their surgeries, and treating hormonal changes from puberty to menopause, I lived my own life as a maturing woman. I had a second child, had surgery, went through a divorce, began a wonderful second marriage, and suddenly realized that I was no longer too young to be that "real doctor," but certainly was too young to get old.

Personally, my fortieth year was possibly the worst year of my life. I had so much to deal with as a newly single woman—the need to support myself and my children (one of whom was a teenager), the breakup of an old relationship and the development of a new one, my medical practice, and, of course, the anticipation of turning 40. I felt that I had not had enough time to be 30 and certainly did not deserve the burden of being 40. I anticipated the rise and fall of my own Fourth Reich! I was wrong. My husband-to-be invited all of my friends to a fortieth birthday party and, despite my threat to sit *shivah* (Jewish mourning for the dead), we celebrated. As I stabilized my life, not only with our marriage but with the knowledge of who I was and what I wanted to become, I realized what a wonderful decade this is. Yes, there may be some changes in our bodies, cycles, and hormones, but they are only changes; they do not represent total physical or mental decline. There is no need to panic or mourn.

My patients have matured with me, and I currently treat far more women over the age of 40 than below it. Many of my patients struggle with their health as they age, while others seem to mature with vibrancy, pleasure, and an increasing appreciation of their lives. What explains these differences? I've looked at all the implications of hormonal therapy, psychotherapy, nutritional therapy, exercise therapy, and no therapy. I've also tried to learn about alternatives to conventional medicine.

The women I treat are unique individuals. However, we share a universal desire to take control of our future health—and that desire only grows stronger once we reach our forties. I've written this book to provide the latest medical information about our midlife bodies and our woman-care needs. We traverse a complicated passage from our forties to our fifties. Some of us need reliable contraception that suits our lifestyle; others want to get pregnant. Many of us have worsening PMS, or our menstrual cycles become irregular. Some of us feel great; others have just a few good days each month. Our hormones fluctuate, and so do our moods, body temperatures, and sleep patterns. We have to make choices about birth control, then hormone control. We should be concerned about cancer prevention and detection, heart disease, osteoporosis, joint problems, and thyroid problems. We want to control our weight and our wrinkles. In the midst of all of this, we are taking care of aging parents and aging children (whom we want to help take care of themselves), dealing with our mates' midlife problems (both physical and psychological) or possibly going through divorce, getting back in the job market or leaving it, and wondering how our twenties and thirties sped by so fast.

I am no longer the young, inexperienced doctor trying to look older so that my male colleagues and female patients will somehow have a greater respect for my diagnostic and surgical skills. I deeply resent that we were taught to treat women in terms of their reproductive functions and that other aspects of our health care were neglected. I currently delight in caring for my "older" patients, who, like myself, suddenly find the need to learn about current medical facts, theories, and research as they apply to women who still have half of their lives to look forward to.

This book has given me a wonderful opportunity to share the medical information that impacts this unique period of our lives. Our concerns are so very common! It's time we become as informed about our health as we are about our finances and cars!

No book can substitute for our own physicians' one-on-one care. But once we're active, informed participants, we can work more effectively with our doctors.

Chapter 18 provides a woman-care checklist to help you organize what you need to know about your family's health history, your past history, and your present health patterns. The list specifies which tests you should have performed, at what age, and how often. I hope you'll use this checklist to discover your individual risk factors and the newer tests that can be used to assess them.

Being a woman in these times is wonderful. We are in a majority; we have grown up; we know who we are, we are vocal, and we have the right to demand that our total health be taken seriously. This book on health care for women over 40 will help us keep our bodies and our psyches healthy, despite the inevitable wear, but not necessarily tear, that comes with the passage of time. We are all "too young to get old."

—Judith Reichman, M.D.

Contraception, Fertility, and Pregnancy After 40

1

CHANGES AFTER 40
Our Bodies, Our Cycles,
Our Hormones

As female baby boomers, we have spent the last twenty-five years being issue-oriented. The issues were, of course, those that affected us intimately: our sexuality, our relationships, our parenting abilities, our careers, our environment, and our health. We tried to redefine our roles as women in the '70s, '80s, and '90s, knowing we couldn't just accept the ones our mothers had. We surged through our twenties—continuing education, working, exploring our sexuality, dealing with contraception, and often subjecting our bodies to abuse, believing we were immortal. We stampeded through our thirties—working on relationships, having and raising our progeny, establishing our careers, and taking better care of our bodies because we knew we could, on occasion, get sick.

These decades flew by, and we're surprised to find ourselves in our forties. How did this happen? This is the "middle age" that we associate with our mothers. Many of us expect that the fifth decade of life will be one of decline. We're not quite sure what goes first, but our fetish for youth has negated our appreciation of maturity. Actresses in their forties have difficulty finding "suitable" roles. (Believe me, I know. As a gynecologist in Los Angeles, I treat many of them, as well as their agents.) They are no longer cast as "femmes fatales," and Hollywood has not figured out how to make them interesting protagonists. It's amazing how

3

the movie industry has been able to portray our "coming of age" during puberty and adolescence but has failed to deal with our true "coming of age" as we enter our middle and perhaps most important years—the gateway to the second half of our lives. We and the media had better wake up to some demographics. Our middle age is, and will continue to be, the age of "majority" as over 40 million women enter their forties and fifties over the next two decades. Hollywood may procrastinate in defining our roles, but we won't. We have not been silent in the past two decades; why should we start being silent now as we add experience and new issues to our midlife agendas?

Our Bodies: What Have They Done for Us Lately?

Our bodies have continued their truly amazing functions for four decades. What they do for us now and in the future depends to a large extent on what we've done to ourselves through our childhood, adolescence, and early adulthood.

Our weight is very much a function of our past. Poor nutrition, overeating, and genetics have made 35 percent of us overweight, and our old jeans no longer fit. But 65 percent of us feel that no matter what we do, the fit has changed. Is this a normal part of getting older? To some extent, yes. Pregnancy certainly didn't help! It stretched our muscles and our skin. If we didn't lose our pregnancy weight within the first six months after delivery, we reset our internal weight standards and this created new weight-loss obstacles. And now we have to find time to balance our care for the results of these pregnancies, work (70 percent of us work outside our homes, and of course all of us work in them), and weight control, "control" being a luxury at this point in our lives.

We lose bone mass with age (our peak, bone density–wise, occurs at age 30), and we also lose muscle mass unless we exercise regularly and vigorously. If muscle is replaced with fat, we add insult to injury (or fat to fat). "Lazy" fat requires less "fuel" to function than more active muscle tissue, and even if we don't change our diets, our changed body composition causes us to burn fewer calories. The leftover calories are converted to additional fat, and a vicious cycle results in middle-age spread (the "middle" is very apt here because the fat deposition occurs in the mid-portion of our bodies). The heavier we get and the more fat we have, the lower our rate of metabolism and the harder it is to lose that weight—a common complaint in our forties. But once we understand that loss of muscle is a major culprit, we can choose to combat this process with exercise. Few of us will wear the same jeans that fit us in our twenties. I, like many other women, keep my old tight jeans in the closet—just in case—but the case (or my body) has not returned to its original form! That doesn't mean we can't reach a weight equilibrium where we maintain a stable, comfortable jean size in our forties.

Our Body Systems

Our bodies' organs and systems have been changing from our childhood throughout the last decades of our adulthood. What makes our forties different is that we are becoming aware that we even have "systems" and that they can malfunction and develop disease. Not looking the way we used to may be a nuisance, but not feeling the way we used to can be a sign of a real problem. Here is a brief review of these systems and the changes they may undergo in our fifth decade.

CARDIOVASCULAR SYSTEM:
THE PUMP AND DRIVE OF OUR BODIES

Our hearts have been pumping and our vessels expanding to meet our demands through our adolescent growth spurts, our subsequent pregnancies (when the volume of fluid in our blood vessels increased by 50 percent!), and our pursuit of physical activities (or lack thereof). Unlike men, women in their forties see little change in this system because we are protected by our estrogen. We can, however, begin to develop high blood pressure, or *hypertension*. Up to 40 percent of black women and 23 percent of white women are hypertensive in their forties. This makes us four times more likely to face future heart disease and stroke. We can no longer "pooh-pooh" blood pressure readings; they are not just for the old or for men. The earlier we treat elevated blood pressure (140/90 or above), the less likely we will succumb to its complications.

MUSCULOSKELETAL SYSTEM:
SUPPORT AND FORM DO NOT MEAN A GIRDLE!

In our forties our bones are the result of an ongoing tug-of-war between our bone-building cells and bone-destroying cells. These cells have either coexisted or have fought and partially destroyed the arena of battle. Our past calcium consumption, exercise, smoking, caffeine intake, and use of medications have aided and abetted one side (bone building) or the other (bone resorption). Our frames may not feel or look poorly supported, but 5 percent of us already have significant bone loss, or *osteoporosis*, and are at risk for fracture. For most of us, it's not too late to help prevent this disease. Simple measures that we institute in our forties can make huge differences in our present and future "support."

Our bones are not the only support in flux. "Use it or lose it" applies to our muscle quality and quantity. Lifting kids is not enough to maintain good muscle support, but walking two miles while pushing or pulling them is. If we lose muscle, we burn calories less efficiently and add fat to our less-than-fit form.

DIGESTIVE SYSTEM:
EAT, DRINK, AND FEEL BLOATED

We've spent the last forty years expecting to digest anything, and usually did. Our gastrointestinal tract is truly a remarkable system. The cells of its lining are regenerated every twenty-four to seventy-two hours. This allows our intestines to recover rapidly from acute "insults" (bacteria, viruses, and some of the junk we send there). This constant "resurfacing" also reduces the chance that cells will become malignant. They are simply not there long enough to be affected by the potential cancer-causing agents we ingest. Although it's the surface cells that are responsible for the resorption of our food and formation of our waste, the deeper muscle of the bowel is necessary to push things along (bowel motility).

We may find that after four decades, our digestive system begins to become more sensitive and may react to certain foods or emotional stresses. Milk and milk products are our best dietary source of calcium, yet many of us (up to 25 percent of whites and 80 percent of African-American and Asian women) develop some milk intolerance in our thirties and forties; we just don't produce enough lactase, the enzyme needed to break down milk sugar, or lactose. As a result of this lactase deficiency, this sugar is not "enzymed," so it's not absorbed and remains in the intestine, where it causes gas, bloating, cramping, and even diarrhea. Using lactated milk, enzyme tablets, or eating yogurt (which has bacteria that makes a lactase enzyme) may allow us to enjoy and benefit from "natural" calcium in our forties.

We are four times more likely than men to develop irritable bowel syndrome, and if we do, this often occurs in our forties. This chronic syndrome is due to changes in our bowel's motility. The muscles push the bowel content either too quickly (causing diarrhea) or too slowly (causing constipation, bloating, and abdominal pain) or alternate between these two extremes so we go from one set of symptoms to the other. There is no question that stress activates irritable bowel syndrome. Some of the stress may have occurred more than thirty years ago; there is a high incidence of childhood sexual abuse associated with irritable bowel syndrome.

Another cause of bloating and stomach "upset" is gallbladder disease. Our risk of developing gallstones increases in our forties. Twenty percent of us will now begin to develop this problem as compared to only 8 percent of men. High fat consumption (the stones are made of cholesterol), high weight, or high estrogen levels from our previous pregnancies can make our gallbladders become stone producers.

As we become aware that our digestive system reacts to adversity, we need to become better consumers (of food) and managers (of stress). Our guts in our forties now have "the guts" to tell us to treat our bodies with more respect.

ENDOCRINE SYSTEM:
THE SILENT CONTROL CENTERS OF OUR WELL-BEING

When we think of our glands and hormones, we invariably consider our ovaries and female hormones. Let's not make the mistake of defining ourselves (or our glands) in such a restrictive, sexist fashion. Our endocrine glands produce substances that are secreted into our circulation and act on other cells and tissues. These are our hormones. Our bodies produce almost one hundred different types of hormones, estrogen and progesterone being just two of so very many. In our forties, most of these hormones continue to be secreted and are "accepted" by the target cells without change. Our birthdays come and go and are greeted with endocrinologic indifference.

There are, of course, exceptions. One is our thyroid. This important gland seems to be much more sensitive and easily disturbed in women than men (by as high a ratio as 10 to 1), and this sensitivity begins to peak in our forties. This gland can become underactive (hypothyroidism) and cause fatigue, poor memory, cold intolerance, and weight gain. If it becomes overactive (*hyperthyroidism*) we can develop heat intolerance, hot flashes, palpitations, rapid heartbeat, and sleep problems. Both sets of symptoms mimic those we associate with menopause. Not all hot flashes (especially if they occur in our forties) are due to "inadequate" ovaries, and a litany of so-called menopausal complaints may indeed be due to a beleaguered gland—in our neck, not our pelvis.

Another gland that may have been overworked over the past four decades, especially if we were obese, is our pancreas, which produces insulin. This hormone is our "energy converter," allowing the cells of our body to assimilate and utilize glucose as fuel. We may begin to develop a type of diabetes called Type II, or non-insulin-dependent, diabetes, in our forties. This probably starts with insulin resistance. Our tissues are presented with insulin, but they ignore it and resist its normal action. Weight gain and the presence of fat encourage this resistance. The pancreas works harder to make more insulin, trying desperately to cope with rising "nonresponsive" glucose levels. We then enter a vicious cycle. High insulin levels stimulate fat production in our liver (and also increase our production of low-density lipoprotein, the "bad" cholesterol, which can encourage heart disease). This fat is stored in and replaces our muscle. The more fat we have, the less we utilize our energy source—glucose. So now we have insulin resistance, underutilization of glucose, and a tired pancreas. All these lead to elevated levels of glucose in our blood and the development of diabetes. We are not sure which comes first: obesity, which causes insulin resistance, or high insulin production, which causes obesity. But those of us who find we're losing the weight battle in our forties may also be embarking on a lifelong struggle with control of our inner energy—our glucose metabolism.

IMMUNE SYSTEM:
KNOWING THYSELF VERSUS REJECTING THYSELF

Our immune system has had to perform a phenomenal feat of recognizing and responding correctly to millions of cells, proteins, and tissues during our last four decades. The cellular and molecular basis of our immunity is extraordinarily complex and includes antigens, antibodies, cytokines, T cells, leukocytes, lymphocytes, macrophages, complements (not the congratulatory kind), and our genes. We've managed to fight off infectious diseases, mutated precancerous cells, and foreign substances and, through this, we have developed protective immunities. Our bodies rejected what was foreign (except our pregnancies, although our children may sometimes seem like foreigners) and accepted what was ours, our "normal" cells and tissues.

As we enter midlife, our immune system becomes more prone to "recognition fatigue." It forgets the coding for normal cell acceptance and begins to attack or reject normal cells and the systems to which they belong. Nearly all of these so-called autoimmune diseases occur in women, and they may be influenced by our female hormone production (or declining hormonal production). Seventy-five to 90 percent of the patients whose immune systems self-destruct—causing diseases such as lupus erythematosus, rheumatoid arthritis, Sjögren's syndrome, multiple sclerosis, and Hashimoto disease—are women. At least 1 in 10 of us will develop an autoimmune disease in our lifetime. These diseases may begin during our childbearing years and often increase in our forties. Although their occurrence is usually beyond our control, recognition of symptoms and appropriate therapy can be our "control" objective.

Our Fourth Decade Equation

Does 40 herald major changes in our lives? As far as our bodies are concerned, this birthday is not special. We're in a continuum of life, and what happens to our physical status can be summed up as a mathematical equation:

Age-related changes + Genetic factors
+ Body abuse × 40 years
− Body care × 40 years
= Body "wear" in our forties

Poetically, knowledge of "wear" should lead us to improved future "woman care."

Our Cycles: Inner Rhythms That Can Change

We spend nearly thirty years "cycling"—our periods, our ovulations, and the concomitant rise and fall of our hormones are a familiar and integral part of our beings. From puberty to menopause, any complaints from the waist down are invariably linked to our cycles by our doctors and ourselves. Men have abdominal discomfort or pain; we have cramps. If these pains coincide with the middle of our cycle, we are told (often with only the most cursory examination) that we have ovulatory pain. (The German term *Mittelschmerz* is used; it makes this diagnosis sound much more official!) If the pain occurs during our periods, it is, of course, menstrual cramps. So we are "covered," diagnostically speaking, for about seven to ten days each month. Obviously, we know our own cycles and the usual degree of discomfort, if any. Unusual pain, no matter when it occurs, should be evaluated. We can get appendicitis while we have our period or a gallbladder attack in midcycle.

We've each become experts on how our bodies feel during the different phases of our cycle, but it behooves us to know why and to understand the process of these familiar cycles. We need to be comfortable with what I term Biology 101 through 303 (our cycles between our teens and our thirties) before we can understand the changes that are a part of Biology 404 (our forties).

The Saga of Our Eggs, Hormones, and Periods

Our ovarian supply of "eggs," or more accurately, *oocytes*, has been dwindling since before we were born. Oocytes are present in our ovaries and have the capacity to mature and develop as follicles and eventually release an egg, which can undergo fertilization. Our ovaries start to "lose it" (from an oocyte point of view) from the fifth month of our embryonic life! Halfway through our gestation, when we still reside in our mother's uterus (and probably could not survive outside), our ovaries contain about 7 million oocytes. Most die (a process called *atresia*), and we're born with "only" 1 million to 2 million. Atresia is unaffected by our newborn life and continues relentlessly; by the time we begin our periods (*menarche*), our oocyte number has fallen to 400,000. Over the next twenty-five years, this loss continues, and it accelerates after the age of 40. By the time we reach menopause, we are left with a paltry few thousand oocytes. So it's not our monthly ovulation that depletes our millions of oocytes, but the process of age-related cellular death. Fewer than 0.001 percent of our ovaries' original oocytes ever reach ovulation. The eggs that "make it" are truly among a very select few.

Our cycles are defined by the hormones (estrogen and progesterone) produced by the follicles as they develop and die each month.

Figure 1.1
The "Control Panel" of Our Reproductive Hormones

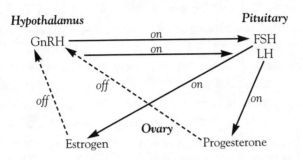

They, in turn, are under the control of a "greater force"—*FSH*, or *follicle-stimulating hormone*, and *LH*, or *luteinizing hormone*—produced in a gland in our brain called the *pituitary*. Finally, the "highest" force controls the pituitary. This is an area in our brain called the *hypothalamus*, which is adjacent to the pituitary. It produces GnRH, or *gonadotropin-releasing hormone*, which turns the pituitary "on."

It sounds complicated, but it is really just a circular control panel with on and off switches (see Figure 1.1). If levels of estrogen and proges-terone are high, the whole system is suppressed ("off"). Production of GnRH, FSH, and LH is inhibited (why start a cycle to produce more hormones if we already have enough?). However, if we need more estro-gen and progesterone, the system cranks up: GnRH production is stimu-lated, causing the pituitary to release FSH and LH, which work on the ovary and tell the oocytes to start developing and producing hormones.

There is one more hormone we should know about that affects our cycle control: *inhibin*. Although it was isolated only a few years ago, doc-tors and researchers had theorized its existence long before. Inhibin is produced by cells in the developing follicles in response to FSH. Like es-trogen, inhibin "inhibits" (hence, its name) FSH production. This sub-stance may also have local regulatory functions within the ovary. The follicle that grows the fastest and produces the most inhibin may prevent other follicles from competing in its race to produce the "egg of the month."

So let's look at our "normal" monthly cycle: We just got our period, and we're at a "low" (subjectively, this is how we may feel) in terms of es-trogen and progesterone levels. This "low" triggers our hypothalamus to produce GnRH, which nudges the pituitary to release FSH (GnRH, in the absence of good estrogen levels, stimulates FSH but very little LH). FSH lives up to its name; it stimulates a follicle, which develops from an oocyte. Actually, a whole bunch of follicles start to grow, but only one becomes dominant and makes it. The rest die before they reach any degree of maturity (atresia is a sad process). The dominant follicle is now producing estrogen, and the levels rise over the next 14 or so days as it "blooms." But more than a follicle is now blooming. Estrogen feeds the lining of our uterus (*endometrium*), causing the glands to grow and the lining to thicken. At midcycle, the estrogen reaches a critical peak and then drops just a bit (as if the follicle is pausing for breath).

GnRH is once more stimulated, and when it reaches the pituitary, which has been bathed in estrogen, it causes an LH surge. The LH goes back down to the ovary and works on the mature dominant follicle and—wow!—does it transform it! The capsule of the follicle ruptures, the egg is released (and, if all goes well, is picked up by the fernlike *fimbria* on one of two Fallopian tubes, where it can be fertilized by a sperm if it happens to be there at the right time), and the follicle is transformed into a *corpus luteum* (or "yellow body"). This new corpus luteum continues to produce estrogen and also produces our second hormone, progesterone. It now reigns supreme. It will live for 14 days and during that time continue to produce ever-rising amounts of progesterone. The progesterone augments estrogen's effect on the uterine lining: The glands grow thicker and the blood supply increases, creating a lush, rich bed capable of enveloping and nourishing an embryo. At the end of 14 days, and in the absence of a pregnancy, the corpus luteum dies. It stops producing hormones, and the levels of estrogen and progesterone fall precipitously. Without its hormonal support, the uterine lining literally collapses. The glands break down, the lining sheds: We get our period.

And so we begin again. Another low (hormonally and endometrially) is now stimulating our system to begin a new cycle, continuing a renewal of our extraordinary ability to ovulate and procreate for the decades of our reproductive lives.

Should we expect this wonderful rhythm to be changed or interrupted in our forties? The answer is yes, but it must be modified by the adverb "gradually." Not every late or missed period in our forties is a sign of approaching menopause! Much of our ovarian function is controlled by the centers in our brain, and these are vulnerable to other stimuli. Our awareness of our world and body is processed through these brain centers, which, in turn, send signals to our hypothalamus and pituitary. New and very strong stimuli can mix them up. This is not just a phenomenon of our forties; we experienced abnormal cycles in our twenties and thirties, when we were perhaps more mixed up (or messed up) from a brain center point of view. So before we blame perimenopause, let's look at our signal input.

Stress is the major upsetting signal and can cause a change in our cycles. Yes, this is the ultimate catchall term, but if we're moving, or we or our husbands have lost our job (or wish we could), or the kids are piercing parts of their bodies other than their ears, we know this is stress. Sudden weight loss (we might be happy with the cosmetic results of our starvation diet, but our brain centers are not), sudden increase in rigorous exercise, travel, illness, and medications (especially steroids) can interfere with signals across our brain-ovary network and result in an abnormal cycle. Our bodies and our cycles are often "smarter" than we are. They function right when we treat ourselves right; they go "off" if we abuse our health.

Our cycles do become shorter in our forties; they average 26 days at the age of 40 compared to 28 days at age 20 (being two days off isn't much for twenty years of monthly repetition). As we continue into this decade, we may start to be late, miss periods, or have more frequent periods. This simply reflects the fact that our remaining follicles are either tentative in their development and may start and quit (an early period) or be recalcitrant (a delayed period). Finally, on occasion, no follicle picks up the FSH "gauntlet," none develops and takes off hormonally, and, hence, we miss a period. These are the cycle changes of the perimenopause (see chapter 5), which generally start four years prior to our menopause. So, if in our mid- to late forties, we have a recurring pattern of irregular cycles, we may not be immediately menopausal (four years is still a long time), but we *are* undergoing hormonal changes. Understanding them makes it easier to know when to seek treatment.

OUR HORMONES: A LITTLE OFF, BUT MOSTLY ON

Once we understand our cycles, we get the concept of our hormonal rise and fall (see Figure 1.1). As we pass through our fifth decade, the hormonal changes may at first be silent. Our inhibin levels are lower and our FSH levels higher. There is no magic here; these changes simply reflect the accelerated depletion of the follicles in our ovaries. The less follicles we "possess" after 40, the less inhibin we produce. The lower the inhibin, the lower the "inhibition" of FSH production.

Initially, our estrogen and progesterone levels are maintained at "pre-40" levels. As we continue through this decade, there may be a gradual decrease of estrogen in all phases of the cycle. The lower the estrogen—you guessed it—the higher the FSH. With time, LH also "breaks through" and "rises," but this usually occurs ten years after a rise in our FSH.

I call our forties the "try harder" period of our hormonal lives. So many of our ovaries' population of oocytes have been lost through years of atresia that the challenge to the pituitary is accelerated. It gamely attempts to "make good" by pushing more FSH and, later, LH to get the leftover follicles to rise up, develop, and secrete estrogen and progesterone.

HORMONAL "FEELINGS" IN OUR FORTIES

Expanding Our PMS Experience

Since few of us are endocrinologists, the real question is not what happens to the exact laboratory readings of our hormonal levels, but how we feel. Most of us feel just fine, even with 26-day cycles. Some of us may want to conceive (see chapter 3), but most of us shudder at the thought and need contraception (see chapter 2). Our chief complaint seems to be an increase in PMS (premenstrual syndrome). There is an adage that may regrettably apply to many of us: "First there's PMS, then there's menopause." We outgrow (or outlive) our PMS when we no longer have monthly fluctuations of our hormones, so indeed it does disappear with menopause.

We were once told that PMS was not really a syndrome, nor was it even worthy of medical investigation. Sexists pointed to this as a "female cop-out phenomenon"; feminists deplored its existence or its public acknowledgment. The most insulting slur was the lack of interest in research and the misinformation on cause and treatment promulgated by the medical profession.

Twenty-four hundred years ago, Hippocrates noted that "women are subject to intermittent agitations, and as a result, the agitated blood finds its way from the head to the uterus whence it is expelled." Frankly, not much more was known for the next 2,370 years. At least we now have a definition for PMS: unpleasant physical and psychological symptoms that recur regularly during the second phase of our hormonal or menstrual cycle. Scientists currently argue as to which symptoms are allowed entry into this syndrome, but they generally agree on the most common: mood swings, swelling and bloating, weight gain, irritability, fatigue, and depression.

The cause of our PMS is still not clear. At one point, it was thought to be due to inadequate progesterone production by the corpus luteum. The only problem is that we've never measured lower progesterone levels in women with PMS, whereas women undergoing fertility workups who do have documented "corpus luteum insufficiency" and low progesterone do not demonstrate an increase in this syndrome. Double-blind studies have been done in which one group of women was given natural progesterone (usually suppositories) and another group given a "dud," or placebo, and then had their medications switched (they and the researchers were "blind" to which medications they received). The studies have not shown improvement in PMS symptoms with use of progesterone. We also know that in cycles where we don't ovulate and produce progesterone, we don't have PMS. Adding progesterone to hormonal therapy during menopause can also reinstitute these symptoms. It's not difficult to deduce from all of this that progesterone is probably a cause of rather than a cure for PMS.

Let's look at another PMS theory. It offers a better correlation with our increasing susceptibility in our forties. PMS may be caused by fluctuations in our hormones and estrogen withdrawal. Before we ovulate, our estrogen reaches its maximum peak, and we often feel better than at any other time of the month. After ovulation the level comes down. In addition, progesterone levels go up. The dominance of progesterone has been established, and to ensure this "victory," progesterone has one more effect. It knocks out estrogen receptors in our target organs. The estrogen may be there, but it just isn't "recognized." If this occurs in our brain centers, we have a relative "central" estrogen low. We can even develop hot flashes similar to those of menopause. It would appear to be the decrease in actual estrogen levels, abetted by progesterone's dampening effect on estrogen's receptors, that affects our mood and sense of well-being. As we get older, there is a gradual decline in our overall estrogen levels. Our system may also become more sensitive to progesterone's dampening effect on our receptors. This would explain the fact that PMS seems to affect more of us and with increasing severity. Indeed, 20 percent of us have some significant "disruption" of our normal lives.

Our treatment options include therapies that are proven to work (but we're not sure why), therapies that *might* work for some of us (and researchers argue over their results and proven efficacy), and doubtful therapies that don't withstand scientific scrutiny but are touted by their producers and their patient advocates.

MEDICAL THERAPIES

Giving women with PMS small doses of non-oral estrogen in the form of a patch, implant, or pellet has gained popularity in Europe and has been shown (in double-blind studies) to reduce PMS symptoms. Doctors are concerned, however, about the long-term effect of added estrogen on women who are not yet menopausal. Could this increase their risk of breast cancer? Partially because of this concern, and also because of the lack of long-term follow-up, this therapy has not been the medication of choice in the United States. In all fairness, we really don't have a medication of choice. It would appear that natural progesterone doesn't work (although some women feel it does and don't want to be confused or bothered with so-called scientific data).

Birth control pills do stop natural ovulation and, as such, should stop the estrogen-progesterone imbalance of the second half of our cycle. I prescribe them for women in their forties whose PMS seems to be getting worse, especially if this is accompanied by menstrual irregularity. The PMS-free existence I would like to promise does not always follow this therapy. Although many women get relief, at least initially, others find the Pill makes no difference or may even worsen their symptoms. There are two possible reasons for this: (1) The progesterone in the Pill might be a PMS-causing culprit. (2) The Pill-free week (when we get our periods) allows the ovary to produce some hormones that promote PMS.

A much more radical approach is to totally suppress ovarian function with GnRH *agonists*. These are like our own GnRH hormone but sufficiently different to prevent pituitary production and release of FSH and LH. Ovulation and hormone production is stopped and, *voilà!*— there are no periods and no PMS. Great, but this drug has now also rendered us menopausal! We have traded one set of symptoms for another. In order to stop the menopausal symptoms and to prevent osteoporosis, we give back hormones using low-dose birth control pills or estrogen replacement therapy. The unfair then happens—PMS may return!

Many physicians are using antidepressants such as Prozac to help treat women whose major PMS symptom is depression. Their results have been quite good. We have to remember that if we suffer from depression, it often worsens during the second half of our cycle. Our fluctuating hormones are affecting an underlying problem. In these circumstances, antidepressant drugs may be ideal. Anti-anxiety medications such as Xanax have also been given during the symptomatic period of PMS with "better than placebo" results.

So much for medication. Let's consider other forms of PMS aid.

NONMEDICAL THERAPIES FOR PMS

We've become so accustomed to quick-fixing our body's problems with medicine (or even surgery) that the idea that a prolonged commitment to a change in lifestyle and diet might accomplish the same goal is often unacceptable. But what should be unacceptable is one to two weeks of "poor-being" when we can get to a state of "well-being" with individual effort.

Regular aerobic exercise can diminish PMS, as can abstinence from caffeine, sugar, and alcohol. If we use coffee to "energize" during a PMS low or give in to our craving for chocolate or other sweets (I especially want chocolate-chip ice cream), our PMS becomes worse.

Vitamin and supplement therapies have been proposed to help PMS symptoms (we're back to pills again). The vitamins formulated for PMS (and distributed under a lot of brand names) generally include fairly high doses of vitamin B_6. We need to exert some caution here. When B_6 was first promoted as an anti-PMS vitamin, many women consumed it in huge doses, in the mistaken belief that if a little works, a lot would be better. Some of these women took doses of 600 milligrams or more of B_6 and developed neurologic symptoms. Since vitamins are still not under "FDA guidance," there is no warning on the bottle. Always check with your doctor before taking this or any other supplement.

Evening primrose oil, which is a fatty acid, has been promoted as a beneficial supplement for the treatment of PMS. Although many of my patients concur, we don't have good scientific supporting data.

Minerals such as calcium and magnesium have also been pushed for PMS control. These do help menstrual cramps, and since we tend to be "under calciumed," I won't protest—at least we are helping to prevent osteoporosis.

None of these therapies works for all symptoms or for all women. The understanding and treatment of PMS need to be advanced from the days of Hippocrates to the world of hormonal molecular biology. I hope this doesn't take another twenty-four hundred years.

Menstrual Cramps: If They're Getting Worse, It Could Mean Disease

Why do we get cramps? As our hormone levels drop and the integrity of our built-up endometrial glands is interrupted, we produce a substance called *prostaglandin*. This is one of the chemical mediators of pain and menstrual cramps (*dysmenorrhea*). It also "encourages" the uterine muscles to contract (which is definitely beneficial, because the contracted muscles close the blood vessels coursing through them and limit menstrual blood loss). Prolonged or strong uterine contractions hurt (we know that from labor pains). Any process that increases prostaglandin production or muscle tension will lead to pain and a worsening of our "usual" cramps.

After dealing with it for over twenty-five years, we have become accustomed to our menstrual discomfort. Pregnancy eliminated our cramps, as did breast-feeding and the subsequent *amenorrhea* (lack of periods). These are no longer options for most of us, but we do have others: Exercise helps. Birth control pills decrease both prostaglandin production and endometrial buildup and have become a mainstay in the treatment of dysmenorrhea. Antiprostaglandin medications (ibuprofen and its anti-inflammatory relatives) are a godsend for cramps, and we no longer need prescriptions for this quick relief. But if our usual therapy stops working and our cramps get worse, we may be developing uterine or pelvic disease. These are some of the conditions that can occur in our forties:

Fibroids More than 20 percent of women over the age of 35 develop fibroid tumors. As they grow, they can cause increased menstrual pain and bleeding.

Adenomyosis This is a common age-related uterine disease. The glands of the endometrium forget that their "limit" is the uterine lining.

With years of monthly hormonal stimuli, they grow and develop in the wrong direction into the uterine muscle wall (the *myometrium*), causing the uterus to become enlarged and soft. When we menstruate, these glands bleed, not just into the uterine cavity, but also into the muscle. The resulting pain can be quite severe.

Endometriosis This is the dreaded "E" word for women who have postponed childbearing and find that they now suffer from both infertility and pelvic pain. Endometrial cells that normally are shed with our menstrual blood can back up and out of our Fallopian tubes (*retrograde*, or backward, menstruation) and "seed" onto our other pelvic organs, including the *peritoneum* (pelvic lining), ovaries, Fallopian tubes, bladder, and bowel. These cells continue to react to our hormonal cycles. They swell, release irritating substances, bleed, and cause scarring. The scar tissue plus chemical and cellular changes in our peritoneal fluid can block the release and tubal pickup of our eggs and result in infertility. This monthly reaction of these misplaced cells will also increase our pain before and during our periods.

Unusual severity of menstrual cramps is a warning sign and mandates a thorough pelvic examination. We should not simply assume that because we are over 40, our periods will be "harder." Our fifth decade should not be synonymous with monthly pain.

2

CONTRACEPTION
AFTER 40
Yes, We Still Need It

Only 6 percent of sexually active, forty-something women who have not had permanent surgical sterilization (or whose partners have not) do not need to worry about contraception; they are trying to conceive. The rest of us have either completed our childbearing (but not child rearing) or have decided we don't want to make this life commitment. The average age of menopause is 51, but natural menopause occurs in 11 percent of women between the ages 45 and 49. By the age of 50 to 54 years, 43 percent of us have gone through natural menopause and another 28 percent have undergone *surgical menopause* (our ovaries have been removed), or had a hysterectomy. That leaves 30 percent of us who are still theoretically fertile from 50 to 54!

I don't want to predict an impending contraceptive crisis for the 13 million women who are currently in their forties, but our unintended pregnancies are a significant problem. They increased from 24 percent of all pregnancies for women between 40 and 44 in the early 1980s to 53 percent for the same age group in the late 1980s, and the proportion continues to rise. A third of all of these unintended pregnancies end in spontaneous miscarriage, and as many as 50 percent of women over 40 undergo elective abortion (this rate is second only to the rate of teenage abortion!).

Unintended pregnancies have other consequences for the health of many women in this age group, especially if they have poor access to health care. The mortality rate during pregnancy or childbirth can be eight times higher for women in their forties than for those under the age of 25 (but who had time to finish having babies by then?) and four times higher than for women in their late twenties and early thirties (a more reasonable time frame). There is a rise in ectopic or tubal pregnancies, which can rupture, causing fatal hemorrhage if not treated with early surgical or chemical intervention. The prevalence of chromosomal abnormalities of the offspring of over-40 pregnancies increases with age, and rises from 2.5 percent at age 40 to 8.3 percent at age 45. (These numbers are obtained at amniocentesis.)

We decry our "aging ovaries." We resist the idea of our so-called biological clock, but as the ticking goes on, so does the monthly release of our remaining viable eggs. They continue to be a target of fertilization by obliging sperm. Our fertility at age 40 is about half that at 20 and will continue to decline, yet this is not "ground zero." Neglecting contraception is as stupid in our forties as it was in our previous three decades (or to hit home more poignantly, as inexcusable as our daughters' being "unprotected"). We should know better.

The contraceptive methods available to us in our forties do not differ greatly from those we used during the preceding decades of our lives. Modern contraceptive technology has improved and modified the old basics (birth control pills and the IUD) and developed some new ways of using hormones such as subdermal (under-the-skin) implants and vaginal contraceptive rings. The major changes we should consider are those of our own concepts of what is safe and effective. We should not bring thirty years of inaccurate perceptions and bias to our current contraceptive choices.

Tubal Ligation: Is It Worthwhile This "Late"?

We may prefer not to deal with reversible contraception and opt for permanence. After all, one of the virtues of reaching our middle years is that we know when we've had enough (pregnancies and children included). About 67 percent of women between 40 and 44 have undergone sterilization. Many women chose this method in their thirties, when they were facing a full twenty years of unwanted fertility, but the specter of "just" eight to ten years of birth control need is sufficient for some of us to seek this surgical "fix" at a later age.

HOW TUBAL LIGATION IS PERFORMED

There are several ways of performing tubal ligations. If the ligation is done right after a delivery, a small incision, 2 to 3 inches in length, is made under the belly button; through this, the abdomen is opened and the Fallopian tubes on the enlarged uterus are exposed and tied (*ligated*). If the procedure is done electively (when we haven't just had a baby), it can be performed through a transverse 2- to 3-inch incision in the lower abdomen, just above the pubic hairline (the *"mini-lap"*). Some physicians prefer a vaginal approach, opening the area below the cervix to expose the tubes.

Currently, laparoscopic tubal ligation is the most common sterilization method for women. During this procedure, a small incision $1/2$ inch long is made in the skin under the belly button, and a special needle is inserted. Carbon dioxide gas is instilled through this needle to "inflate" the abdominal cavity. This balloonlike distention causes the abdominal wall to move away from the internal organs. A *trocar*, an instrument consisting of a hollow tube the width of an index finger into which a sharp, pointed metal rod is placed, is then pushed through the small incision (distending the abdomen prevents the physician from "stabbing" the bowel during this part of the procedure). The inner rod is removed, and a laparoscope is put through the hollow tube. This scope allows the surgeon to view the abdomen and pelvic organs. Another, smaller incision is then made by the pubic hairline, and a second trocar is pushed through. An instrument is then placed through this second trocar to grasp a portion of the tube and "burn" it with electric current. Some surgeons prefer to place a permanent clip or band around a loop of each tube. All these methods effectively block the tube, and the occluded portion eventually scars.

A decision to undergo this type of permanent contraception should not be based simply on a description of the procedure. Understanding how it works, how well it works (or conversely, the failure rate), and the benefits, as well as side effects, of this and other contraceptive methods should figure into our choice at any age.

HOW TUBAL LIGATION WORKS:
WHAT HAPPENS TO THE EGG

After ovulation, an egg enters one of the Fallopian tubes, where it remains in hope of meeting sperm and becoming fertilized. If the tube's channel is blocked, fertilization cannot occur. The egg simply withers, dies, and is eventually reabsorbed. Many of my patients express great "egg concern," worrying that these unused eggs somehow will accumulate and cause problems. Each human egg is microscopic and in no way resembles the more familiar chicken egg. Billions of cells die in our bodies daily—this is just one more. Even if our tubes are not artificially blocked, in the absence of pregnancy, our monthly egg undergoes the same cellular death.

THE FAILURE RATE OF TUBAL LIGATION

In an ideal world, the failure rate would be zero; it's not. We have to contend with human error. If a ligament near the tube (the round ligament) is mistakenly cauterized or banded rather than the tube itself, pregnancy is not prevented. Other causes of failure include insufficient cautery or burning so that the tube's central canal is not destroyed. Bands and clips can fall off if not securely placed. Overall, most follow-up studies have shown about a 1 in 1,000 failure rate. (In other words, if a thousand women get sterilized, one will get pregnant.) However, this is still lower than the failure rate of any other contraceptive technique. If a pregnancy does manage to develop, we have to remember that the tube is now damaged, and there is a possibility of ectopic pregnancy. It's rare, but if you have had a tubal ligation, missed a period, and have pelvic pain, consult your doctor immediately!

THE BENEFITS OF TUBAL LIGATION

You've taken a day out of your life, had a surgical procedure, spent two or three days recovering, and, for all practical purposes, need never again worry about contraception. You also get a hidden benefit: Tubal ligation has been associated with a 33 percent decrease in the risk of developing ovarian cancer.

THE DISADVANTAGES OF TUBAL LIGATION

Surgery is expensive, and since most of the laparoscopic procedures are done with general anesthesia, your bill will include your surgeon's fee and use of the operating room, instruments, and anesthesia. This can cost thousands of dollars. Most insurance companies will pay, not out of altruism but because they figure this is cheaper than prenatal care and delivery charges, plus the cost of insuring one more family member. In terms of cost effectiveness, we have to weigh this against the years of cheaper birth control. If we need contraception for only five years, birth control pills would cost about $1,500, an IUD less than $400, and a diaphragm $100 (assuming we get a new one every two and a half years).

In terms of "soul-effectiveness," if we psychologically can't deal with abortion once another nonpermanent method has failed, the monetary cost should not be an issue.

There are also potential side effects. On very rare occasions (0.6 percent of procedures), a major complication can occur. The bowel, the bladder, or a blood vessel can be perforated by the trocar. Once the surgeon recognizes this, she or he has to open the abdomen (*laparotomy*) and repair the damage. Suddenly a relatively minor mini-procedure has become major surgery that could require multiple blood transfusions and result in the possible complications of any surgical procedure (infection, etc.). Our consent for any surgical procedure should be made only after we are aware of what can go wrong. (For a complete list of questions to ask your doctor, see page 366).

Remember, there is no consent for the complications and even fatalities that occur when we continue an unwanted pregnancy and delivery. These occur much more frequently than those of elective tubal ligation.

There has been some concern over menstrual abnormalities in women after tubal ligation. This problem has even been elevated to the status of a "syndrome"—the so-called post–tubal sterilization syndrome. Many of us were on the Pill before we had our tubes tied, and when we stopped, we unmasked irregular cycles that would have been apparent had we not been "fixing" them with contraceptive hormones. We are also getting older, and our ovarian function is changing. This, rather than our tied tubes, is probably the chief culprit in our menstrual changes. Recent studies tend to report no real changes in menstrual patterns, and we can conclude that if post–tubal sterilization syndrome occurs at all, it affects only a very small minority of women. If we do develop irregular perimenopausal cycles, we might decide to use low-dose birth control pills to regulate them. Having our tubes tied *and* taking the Pill is contraceptive overkill! For this reason, I encourage my patients who are over 40 and experiencing cycle irregularity to put off surgical sterilization and try the Pill.

One last sterilization "failure"—it doesn't protect us from STDs (sexually transmitted diseases), although once the tubes are blocked, they are less likely to "conduct" bad microbes from the uterus to the abdominal cavity, and we're less likely to develop pelvic inflammatory disease (PID).

Reversible Contraception: Birth Control Pills, Hormones, IUDs, and Barrier Methods—Should Our Choices Change in Our Forties?

BIRTH CONTROL PILLS

"The Pill"

How appropriate that we and the Pill have both entered our fifth decade of "use"! We've grown; the Pill has shrunk. Gone are the superdoses of the 1950s and '60s. Current low-dose birth control pills contain one tenth the estrogen of their original predecessors. We found that less worked as well contraception-wise. This means that the side effects and warnings we associated with our old pills have to be diminished by at least a factor of 10; in many cases, they are no longer valid.

HOW BIRTH CONTROL PILLS WORK: NO EGG, NO PREGNANCY

Birth control pills contain both estrogen and progestins (progesterone-like hormone). The estrogen is "synthetic"—this means it is not one that we manufacture in our bodies. In addition, this form of estrogen is not broken down by the liver (as are our natural estrogens). The estrogen in birth control pills, therefore, remains more potent than our own hormone and it preferentially asserts its influence on our estrogen receptors. The combination of estrogen and progestins in the Pill will shut off

GnRH and pituitary production of FSH and LH. If we turn the pituitary off, we suppress ovulation. If we don't ovulate and release an egg, we can't get pregnant.

WHAT ARE LOW-DOSE BIRTH CONTROL PILLS?

The new low-dose Pills contain less than 50 micrograms of estrogen (usually between 20 and 35 micrograms). In comparison, the "old" Pills had 50 micrograms or more. The dose of progestins has also been lowered, and new types have been introduced. (The original progestin compounds shared some chemical features with male hormones and could have a very mild *androgenic*, or male hormone, effect.)

Modern technology has been marked by shrinkage—in computers, memory chips, telephones, and birth control pills. These "teensy" innovations have created a new telecommunications superhighway. The low-dose Pill can be our "turnpike" to cycle control, as well as disease control.

BENEFITS: THE PENDULUM HAS SWUNG; THE PILL IS NOW SOCIALLY AND MEDICALLY WELCOME

Cycle Control   The low-dose birth control pill acts as an ovarian disciplinarian. As our follicle numbers dwindle and our hormones and cycles change, we are at the mercy of inconsistent ovarian function. The Pill shuts down the ovary (or, less politely, shuts it up) and "takes over," providing a consistent level of estrogen and progestin. During the 21 days we take the active pills (28-day packs have 7 inactive, or placebo, pills), the uterine lining builds up. Because the hormone doses are low and progestin is always there to counteract estrogen's effect on our endometrial glands, the glandular buildup is often less than that of our "normal" cycles. This means there is less lining to slough when we cycle off the Pill (or take the placebo) at the end of the month. Not only do we get contraception, but we enjoy lighter periods and fewer or no cramps! We are (or more precisely, the Pill is) now in control of our cycles.

Hormone Control   Our estrogen levels diminish years before we are menopausal. We don't need an advanced endocrinologic degree or expensive lab tests to realize this as we develop hot flashes, mood swings, worsening PMS, vaginal dryness, and skin changes (see chapter 5). The estrogen in the Pill can "right" this physically "wrong" situation and set our hormone levels straight. Ongoing use of low-dose birth control pills will prevent many of our perimenopausal symptoms.

Cancer Prevention   The Pill suppresses ovarian function. "Hushed," inactive ovarian cells are far less likely to undergo the mutations needed to initiate ovarian cancer. Just one to two years of birth control pill use can decrease our lifetime risk of ovarian cancer by 30 to 40 percent, five years by 50 percent, and twelve years by 80 percent!

Birth control pills exert a similar effect on our uterine lining. The monthly stimulation of the endometrial glands is gentle and controlled. Gone are the months of unopposed estrogen (in nonovulatory cycles) that occur with increasing frequency in our forties and early fifties. The small amount of daily progestin in the Pill inhibits any tendency to glandular "wildness." Birth control pills prevent 98 percent of pregnancies and, after four years of use, 60 percent of cancers from developing in our uterine lining.

The minute we take a pill that contains hormones, we clutch our breasts: What's going to happen to them? We assume that since the Pill contains hormones, we're putting ourselves at risk for breast cancer or breast disease. In fact, the opposite may occur. In Pill users, benign diseases of the breast seem to decrease. There is a 30 percent reduction in fibrocystic disease and a 60 percent reduction of benign tumors called *fibroadenomas*. Most of us are more concerned about breast cancer than benign disease. More than twenty-two studies examining the possible relationship between Pill use and breast cancer have been published. The preponderance of evidence indicates that birth control pills do not increase our breast cancer risk. Indeed, a recent study has shown a fall in the incidence of breast cancer in women over 45 who have used birth control pills in the past.

Pelvic Disease Control   The use of birth control pills has been associated with a decrease in serious pelvic infections. The hormones change the secretions of the cervix and make it harder for bacteria to get from the vagina up into the uterus and tubes. Remember, however, that although this "swim-up" may be more arduous, the Pill will not protect us from the consequences of sexually transmitted diseases.

The Pill decreases our risk of endometriosis by lessening potential backward menstrual flow and stimulation of pre-endometriosis cells.

Fibroid tumor growth does not seem to be promoted by the Pill, and indeed the heavy periods often associated with these benign growths may be appreciably lessened, allowing us to "reach" menopause without a hysterectomy. The fibroids may diminish in size because we are not exposed to long periods of unopposed estrogen stimulation. The small amounts of progestin we get in our daily Pill can decrease the estrogen receptor activity of fibroids and stunt their continued enlargement.

Throughout our reproductive lives, our ovaries are potential cyst formers. As our follicles develop, they accumulate fluid—an exaggeration of this process causes an overabundance of fluid production and cyst formation. The same event can occur once we release the egg and develop a corpus luteum. Blood can collect, and a hemorrhagic cyst results. These are "functional" cysts; they are not malignant tumors, and they go away once they are deprived of the hormones produced during their formation. By suppressing ovulation, the birth control pill helps to prevent the development of these functional cysts.

Prevention of ovulation is also our best protection against one more pelvic disease—ectopic or tubal pregnancy.

Disease Prevention   Osteoporosis is not just a disease of menopause. Many of us lose considerable bone density in our forties and early fifties (see chapter 11). The lower estrogen levels we experience during our mid-decades have depressed our bone-building cells and motivated our bone-destroying cells. Birth control pills even the estrogen score. We can win back a 2 percent annual gain in bone protection.

Recent studies not only have discounted our worries about an association between birth control pills and heart attacks, either while we are taking them or years later, but they've also shown that the low-dose pill may ultimately be good for our hearts (provided we don't smoke)! Pills with less than 35 milligrams of ethinyl estradiol decrease plaque formation and subsequent coronary heart disease in both monkeys (they got tested first) and women. Moreover, the newer forms of birth control pills with progestins that are not like male hormones have an additional positive, rather than negative, effect on our cholesterol and lipids.

Heavy or frequent periods are not just messy inconveniences; they ultimately cause us to become anemic (with symptoms of fatigue, headache, dizziness, and palpitations). Birth control pills control excessive blood loss and prevent anemia. This makes a lot more sense than continuing to bleed and trying to rebuild our blood count with iron supplements. Oral contraceptive advances have allowed us to do more than just put a finger (or a tampon) in the proverbial dam of excessive blood loss. (I could not pass up this analogy!)

The risk of severe rheumatoid arthritis has been found to be reduced by use of oral contraceptives. Perhaps preventing swings in our cycling estrogen levels diminishes stimulation of the self-destructive immune reactions that are so common in women (and not in men).

We've come a long way in the saga of oral contraception. We loved the freedom the Pill gave us in our late teens through our thirties, but we worried. We worried that the facilitator of our sexual revolution had to be inherently bad. We worried about the chemicals we were putting into our bodies (although God knows what else we were putting into our bodies!). What a waste of worry. It turns out that these "chemicals" did more than just stop unwanted pregnancies. They stopped cyst formation and helped protect us from pelvic infections, anemia, cancer, and infertility. They can continue to help preserve our well-being through our forties and even benefit our health for the rest of our lives.

RISKS AND SIDE EFFECTS: REALITY VERSUS "I'LL HAVE A STROKE OR A HEART ATTACK OR GAIN WEIGHT IF I TAKE THE PILL IN MY FORTIES!"

Heart Attack   The ever-decreasing hormonal content of birth control pills has reduced or eliminated early concerns about the risk of Pill-related heart attack and stroke (particularly in women over 35). While "age restriction" warnings have been taken off the Pill, "smoke restriction" warnings remain. A study from England has shown that current users of oral contraceptives who do not smoke have no increased risk of heart attack. Current users who smoke fewer than fifteen cigarettes a day have more than a 3-fold increase in risk, and those who smoke fifteen or more cigarettes a day have a 21-fold increase! The experts have made a case for making oral contraceptives available over the counter and cigarettes available by prescription!

Blood Clots   The new, less androgenic birth control pills containing the progestin desogestrel were recently blamed for a rare, nonfatal increase in clot formation (thromboembolism) by the Committee on Safety of Medicines in the United Kingdom. There was an ensuing Pill uproar when the Committee suggested that women taking these pills be switched to other brands. They cited three unpublished studies that indicated a twofold increase in the risk of clots when contraceptives containing desogestrel (and gestodene, which is not available in this country) were compared with products containing other progestins.

There is a very small increase in risk for clot formation with all birth control pills. The lower the estrogen content, however, the lower the risk. If we look at the numbers for women in their reproductive years, they are as follows:

The average risk of nonfatal thromboembolism per 100,000 women per year	Status
4	Healthy, not pregnant, not taking hormones
10–15	Taking "older" low-dose birth control pills
20–30	Taking desogestrel-containing products (Orth-Cept or Desogen)
50	Pregnant

The FDA has reviewed these numbers and at this time does not feel that the risk is great enough to justify switching to other products. Some researchers also feel that the lower male hormone–like qualities of these pills may ultimately protect us from future heart attack. Based on the FDA guidelines and the positive qualities of these newer pills, I've continued to prescribe them when I feel they are a good "match" for my patients (and myself).

Now that we've dealt with life-threatening issues, let's look at our more mundane concerns.

Weight Gain   This occurred more frequently with the old pills, which contained fairly high levels of progestins. With the new low-dose pills, especially those containing the "purer" progestins, we find this is a "weightless" issue. In clinical studies with these new pills, the maximum mean weight gain after one year of use was only half a pound. (For most of us, a half-pound difference is less than what we gain premenstrually when we don't take the Pill.)

Acne and Skin Changes　The right Pill with non-male-like prog-estins such as levonorgestrel, desogestrel, and mestranol (brand names are Demulen, Ortho-Cyclen, Ortho-Cept, and Desogen) reduces acne. For some of us, pimples are a lifelong problem or can even "crop up" in an embarrassing fashion in our middle years. The estrogenic qualities of these pills are also good for the collagen content of our skin (estrogen has been shown to protect us from collagen loss).

On the "brown" side, estrogen can also cause increased pigmenta-tion and brown spots, especially if we are fair-skinned and we add the in-sult of sun damage. Sunblocks (worn constantly under our makeup) and bleaching creams help, but may not always be enough. Having freckles expand to one big blotch on our cheeks is not esthetic.

Nausea　One of my assistants would just look at her pack of pills and develop nausea! Some of us are very sensitive to estrogen; we vomit the minute we get pregnant, and we react to the estrogen in oral contracep-tives. My nurse overcame her problem by taking a pill with only 20 mi-crograms of estrogen (Loestrin 1/20) and ingesting it at night before she went to sleep. In this way, she literally slept through any reaction. It worked! If you are a new Pill taker, you may have mild nausea the first week or so. Take the pills at night, and if the nausea persists, ask your doctor to switch you to the lowest dose of estrogen.

Breakthrough Bleeding　One of the reasons we choose the Pill for contraception is to control our cycle. We are not going to be overly tol-erant of breakthrough bleeding and spotting.

This will occur more frequently when we first start using oral con-traception (as many as 18 percent of us will bleed the first cycle, but the number falls to 8 percent the second cycle and comes down to 2 to 3 per-cent by sixteen months of use). To minimize this problem, we should be sure we don't miss any pills (especially in the beginning of the pack; these start-up pills are the most important in controlling our cycle and our contraception) and that we take the Pill at approximately the same time every day. The lower the estrogen, the more critical this timing be-comes. If a pill is missed, two should be taken the next day to catch up. I know; I, the most informed of "patients," would miss a pill every few weeks and sometimes wake up at 3:00 A.M. to run to the bathroom and guiltily swallow the poor forgotten thing.

I generally have my patients "double up" and take two pills instead of one if they have breakthrough bleeding until the bleeding stops. They need a second pack of pills to do this (otherwise, they use up their current pack and start to bleed again with an early period). But doubling up should be an exception, not a rule. The idea is not to go to high-dose contraception. If bleeding continues on 20 micrograms of estrogen, I raise the dose to 35 micrograms or—rarely—to 50 micrograms (I'm not happy using this dose in women over 40). I also try changing the type of progestins in the Pill, using a higher-potency formulation. If bleeding continues despite these changes, we have to look for uterine pathology (fibroids and polyps) and consider diagnostic testing such as ultrasound or hysteroscopy.

No Period   The amount of blood we lose with each period is proportionate to the amount of endometrial buildup during our cycles. The lower the dose of our birth control pills, the less the lining is stimulated. On occasion, this buildup is so minimal that there is nothing to slough off, and we don't bleed. This lack of a period (*amenorrhea*) can occur in less than 2 percent of women on the low-dose Pill and often corrects itself with time. If you don't get a period, don't assume you're pregnant and stop the Pill, because the next month, you can get pregnant. Restart your new pack and if you are concerned, do a home pregnancy test. If you took your pills correctly, it should be negative.

Headaches   We all get headaches and most have no effect on our use of birth control pills. Looking at "the headache" neurologically (I now sound like a doctor in a white coat advertising pain remedies!), there are two kinds: *vascular,* or migraine, headaches and *nonvascular,* or muscle tension, headaches. The nonvascular ones are more common and cause a steady ache without throbbing on one or both sides of the head. They can be recurrent and often start in the afternoon or evening (when the day's tensions have accumulated in our muscles). These headaches are not increased or decreased by birth control pills.

The vascular headaches are divided into two groups: common and classic. Common migraines are recurrent and severe, and often occur on just one side. They may be accompanied by nausea, a general feeling of being sick, and sensitivity to light. Approximately 17.6 percent of women have one or more migraine headaches each year, and the highest prevalence is between the ages of 35 and 45. Seventy percent of these women have relatives who suffer from migraines. "Classic" migraines are less "common" than common migraines (that's a brilliant deduction!) and are preceded by neurological symptoms such as vision change, numbness, paralysis, or even an inability to speak. (Thank goodness, few of us are rendered speechless by our headaches; we just don't *want* to talk.) Up to 70 percent of women who suffer from migraines get them just before or during their periods. We've even given them the official term of *menstrual migraines*. They seem to be brought on by the same cyclical fall of estrogen that causes us to get our periods. These headaches often get worse in our forties as our estrogen levels reach new "lows." Our monthly estrogen decline can activate a release of chemical messengers in our brain that in turn cause adjacent blood vessels to dilate, sensitize nerve endings, and create muscle spasm. Add to this a reduction in the brain's endorphins, which in better hormone times helped us deal with pain, and we develop the dreaded migraine. We may also produce more uterine prostaglandins as we get older (and our uterine walls get thicker). This substance causes menstrual cramps and, you guessed it, menstrual headaches.

So how do birth control pills enter the migraine picture? There seem to be both contraindications and indications for their use. Early studies (in 1978) showed that higher-dose birth control pills increased migraine headaches by 15 to 50 percent. Most of these headaches occurred during the Pill-free week, probably as a result of the rapid fall of estrogens from their artificially high level. Some women develop migraines for the first time when using the Pill, and these may continue for several months after stopping. A study from 1975 suggested an association between migraine headaches and stroke. Whether birth control pills make this risk even greater is still not clear. What is clear is that if we have classic (or neurologic) migraines, we may be at risk. There is no sense in taking any chances with regard to worsening this condition or its associated risk of stroke with birth control pills. If we suffer from common migraines, we can use the birth control pills to stabilize some of our estrogen variations and see how we feel. A low-dose formulation that has constant doses of both estrogen and progestin (monophasic pills) should be used. Since synthetic progestins have been shown to increase the severity of migraines, pills with a low progestin content are preferable;

these include Ovcon 35, Modicon, and Brevicon. I have also had success with LoEstrin 1/20, a pill with a very low estrogen content. Because the headaches may rear their ugly heads when we take the placebo pills and withdraw from estrogen, I suggest shortening this "rest" period from seven to three days. Rarely, even this estrogen-free interval evokes a headache. It may be necessary to add estrogen replacement to overcome this hormone sensitivity, and I've had some patients use an estrogen patch for three days with "migraine success." (Note: The estrogen patch can also be used for menstrual migraines during the natural estrogen lull of the period in women who are not taking the Pill).

A word of caution: If we develop new migraines on the Pill, we should stop, consult our physician, and consider other modes of contraception. Nonvascular, or tension, headaches are okay (not necessarily for us, but for use of the Pill). Indeed, a German study showed that women who use low-dose birth control pills were able to reduce these types of headache, especially if they were premenstrual, by half. For most of us, one source of headache will be banished by the Pill, that of "contraceptive worry."

FAILURE RATE OF ORAL CONTRACEPTION

If we lived in a perfect world or, more objectively, if we ourselves were perfect oral contraceptive users and took those little pills consistently and correctly, the annual failure rate would be 0.1 percent. But the reality is that we forget pills, start the cycle a day or two late, or use antibiotics, which can affect the absorption of the Pill by our gastrointestinal tract. That brings the oral contraceptive failure rate up to 3 percent a year among married women of all ages. However, if we then calculate our diminished fertility over 40, we "gain" a margin against failure and bring the odds down to 1.9 percent. This is low when compared to barrier contraception (see Table 2.1).

"YOU CAN'T TAKE THE PILL": ABSOLUTE, RELATIVE, AND UNSUBSTANTIATED CONTRAINDICATIONS TO ORAL CONTRACEPTIVES
ABSOLUTE CONTRAINDICATIONS: WHEN THE PILL IS "OFF LIMITS"

Previous Clotting Disorders Leading to Stroke, Heart Attack, or Clots in Our Major Deep Veins The Pill does affect clotting factors

TABLE 2.1 FAILURE RATES
(UNWANTED PREGNANCY) FOR WOMEN
OVER 35 (35 TO 44) ACCORDING TO
CONTRACEPTIVE METHOD

IUD	1.7%
Birth control pills	1.9%
Condoms	3.3%
Periodic abstinence	6.2%
Spermicides	9.1%
Diaphragm/Cervical cap	10.3%
Sponge	13.7%

Harlap, Kost, Forrest. 1991

(although the low-dose pills are less likely to cause clot formation), and we don't want to add to established clotting risks. However (I love using that word!), if you have a bleeding (not clotting) problem you can use the Pill to diminish blood loss during your period. Moreover (another great word!), women who have a history of clotting from trauma or injury or a brain hemorrhage from a vascular malformation (which was corrected) may use birth control pills.

Abnormal Liver Function   The hormones in the Pill are metabolized in the liver. Without normal liver function, the actual levels and effects of these hormones will change. If you have acute infectious hepatitis, you should not take the Pill. Once your liver function returns to normal, you can resume using oral contraception with your doctor's okay.

Estrogen-Dependent Cancers   We do not want to "feed" any residual tumor cells with estrogen (although the progestins in the Pill might be helpful, and pregnancy provides much more estrogen than the Pill). So women who have had breast cancer or uterine cancer should not take birth control pills.

Abnormal Vaginal Bleeding   Although the Pill will generally cure this problem, we should be certain abnormal vaginal bleeding is not caused by pregnancy or endometrial cancer. Our new sensitive pregnancy tests and endometrial sampling in high-risk women will give us this information.

Known or Suspected Pregnancy   If your period is late, make sure you are not pregnant before starting the Pill. If you know you're pregnant, stop taking the Pill. If you do take the Pill by mistake in early pregnancy, don't freak; there is no solid evidence that birth control pill use during pregnancy adversely affects the developing fetus.

Smoking over the Age of 35   When we mix the Pill and smoking, we "brew" heart attacks. What a shame: Women who smoke have lower estrogen levels, higher rates of osteoporosis, and an earlier menopause. The Pill would have helped these problems, but smokers over 35 are not "Pill-eligible."

RELATIVE CONTRAINDICATIONS

A "relative contraindication" means that you should discuss your problems with your doctor. If the benefits of the Pill outweigh other health concerns, you can use oral contraception with careful monitoring.

High Blood Pressure   If your blood pressure is controlled and doesn't become unstable on the Pill, you can probably use oral contraceptives. I have a patient who is a well-known performer, and her irregular and heavy periods have made it difficult for her to adhere to a preset schedule. Her blood pressure is labile; it rises in my office (I guess it's me) but returns to normal at home. The Pill has not affected her home readings and has allowed her to carry on with her demanding performances. Her periods are now timed, light, and totally unobtrusive.

Cardiac Disease   Many women (13 to 17 percent) have a condition called *mitral valve prolapse* (MVP). The edges of this heart valve don't close cleanly, and we can hear a characteristic murmur or click or see this "floppy" closure on ultrasound. There may be a higher incidence of heart palpitations with MVP. Most of us are unaware of our condition. Simple MVP without cardiac-flow problems should not prevent us from using birth control pills. If more severe MVP or abnormalities of other valves are found, doctors worry about clots forming in these "faulty" valves and hesitate to prescribe the Pill.

Diabetes Type II, or non-insulin-dependent, diabetes increases after we turn 40. Our concern about oral contraception relates to whether or not plasma insulin levels or glucose tolerance will be affected. The estrogens in the Pill will have no effect on either. However, the older, more potent progestins derived from male hormones may increase insulin and slightly decrease our tolerance of sugar. With the new low-dose birth control pills and the new progestins, there is little, if any, impact on insulin requirements or any of the complications of diabetes. However, if your diabetes requires insulin and you are known to have blood vessel complications, you may already be at risk for clots and should not add to this by taking birth control pills.

Gestational diabetes (which develops during pregnancy) can occur in 4 percent of women and is certainly more common in our late thirties and forties. More than half of us who had gestational diabetes will develop overt diabetes within fifteen years of our pregnancy. There is no evidence, however, that the Pill will hasten the appearance of diabetes or increase this risk. If you have a history of previous gestational diabetes, you can use low-dose birth control pills that contain a low-activity progestin. Just don't forget that you need annual blood sugar screenings (whether or not you use oral contraception).

Uterine Fibroids Estrogen may cause fibroid growth, but a balance of low-dose progestin and estrogen usually will not stimulate these benign tumors. In fact, we can use birth control pills to reduce the heavy bleeding associated with fibroids.

Gallbladder Disease Long-term use (ten to fourteen years) of birth control pills has been associated with a "modest" risk of our developing symptomatic gallstones (a relative risk for women of 1.5 versus 1 for nonusers). Because the Pill can influence the components of bile, we need to consider whether this will affect an already compromised gallbladder.

Epilepsy This neurological condition occurs in 1 percent of our population. Estrogens and progestins do not seem to have an effect on the course of epilepsy. We know that the sensitivity of the brain to seizures is decreased by progestins and increased by estrogen, so the Pill, which combines both, is balanced and should have no effect. Our main concern is the efficacy of the Pill when taken together with antiseizure medications. These drugs can increase liver enzymes, so that the hormones in the Pill are broken down with "greater enthusiasm" and the affected blood hormone levels become too low to be effective. This is the one instance when the higher-dose Pill (containing 50 micrograms of estrogen) is recommended.

MYTHICAL CONTRAINDICATIONS:
"YOU'RE TOO OLD FOR THE PILL"

We are not! Forget age restrictions; the Pill not only will provide us with birth control but will also provide numerous benefits for our hormones, our cycles, our diseases, our cancer risks, and our perimenopausal symptoms! These little unobtrusive packs (pharmaceutical marketing experts felt that we didn't want to acknowledge our use of the Pill and made them and their packages as minuscule as possible) can "pack" amazing benefits into our middle decades. They help keep us too young to get old.

The Morning-After Pill

Publicity has made most of us think that the only morning-after pill is the controversial RU-486, also called the "abortion pill." It has anti-progesterone activity and deprives an early pregnancy of progesterone "support," causing the pregnancy to detach from the uterus and spontaneously abort. RU-486 has other important effects for women. It can shrink uterine fibroids and may help prevent recurrence of breast cancer, endometrial cancer, and ovarian cancer. Due to political pressure from anti-abortion groups, it is currently not available for clinical use in this country.

When given during the second half of our cycle, RU-486 interrupts the progesterone-controlled buildup of the endometrial lining and prevents conception. This may be our morning-after (or at least ovulation-after) pill of the future, but we've had morning-after contraception available to us for over twenty years. It was and is our "plain old" birth control pill! If used within seventy-two hours after unprotected intercourse, two high-dose birth control pills (with 50 micrograms of estrogen), followed by two more pills twelve hours later, will effectively prevent most pregnancies (the failure rate is just 2 percent). If you use the low-dose pill (30 to 35 micrograms of estrogen), you need four pills initially and four more twelve hours later.

I must stress that this is "off-label" use, which means that the drug companies won't accept responsibility for side effects, and the FDA hasn't given official approval (or instructions) for this use. There are several good reasons. These high doses of hormones are hard to take and may sometimes be dangerous. They can cause nausea, vomiting, and bloating, and, more important, may rapidly increase clotting factors and blood pressure, which could lead to stroke. For the young and impetuous who have "unexpected" sex, it certainly can prevent the need for many abortions. Planned Parenthood organizations and many private physicians prescribe the Pill for this purpose.

WARNING! You should use morning-after birth control pills *only* after you've consulted your doctor! If you have any risk factors for stroke or heart attack (high blood pressure, high cholesterol, high triglycerides, diabetes, obesity, or you smoke), I would strongly advise against this last-minute "way out." By our fifth decade, we should be wiser and better able to plan ahead without having to scramble to clean up spilt milk (or in this case, sperm).

The "Mini-Pill": If Estrogen Is "Out," the Progestin-Only Pill May Still Be "In"

The progestin-only pill had almost twice the failure rate of combined oral contraceptives (pills with estrogen and progestins) when we were younger. But as our fertility diminishes, this mini-pill gets better, and after 40, its contraceptive efficacy is the same as that of low-dose (combined) birth control pills. So if estrogen is deemed unacceptable by us or our physicians, we can try the mini-pill. This would certainly apply to women who smoke, have a history of clots or classic migraines, or just don't feel well on combined oral contraception.

HOW THE MINI-PILL WORKS

Constant small doses of progestin have a strong negative effect on the hypothalamus and pituitary in our brain, preventing signals that stimulate ovulation. The ovary is not entirely shut down, but the progestin "atmosphere" downgrades the quality of ovulation. Progestin also adversely affects the mucus produced by the cervix. This very thick, "hostile" mucus prevents sperm from swimming up into the uterus and out into the tubes.

FAILURE RATE

If we don't forget to take the mini-pill, its failure rate falls to less than 0.5 percent.

POSITIVE BENEFITS

We are protecting our uterine lining from perimenopausal spurts of un-opposed estrogen, so this mini-pill may help prevent endometrial cancer.

LACK OF POSITIVE BENEFITS

Since ovarian function is not suppressed to the same degree as with combined birth control pills, we probably will not get the same ovarian cancer protection. Also, since we are not "upping" our falling estrogen levels, our bones may not get bone-density protection (although progestins have been shown to help bone-building cells). The mini-pill fails to protect us from sexually transmitted diseases, including AIDS.

SIDE EFFECTS

This "harmless" mini-pill (harmless with respect to its lack of estrogen and all of the angst that goes with the E-hormone) sounds too good to be true—and, of course, it is. Its chief side effect is cycle irregularity. Some women stop having periods with the mini-pill and then worry that they are either pregnant or menopausal. Others develop erratic bleeding, and their worries switch to miscarriage, cancer, or perimenopause. No matter what reassurance we get, bleeding without cycle or reason is less than acceptable in our forties. Finally, ovarian cysts may be more common in mini-pill users. They are not permanent but can cause pain and result in expensive and even invasive workups.

INJECTED PROGESTERONE: LONG-ACTING SHOTS AND IMPLANTS

A Shot Every Three Months: Depo-Medroxyprogesterone Acetate (DMPA or Depo-Provera)

Our personal-responsibility quotient is dramatically reduced with this form of contraception. All we have to remember to do is show up

four times a year for our prescribed shot. This product, similar to naturally occurring progesterone, is injected deep into the muscle (in our
buttock or arm), and from there it is slowly released into our bloodstream. It stops ovulation, but it does not completely shut down the
ovary, which continues to produce estrogen levels similar to those produced at the beginning of our cycle. These are lower overall than if we
ovulate, but higher than if we're menopausal, so we won't get hot flashes.

FAILURE RATE

The failure rate of DMPA is very low, ranging (for all ages) from 0.1 to
0.7 percent.

POSITIVE BENEFITS OF USE

The level and efficacy of the hormone are not affected by ingestion and
absorption. Antibiotics and antiseizure medications won't lower or raise
the level as they do with oral birth control pills. Indeed, DMPA seems to
have a quieting effect on brain seizure activity, enabling women with
epilepsy to have both contraceptive control and better seizure control.

Use of DMPA is associated with an 80 percent reduction in the risk
of endometrial cancer. This is not surprising, because the uterine lining
is subjected to less estrogen and more progesterone.

Also, women who use DMPA may have fewer pelvic infections (or
pelvic inflammatory disease, PID) because the progesterone thickens the
cervical mucus and thins the uterine lining, making it difficult for bacteria to swim up and infect the uterus. This, however, has no beneficial effect on the STD we fear most—AIDS.

Periods often stop or are very light, so we won't have to worry about
heavy bleeding, cramping, or anemia.

Smokers and women with previous clotting problems can use this
contraceptive. It does not increase clotting factors or adversely affect
their risk of heart attack, stroke, or thrombosis.

DMPA doesn't clinically change liver function or affect the
gallbladder. If we have problems related to these organs (hepatitis, gallstones) and can't use birth control pills, we can probably use Depo-
Provera.

HEALTH CONCERNS AND SIDE EFFECTS

Bleeding   Irregular bleeding is already an "issue" in our forties. DMPA can either cure it by stopping our periods (this occurs in 50 percent of women using DMPA for one year and 75 percent after two years) or can make it worse. Most women experience unpredictable bleeding during the first few months of use. This subsides with time, but it is hard to bleed and maintain our equanimity when we have been taught to be concerned about abnormal bleeding.

Weight Gain   Bleeding is worrisome, but for most of us, weight gain is gruesome. This is probably the greatest drawback of DMPA. Women using Depo-Provera may gain 5 pounds the first year and continue to gain at a rate of 2 to 4 pounds a year with long-term use. I have my patients on DMPA watch their diet and weight, and if the latter creeps up with no apparent change in the former, we do an "over-the-scale" consultation on the possible use of other forms of contraception.

Cancer   The most serious concern about the use of DMPA is breast cancer. FDA approval for this drug's contraceptive use was delayed for many years because of early studies implicating progesterones in breast cancer in beagles. Data from the World Health Organization (WHO) helped convince the FDA that DMPA was breast-okay (please note the rhyme!). Their conclusion was that breast cancer risk was not elevated and was no greater than if we used birth control pills. A New Zealand study disagreed and found that the risk of breast cancer increased 2 to 2.6 times. A review of both studies concluded that women who start to use DMPA have a twofold increase in their risk of breast cancer in the first five years, but that there is no increase in cancer if DMPA is used for longer periods of time. (Translation: The DMPA may accelerate growth of a preexisting tumor but won't cause a new one to grow.)

Unlike birth control pills, DMPA does not seem to confer protection against ovarian cancer.

Bone Loss   Because we are not ovulating and our total levels of estrogen are somewhat lower with use of DMPA, our bone density may be affected. A New Zealand study showed a greater loss of bone density in perimenopausal women using DMPA for five years or more (6.5 to 7.5 percent) compared with nonusers. This was self-limited (it never got worse with ongoing use) and not enough to cause fractures. It also was not permanent; it reversed two years after the shots were stopped.

More Frequent Side Effects   Sometimes we feel "off" with DMPA and wonder if it is the shot or us. Progesterone can be the culprit in bloating, breast tenderness, depression, loss of libido, headaches, dizziness, and even hair loss. The problem is, we have to wait several months for the shot to wear off in order to tell if it indeed caused these symptoms.

Norplant Subdermal Implants

Norplant consists of six Silastic capsules containing a progestin (levonorgestrel) that are inserted under the skin in the fleshy inner portion of the upper arm. The progestin is slowly released (it's so slow that it takes five years to be used up). It prevents ovulation about 50 percent of the time, but its chief effect is to prevent the egg from maturing properly so that it can undergo fertilization. The progestin also changes the cervical mucus so that sperm have a hard time getting up to make their overtures to the underdeveloped egg.

FAILURE RATE

This varies with years of use, but is consistently very low. It starts with the negligible rate of 0.2 percent the first year and may rise to 1.6 percent in the fourth year. For some reason, it then drops to 0.4 percent in the fifth and last year of the implants' effective lifetime.

ADVANTAGES

This is one-stop contraception for five years, possibly just enough time to get us through our last gasp of unwanted fertility. Like any progestin-only contraception, it will probably decrease our incidence of endometrial cancer.

There is a slow, delayed (after four years) beneficial effect on our lipoproteins and triglycerides. This is probably too slight and too late to give us actual clinical benefits against cardiovascular disease (but at least we're not put at increased risk).

DISADVANTAGES AND SIDE EFFECTS

The initial disadvantage is the "start-up" cost. The manufacturer, Wyeth-Ayerst Laboratories, charges $320 for a fancy kit (it even has the antiseptic and gauze) that contains less than $50 worth of progestin capsules. An even higher price is passed on to us as consumers (doctors and nurses have to charge for the twenty or more minutes of their time needed to insert these capsules), so we can end up paying between $500 and $700. Over five years, Norplant is cheaper than Depo-Provera, but our initial "charge" can certainly be jolting.

The main physiological side effect is bleeding. As many as 80 percent of women on Norplant have changes in their cycle, especially in the first one to two years. These include bouts of prolonged or heavy bleeding, spotting between periods, frequent periods, and—on the opposite side—no bleeding (12 percent). Over the five years, this tends to right itself, but bleeding patterns may still be irregular for 30 percent of women. So how do we react to this in our forties? Do we need a "bleeding workup," and is it safe to discount this important sign and chalk it up to those little rods in our arm? Most women (and their uteri) will be fine, but if we are overweight, diabetic, or have a family history of endometrial cancer, we can't be "implant blasé" and should consider endometrial sampling.

Even if we are not at risk for cancer, the bleeding can be very annoying, and it is the reason for half of the requests to get the darn things out now! This is where, in my opinion (as well as that of the women and lawyers who are currently suing the makers of Norplant), the chief side effect occurs: difficulty in the removal of all six rods. If they were not evenly inserted (at the same level in the fatty tissue under the skin), or if they were bent or scarred, their removal can be traumatic. I once spent forty-five minutes trying to get two "lost" rods out of a patient who had had them inserted by someone else. They were positioned at weird angles, the patient was heavy, and I had trouble feeling them. So before you shell out as much as $700, make sure you are willing to cope with bleeding (you may have to always carry a pad or tampon with you) and be aware that you may one day have to request that your implants be "shelled out" before their time.

Being "armed" with Norplant will not protect us against AIDS or other STDs, and since this progestin does not completely inhibit ovulation, we expect little protection against ovarian cancer. There are no good data on any increase or decrease in our risk of breast cancer.

IUDs (Intrauterine Devices)

IUD has become a bad word (or more correctly, a bad acronym) because of widespread publicity over a reputed increased risk of pelvic inflammatory disease (PID) with IUD use. Remember, not all IUDs are (or were) Dalkon Shields, which had a faulty design that caused them to harbor unwanted bacteria. Because of the frenetic activity on the part of many lawyers (and the resulting burden on the liability insurance of the companies supplying this product), most IUDs became unavailable in this country for several years.

Let's face it: Having a foreign body in our uterine cavity is not a great idea if we're going to have sex with even one partner who could expose us to sexually transmitted bacteria or viruses. If these bugs get into our vagina, their entry into our uterine lining may be aided and abetted by this foreign body. Being over 40 doesn't mean we or our partners are "purely" monogamous, but statistics and our maturing wisdom make this a more likely circumstance. So if the definition of monogamy fits— you've got only one sex partner, and that partner has sex *only* with you— an IUD may be an excellent form of contraception.

The ParaGard (Copper IUD)

HOW IT WORKS

ParaGard, the most commonly used IUD, is composed of a polyethylene (plastic) T wrapped in fine strands of copper wire. The top portion of the T fits nicely across the top of the uterus, and the perpendicular body points down toward the cervix. A single-filament string hangs from the lower portion out of the cervix, allowing us to check to make sure the device hasn't "gotten lost" and providing a handle for later removal. The device interferes with pregnancy implantation in some way, while the copper, which is slowly released, again "in some way," enhances the

IUD's contraceptive effect, possibly by interfering with sperm transport, fertilization, and implantation. (I apologize for the vagueness of this explanation, but it's the best the contraceptive "experts" have to offer.)

FAILURE RATE

This is a highly effective contraceptive with an all-age failure rate ranging from 0.6 percent (the first year) to 2.8 percent (by the tenth year of use). But remember, by our tenth year, our fertility will be decreased, so this number is probably much lower for forty-something women. If you do get pregnant with this IUD and decide you don't want an abortion, your doctor should attempt to remove the device. If you continue the pregnancy with the IUD in place, you run the risk of miscarriage, infection, and premature delivery.

POSITIVE BENEFITS

The ParaGard works for ten years. One insertion in our early forties, and that's it. We may begin menopause at the end of its "tour of duty." Although it's initially expensive (a $220 cost to physicians, most of which covers the manufacturer's liability insurance), it's cheap when we consider the years of use.

LACK OF POSITIVE BENEFITS

Unlike birth control pills or even barrier methods of contraception, it doesn't protect us from anything (disease-wise) except pregnancy. Lacking hormones, it bestows no protection against cancer, osteoporosis, or heart disease.

SIDE EFFECTS

It would be great if this intrauterine device would meekly reside as a silent companion within our uterus for those ten years. Sadly, the uterus may "protest," and we may develop heavy or prolonged periods, cramps, and spotting between cycles. When this occurs in our forties, we are never quite sure whether the bleeding is caused by a uterine problem or the IUD. I usually prescribe nonsteroidal anti-inflammatory medications (such as ibuprofen) and see if these symptoms improve. An ultrasound will help determine if there's "something wrong" with the uterus and will also show if the IUD is in the right place. But if abnormal bleeding continues, we have to remove the IUD and consider another mode of contraception.

Bleeding changes are a nuisance but rarely endanger our lives. Pelvic inflammatory disease is another story. A large World Health Organization (WHO) study found a very slightly increased rate of PID in IUD users ("just" 1.6 cases per 1,000 women using the device for one year) compared to nonusers. The risk was six times higher in the first twenty days, probably because bacteria were pushed up into the uterus from the vagina during insertion. To prevent this risk, I and many other physicians prescribe an antibiotic (doxycycline) for a few days after the insertion. An ongoing risk of PID, however, is strongly related to our sexual behavior. Our partners' "flora" (and that of their previous sexual partners) is what will "rise up and infect," not the IUD itself. The IUD may simply create a path of least resistance. If we develop pelvic pain, tenderness, fever, or discharge, we need to be checked and treated. Untreated infections can result in widespread abdominal infection, abscess formation, and even sepsis and death. The monogamy "thing" is more important than ever for those of us choosing this form of contraception.

CONTRAINDICATIONS: WHEN SHOULD YOU ABSTAIN FROM IUDS?

The IUD is contraindicated if you have or have had any of the following:

No Previous Children   If you have not had any term pregnancies, your uterus may be smaller than that of a woman who went through nine months of uterine stretching. You could be at increased risk for perforation during insertion of the IUD, as well as expulsion (the uterus contracts and pushes it out) and bleeding problems.

Unexplained Bleeding   Let's not make matters worse with an IUD.

Uterine Abnormalities (Fibroids, Genetic Malformations)   These distort the uterine cavity, increasing the risk of perforation, bleeding, and cramping.

Previous PID or Uterine Infections Damaged or scarred tissue is more prone to reinfection.

Previous Ectopic Pregnancy This may have occurred as the result of a silent PID and certainly has left the Fallopian tubes or the remaining tube vulnerable.

Conditions Causing Susceptibility to Infections If you are diabetic or have a faulty cardiac valve that is prone to damage by infection, or if you are taking long-term steroid therapy, you should probably avoid the IUD.

Wilson's Disease, or Any Type of Copper Allergy Since the IUD is made of copper, your body will react to it.

Having a Nonmonogamous or "Wrong" (Microbially Speaking) Partner

The Progestasert IUD

Progestasert is a T-shaped IUD containing a reservoir of progesterone in its vertical body. Over a peroid of one year, it slowly releases progesterone, which aids the device in preventing sperm "travel," fertilization, and implantation.

ADVANTAGES

The slow progesterone release makes this IUD less likely to cause abnormal bleeding than the copper IUD. Indeed, it can reduce heavy periods.

DISADVANTAGES

It's good for only one year. We would need ten Progestasert IUDs to equal the lifetime of one ParaGard. This becomes expensive at $90 for each Progestasert IUD (this is the cost to the physician and doesn't include insertion and removal fees).

SIDE EFFECTS AND WARNINGS

Those listed for the ParaGard also apply to the Progestasert.

BARRIER METHODS AND SPERMICIDES: "STRIKING" BELOW THE CERVIX

Many of us (15 percent) prefer barrier contraception. These barriers aren't perfect. Condoms can slip and tear, while diaphragms and caps don't provide "sperm-tight" coverage of the cervix. The good thing is that as we get older and our natural fertility declines, we don't need perfection, and if these barriers afford some protection from sexually transmitted microbes, we've helped ward off more than pregnancy. There are a number of unwelcome organisms that can accompany sperm and cause *sexually transmitted diseases* (STDs).

The most worrisome is, of course, *HIV (human immunodeficiency virus)*, the virus that causes AIDS. Other sexually transmitted viruses include *HPV (human papillomavirus)*, which causes venereal warts and increased risk of cervical cancer, and the *herpes virus*, which causes recurrent painful lesions.

The next group of unwanted sperm escorts is bacteria, which include *chlamydia* (a silent infection that can cause PID and tubal scarring), *gonorrhea*, and *syphilis* (yes, they're both still around). And finally, to complete our microzoo, *trichomonas*, a single-celled organism (which has a tail and looks rather like a sperm) that causes a foul, irritating discharge (probably the least serious of all of our STD worries). When we "block and destroy" with barrier devices and their accompanying spermicide, we protect our uterine cavity from both pregnancy and infection-causing organisms.

Condoms

These should be latex; sheepskin is too porous and won't prevent STD infections. An effective polyurethane condom has been introduced and can be found at "specialty" stores and in catalogues. Condoms with spermicide are obviously preferable. Condoms should be lubricated only with water-soluble substances designed for this purpose; petroleum jelly, baby oil, and the like can break down the latex.

FAILURE RATE

Overall, 2 to 12 percent; this depends on appropriate "penis dressing" (the condom should be put on an erect penis before it touches our body, because the initial secretion of fluid can contain active sperm), "anchoring" (so it doesn't slip off in action), and removal (without spill onto our genitalia). Commercialism has hit the condom market (considering the disease-prevention benefits, we should laud whatever it takes to sell these things). Condoms come in great colors; they can glow in the dark; they have scents, tastes, and variations in surface and texture. We can laugh and leave them to our kids or join in the fun! We're lucky; we and our partners have had two or more decades to learn how to properly use them by trial (and error). Our novice daughters and sons are still struggling to do it right (and in this area—unlike other learning tasks—we're not exactly urging them to increase their practice time).

SIDE EFFECTS

Side effects are few, but some women are allergic to the spermicide or latex. If you develop irritation, swelling, and discharge every time your partner uses condoms, you probably have this allergy. Try switching from latex to polyurethane and changing spermicides, or, if necessary, use condoms without spermicide (but remember you'll have less protection).

Diaphragm

A diaphragm is a soft rubber or latex cup with a round rim. It works only if spermicidal jelly or cream is put into and around it. It's placed over the cervix, but is large enough to come down the vagina and lodge under the pubic bone. It provides a physical barrier to sperm, but not a perfect seal; they can sneak around the edges. That's where the spermicide goes into action, killing the sperm before they enter the cervix. To give this method a chance to work, the diaphragm and jelly should be inserted before intercourse (but no more than two hours before) and have to remain in place at least six hours after intercourse. If you and your partner are feeling amorous (and energetic), and you go at it again before the six hours are up, you have to use a special applicator to insert more spermicide. The diaphragm should not be removed to do this.

FAILURE RATE

The failure rate is from 3 to 18 percent for all ages; this, again, is a function of our proper use (was there only a small dollop of spermicide left in the tube and you forgot to buy a new supply, or did the diaphragm pop out when you went to the bathroom?).

ADVANTAGE

We control our contraception "per event."

DISADVANTAGE

The diaphragm is less effective than condoms in preventing the spread of STDs.

SIDE EFFECTS

The chief side effect of the diaphragm is that it can increase our frequency of bladder infections. If we empty our bladder before and after intercourse, flush our systems by drinking eight glasses of water a day, and add a daily glass of cranberry juice (which decreases bacterial activity), we may be able to overcome this. But if this bladder regimen doesn't work, we should switch to another form of contraception. Some women develop an allergy to the spermicidal jelly or cream. This can result in local swelling, redness, irritation, and chronic discharge. I advise my patients to try switching brands of spermicide, but if all nonoxynol-9 substances cause this, they have to find an alternative nonbarrier form of contraception.

Cervical Cap

The cervical cap is a mini-diaphragm, but thicker and less pliable. It should be filled with contraceptive jelly and cream and then placed directly on the cervix, where it fits tightly.

ADVANTAGES

A cervical cap doesn't fill the vagina, and you and your partner probably won't notice its presence. It is less likely to cause bladder infections, since the rim is not pressing on the bladder or urethra as is the case with the diaphragm. It can be worn for forty-eight hours. You can "premeditate" its insertion, but you have to add the jelly right before intercourse.

DISADVANTAGES

The fit has to be just right; if not, it can dislodge. It's not enough of a barrier (no matter how well it fits) to protect against STDs.

Contraceptive Sponge

The contraceptive sponge—a disposable form of contraception— was convenient, did not require a "fitting," and was simple to use, needing no additional spermicidal gels. Its failure rate was somewhat higher than that of the diaphragm. Alas, it is no longer available, not because it was defective, but because federal regulators demanded changes be made at the factory where it was produced. The manufacturers felt that the cost of these changes would lower or eliminate their profits, so they simply closed shop.

The Female Condom

The female condom is the first barrier contraceptive with proclaimed STD protection which is ours. We buy it, we insert it, and it covers our vulnerable areas. It looks like a Saran Wrap sheath (it's made of polyurethane) with a closed ring at one end and an open ring at the other end. The closed ring is inserted like a diaphragm; the open portion then hangs out from the vagina, covering and protecting our vulvar area. It's prelubricated with silicon; it does not contain spermicide.

FAILURE RATE

This device was evaluated under an expedited FDA study protocol and was quickly released because there was pressure (hopefully, by women) to find new forms of STD protection. So the numbers aren't all in; many of the women testing the device used it for only six months. The pregnancy rate for them was high (12.5 percent), leading to an estimated annual rate of 26 percent (these rates can be compared with an expected pregnancy rate of 28 percent found in women of all ages using *no* contraception!). Most of the failures were due to inconsistent use or inappropriate placement, and the manufacturer feels that with better and correct compliance, the numbers will improve. We also lack current proof that this condom offers the same level of STD protection as the latex male condom.

ADVANTAGES

We are in control; we insert it, and our partner has to insert his penis into the sleeve. Theoretically, there is no skin-to-vagina contact.

DISADVANTAGES

Once inserted, it's not a pretty sight! You have this plastic sheath and ring hanging out of your vagina. During intercourse, there is a crinkly noise from the rubbing of the polyurethane. One of you has to grasp the outer ring when the male withdraws. We're going to need better documented protection rates (from pregnancy and STDs) to persuade us to use it. Male condoms are still more effective and less noisy.

Vaginal Spermicides

Vaginal spermicides are designed to be used alone and do not include the creams and gels that are marketed to accompany diaphragms and caps. They come in several forms: inserts (suppositories), foams, creams, gels, and absorbable films. They either melt or spread in such a way as to form a protective coating of spermicide in the vagina and over the cervix. They contain nonoxynol-9, which immobilizes and kills sperm. This chemical may also be "cidal," killing viruses and bacteria, but not sufficiently to eliminate the need for a physical barrier such as a condom.

FAILURE RATE

This ranges from 2 to 29 percent, again depending on consistency of use. But if our own fertility rate is falling, this could very well suffice.

ADVANTAGES

Spermicides can be purchased without prescription and are inexpensive. No fitting or training is needed. We just insert them, and the heat of our body (more precisely, our vagina) is sufficient to melt and spread the antisperm chemicals.

DISADVANTAGES

The spermicide must be inserted before intercourse, and you may have to allow ten to thirty minutes for it to melt, spread, and coat the vaginal and cervical area. If you have intercourse a second time, you have to insert a new dose. This can end up being messy, and there is no immediate cleanup solution. (You shouldn't try to douche or rinse the stuff out for at least six hours after intercourse, while the spermicide is working—in general, douching should not be necessary for most women.)

Sex, Barrier Contraception, and Our Safety: Pregnancy May Be the Least of Our Worries

This section on barrier contraception would be incomplete without stating the obvious: Although spermicide kills some bacteria and viruses, and diaphragms and cervical caps cause some decrease in the access of microbes to our inner pelvic organs, condoms are the only barrier that permits us to have "safer" sex. The term "safe sex" connotes a reassurance that we have nothing to fear, a definite misnomer. If the "Don't allow sperm to get up there" failure rate is 2 to 29 percent, we can't expect to do any better with smaller penetrating viruses and bacteria. Latex condoms plus spermicide will give us about a 70 percent reduction in STDs, including chlamydia, gonorrhea, herpesvirus, HPV, and perhaps, most important, human immunodeficiency virus (HIV).

Our midlife often includes separation, divorce, and/or widowhood. We find ourselves out in a sexual world that changed while we were gone. The men we see are usually veterans, not of traditional military war, but of a microbial penis war. They may now be endowed with every virus and bacterium to which they exposed themselves during their previous sexual encounters. I'm amazed at how many of my over-40 patients admit to falling into an amorous exchange of seminal fluid without condom protection. The contraceptive issues might have been raised (he had a vasectomy; she had a tubal ligation), but the STD issues were ignored.

At least 15 percent of women diagnosed with AIDS are over the age of 40. We are *more* likely than younger women to become infected with the human immunodeficiency virus (HIV) during intercourse. If a man is infected by this virus, it will be present in his semen. The HIV virus can reside in the body and the semen for a decade or longer before it presents itself with typical symptoms of AIDS. We become infected if it enters our bloodstream. This closed circulatory pathway opens up if we develop minute tears in our vaginal tissue during the stretching process of intercourse. This is far more likely to occur if this tissue is thin or inadequately lubricated. Both of these conditions occur as our estrogen levels decline, or if we've been in a state of coital abstinence.

The best sexual case scenario would be to request that your potential partner have HIV testing prior to your becoming sexually involved. I generally suggest my patients also be tested; that way they can use traditional barter—"You show me yours and I'll show you mine." But one such test is not sufficient. If your partner was recently exposed, he may test negative (we're testing the antibodies that develop against the virus, and it may take three to six months for these to "come out"). So repeat testing should be done six months later, and if at that point he's negative and monogamous, and you don't need or want this form of contraception, the condoms can go, *but not before!*

Our vulnerability is not limited to the vaginal area. Anal sex places us at an even higher risk, since the anus is more likely to develop minute lacerations during sexual activity. Even oral sex poses a risk for STDs, including AIDS, if we have any sores or lesions (cold sores, gum problems, or just cracked lips) that allow the virus to enter our bloodstream. Condoms should still be used, but at least for this purpose, they don't have to be permeated with spermicide.

AIDS and other STDs know no age limits. The advice we know to be mandatory for the younger generation applies to us with equal vehemence.

The Rhythm Method (Timed Abstinence)

The rhythm method is based on knowledge of when we ovulate. We then calculate that the egg has an active life ranging from twelve to forty-eight hours, during which time it can be fertilized. We add to this calculation an estimate of sperm life (in cervical mucus or the uterus) of twenty-four to forty-eight hours. These combined life spans give us only ninety-eight hours a month in which intercourse can lead to pregnancy. So if we abstain during this period, we should not conceive—theoretically, that is. As usual, theory cannot predict biologic outcome. We face several problems. Sperm have been found to live as long as a week in cervical mucus, waiting to pounce after an egg is released, so pre-ovulation intercourse can be dangerous. Indeed, if we simply try to abstain a few days before intercourse, the failure rate for all ages is as high as 48 percent. If we abstain from the beginning of our period until after ovulation, we may drop this pregnancy rate to 7 percent, but we're also decreasing our frequency of intercourse to only two weeks each month. It's also difficult to determine our exact date of ovulation. We can monitor our basal body temperature (it rises after we ovulate), do urine ovulation tests (which are expensive), check our cervical mucus (it's more abundant and fluid before we ovulate), or just figure when our midcycle occurs (14 days for a 28-day cycle). But even in young women, these factors can vary; and in our forties, when our cycles change, we are less able to accurately predict egg release. The minute our cycles become irregular, we lose our rhythm, so obviously it is difficult to avail ourselves of the rhythm method.

The Future of Contraception

Over the last two decades, contraceptive research has been hampered by regulations, political pressures, and liability concerns (the makers of spermicidal jelly have been sued when this mode of contraception didn't work and the resulting infant had a congenital problem!). By the time new devices are approved and available, most of us won't need them, but that doesn't mean we shouldn't care. Here are some of the methods that are in development.

HORMONAL CONTRACEPTION

Implants

Instead of six rods, there will be just one or two. This will make the process of insertion and extraction much easier. In order to totally eliminate removal hassles, biodegradable implants (working on the same premise as dissolving stitches) are also being developed.

Biodegradable Pellets

These are injected under the skin. They are the size of rice grains, contain progestin, and disintegrate after twenty-four months.

Biodegradable Injectable Microcapsules

These are time-released and provide contraception for one to six months.

Transdermal Contraceptives

A progestin gel could be rubbed on and absorbed into our bodies for contraceptive purposes.

Vaginal Rings

These are impregnated with a combination of estrogen and progestin, or progestin alone. The hormones leach out of the ring and are absorbed through the vagina. The ring is the size of a diaphragm (but hollow) and can remain in place during intercourse. But if that's not appealing, it can be removed for a few hours and reinserted without losing its effectiveness.

INJECTABLE CONTRACEPTION

DMPA lasts three months. Scientists are working on other injectables that last six to eight months. Once-a-month shots will also be available; they contain both estrogen and progestin so that bleeding patterns are closer to normal than those with DMPA.

NEW SPERMICIDES

Scientists are working on developing new, stronger spermicides that can inhibit HIV, chlamydia, trichomonas, and other infectious microbes from multiplying or adhering to the vaginal wall. Disposable diaphragms that are prefilled with spermicides are also being tested.

CONTRACEPTIVE VACCINE

This would immunize us against the pregnancy hormone (HCG, or *human chorionic gonadotropin*), which is necessary to maintain early pregnancy growth. Other vaccines could cause immunization against a substance in the developing egg or could work against the pregnancy "instigator"—sperm.

MALE METHODS

Let's not forget that men can and should be as responsible as we are for contraception. Long-term shots to render them reversibly infertile are a future possibility. Condoms will get better. New and thinner polyurethane may allow more sensation during sex while continuing to be leak- and tear-proof.

Whatever contraception we choose now or in the future, we have to be consistent in its use. Four decades of maturity will not necessarily make our eggs impermeable to sperm or our bodies invincible to infection. We're "too old" to make the kinds of mistakes young people do with regard to contraception and disease.

3

I'M READY
I Want to Be Pregnant Yesterday!

Playing Mommy when we were children might not have been politically correct, but it was fun. We knew we could play with our made-up progeny as long as we wanted (and our attention span allowed) and then go on to other things. Pretty soon, the "other things" became more important, and we developed our opportunities, our minds, our psyches, and our relationships, sure that when we were really "old," we would or could become the grown-up mothers who had become a part of our female identity. Meanwhile, our eggs were poised in a state of frozen chromosomal division that would "awaken" with the kiss of a prince and his sperm.

So now that we've entered our forties, we've finished growing up. We may feel and look as good as we did ten years ago, but we're told our eggs are "antiquated." One of the first reactions to infertility at any age is disbelief. After 40, many of us get angry and feel cheated. Surely, if we can put a man on the moon, a woman in a spaceship, and freeze men's sperm, we can find ways to preserve our own fertility until we have time for children.

Infertility After 40

REDUCED PREGNANCY RATES: THE EGG THAT JUST CAN'T

If we look at "natural" populations, where contraception is not used, fertility rates are fairly constant until women turn 30. From this point on, the decline begins, reaching a 50 percent reduction in live births by age 35 and a 95 percent reduction by age 45. In this country (where we have very few "natural" populations), less than 1 percent of all total live births from a spontaneously conceived pregnancy are to women over 40, and this figure drops to 0.01 percent by the age of 47.

Obviously, our goal is not just pregnancy, but the delivery of a live, healthy baby. Fertilization of our eggs is not an all-or-nothing phenomenon. If the completion of chromosomal division and redistribution and pairing that follows fertilization is not perfect, the resulting early pregnancy is faulty. Either it ceases to develop and we miscarry (this is nature's way of handling abnormal or mutated pregnancies) or the baby develops with chromosomal additions (such as Down's syndrome) or deletions. By the age of 45, our miscarriage rate is 50 percent, and our risk of bearing a child with a triple set of chromosomes (Down's syndrome is a triple set of chromosome 21) is 2 percent. Our eggs have been in arrested division (forty-eight pairs plus the X or Y chromosomes have separated, waiting to be paired up again) since we were 20 weeks old in our mother's womb. This "halved" condition of our eggs' chromosomes has made them very susceptible to spontaneous mutations, as well as to the environmental toxins and insults to which we have subjected them and ourselves for over four decades. Feeling good, or even taking care of our bodies and souls, will not protect those fragile eggs from aging.

MECHANICAL CAUSES OF INFERTILITY:
FORTY YEARS OF WEAR AND TEAR

Age has dealt us another blow below the belt or, more exactly, in the pelvis. The longer we postpone pregnancy, the more we are at risk for diseases that can scar our tubes, create cysts and tumors, and even result in surgical removal of part or all of our pelvic organs. Youth (and its accompanying carelessness), experimentation, and the need to try several partners before we or they could commit to a future pregnancy-producing relationship may have exposed us to STDs. If we had pelvic inflammatory disease or the more silent chlamydia, our tubes may be scarred. Damaged tubes don't allow fertilization; the sperm simply can't enter from the uterine cavity, while at the other end, the egg can't be picked up by the the Fallopian tube.

Endometriosis has been termed the "career woman's disease." The longer we put off having our children, the longer we expose ourselves to the factors researchers think cause this condition:

1. "Backward" menstrual flow from the uterus out through the tubes. Endometrial cells seed onto the ovaries and other pelvic surfaces.

2. Multipotential cells (they are confused as to their identity) in the pelvis that change to endometrial-like cells.

In whichever way these abnormal cells reach the surface of our pelvis, they respond destructively to our hormones. They bleed, cause pelvic and tubal scarring and blood-filled ovarian cysts (*endometriomas*), and produce substances that suppress fertilization. This so-called career disease can prevent our second career of natural pregnancy and motherhood.

More than 20 percent of women over the age of 35 develop uterine fibroids. These can distort the uterine cavity and, on occasion, can block the tubes. A *submucosal fibroid* (which grows into the endometrial cavity) can prevent pregnancy implantation or adequate placental growth, causing miscarriage. Large fibroids can rapidly become even larger during pregnancy, outgrow their blood supply, and result in severe pain and even premature labor. We want our uterus to grow in pregnancy with a fetus, not a tumor!

HORMONAL CHANGES:
DO WE HAVE A "REPRODUCTIVE MENOPAUSE"?

Not only are our individual eggs and their chromosomes "losing it" as we get older, but we're rapidly decreasing the sum total of these eggs. This decrease in our egg count and quality affects our hormonal levels, particularly those of estrogen and inhibin. Both may be necessary for the development of a dominant follicle and egg. These two factors also affect the pituitary. The pituitary—"thinking" (after all, it is in the brain) that it has to work harder because estrogen and inhibin are not shutting it off—produces more FSH. Our normal levels of FSH are very low when our cycle begins. If these levels rise, we have a marker for low number, poor quality, and poor performance of our eggs. If we measure FSH on the third day of our cycle (day 1 is when our period starts), levels above 20 milli-international units per milliliter are associated with a decreased pregnancy rate, and levels over 25 indicate little or no chance of pregnancy. This is the measurement of our "reproductive menopause," and it occurs approximately ten years before our true menopause.

INFERTILITY WORKUP AFTER 40: DO WE GIVE NATURE (OR OUR UNTREATED EGGS) A CHANCE?

Do the 6 percent of us over 40 who still want children have to "celebrate" our birthdays at the office of an infertility specialist? This depends on our level of emotional panic. I had one patient who came to see me shortly after her fortieth birthday bemoaning her age, her single status, and her forgetfulness: "I forgot to have a baby!" were her exact words. If you have regular periods, if you've been pregnant in the past or have had a child in the last ten years, and if your partner has caused previous pregnancies, you can probably try on your own for three or four months. (Note: Doctors usually advise couples in their twenties and thirties to try for up to one year before they begin an infertility workup.) Beyond that, I do not suggest a laissez-faire attitude of "Let's wait and see" or postponing trying until you've completed that project or returned from your vacation next spring. From an egg point of view, this is an emergency!

Trying means you have to have intercourse around the time of your ovulation. You can arbitrarily do this by having intercourse at least every other day beginning 5 or 6 days before you normally ovulate. You simply follow your basal body temperature to see when ovulation occurs. Take your temperature the first thing every morning before you get up and out of bed or have your coffee. If it rises about half a degree and stays up, you've ovulated. If the thermometer seems too primitive (you'll need one with a digital readout that calibrates to tenths of a degree), or your schedule too hectic for morning measurements of your temperature, you can use the home ovulatory kits sold at the drugstore to project when you develop an LH surge (the rise in pituitary hormone that causes the egg to be released). These kits cost about $80 a month and may vary as to when they predict ovulation. A kit can also be helpful if it doesn't show an LH surge, indicating you have ovulatory problems. In some cases, it can be counterproductive if you wait too long to see if you're ovulating. The greatest chance of pregnancy will occur with intercourse from six days before, improving until the day of ovulation but not after it has taken place.

If four months of hard work and diligence (coitus-wise) have not paid off, it's time to see your doctor. These are some of the initial tests that should be done to rule out factors other than "aging eggs." (Note: Thirty percent of couples' infertility is caused by more than one factor.)

Semen Analysis

Semen analysis should show more than 20 million sperm per cubic centimeter with 60 percent of them having good forward motion and normal structure (sperm have to conform to certain shapes and sizes in order to perform). There should be no signs of infection, and the final workup includes testing the sperm to see if they can penetrate mouse eggs. Theoretically, male fertility is not racing a biological clock (men continue to produce sperm into their eighties), but if your partner is over 55, his sperm may produce more offspring with triple chromosomes, and he is more likely to have chronic problems such as *prostatitis* (inflammation of the prostate) and *epididymitis* (inflammation of the testicular ducts) that can affect the ability of his sperm to fertilize eggs.

FSH Level

FSH should be checked from a sample of your blood around day 3 of your cycle. If it's over 20 milliunits per milliliter—and certainly if it is over 25—repeat it the following month. If it remains high, you're faced with the very unfortunate fact that your own eggs won't be able to get you pregnant. Your FSH level is an inexpensive and reliable fertility fortune-teller. When "read right," it should prevent you from getting hooked into investing your time, your money, and, most important, your emotions in trying to conceive with your own eggs at all costs. A high FSH doesn't mean, however, that you'll never get to be pregnant or have a baby. Oocyte donation allows doctors to fertilize a donor's egg with your partner's sperm and implant the resulting embryo in your tube

(GIFT, *gamete intra-Fallopian transfer*) or uterus (IVF, *in vitro fertilization*) to grow and deliver (see below). If your FSH is high, you should consider starting rather than ending with this option.

Other Hormonal Testing

Low FSH levels still don't mean you're ovulating or that your eggs will easily be fertilized, but you can at least continue to investigate and work on your ovulation "performance." This can be determined by checking the levels of progesterone in your blood about one week before you are due to get your period. Another test to assess progesterone effect is an *endometrial biopsy*. For that, a small curette is inserted through the cervix, and a strip of endometrium is scraped off. Microscopic sections of this strip can be checked by a pathologist to see if the endometrial glands show the right degree of development. Both of these tests are "traditional" in an infertility workup, but I should point out that over the age of 40, we'll most likely go on to use ovulatory stimulation drugs, and it could be argued that our natural progesterone levels are irrelevant.

Postcoital Testing

Rarely, we develop antibodies to sperm and, more particularly, to our partners' sperm. This problem accounts for less than 5 percent of infertility in couples of all ages. Once the sperm are dutifully deposited in the vagina, they have to quickly swim into the cervical mucus, where they are protected from the natural acidity of the vagina. The mucus has to be secreted in large amounts and can't be too thick or viscous in order to transport the sperm into the uterus. This occurs only during ovulation. If its physical properties are "off," or if it contains antibodies that attack the sperm, it fails as a conduit in that initial journey up the uterus and tubes to the awaiting egg. We check this by sampling the mucus several hours after intercourse. If we see only dead sperm, there may be a transport problem. We treat this with intrauterine insemination. The sperm are washed and separated from the surrounding seminal fluid, treated with special solutions that enhance their activity, and inserted via a thin tube through the cervix straight into the uterus. This process bypasses the cervix and its hostile mucus to place the "good stuff" as close to the tubes as possible. I think of it as a kind of Federal Express for sperm!

Uterine and Tubal Assessment

It's imperative to know if at least one Fallopian tube is open and in good working condition. We usually start with a test called a *hysterosalpingography*, or HSG (translation: uterus = hystero and tubes = salpingies). Dye that is imaged by X ray is injected into the uterus through the cervix and should flow out of the tubes. If the dye doesn't demarcate the tubes, they may be blocked. We can assess this by putting a small telescope (hysteroscope) through the cervix into the uterine cavity to check the lining and openings of both tubes (growths or fibroids would also be seen). A more direct way of checking the tubes is to perform a laparoscopy. This usually requires a general anesthetic. A scope is placed through a small incision under the belly button and, *voilà!*—the mysteries of the pelvic organs are easily visible. Because this procedure is invasive, many infertility experts perform it in conjunction with ovarian stimulation, so that GIFT (introduction of an egg and sperm into the tube) can be performed at the same time, or, if the tubes are blocked, the procedure can instantly be converted to in vitro fertilization (see below). Laparoscopy is important, not only to assess our tubes, but to establish if our years of motherhood procrastination have contributed to the development of endometriosis.

Treatment: It's Time to Do Something About This

If you have one open, apparently normal Fallopian tube, and your FSH levels indicate that you are not in "reproductive menopause," you and your physician should consider an aggressive approach before the options involving your own eggs run out. Success rates for us over 40 are less than one fourth those attained at an earlier age using the same techniques.

DRUG THERAPIES

Stimulatory drugs for women with "normal" hormones may be overused in our twenties and thirties, but it is an empiric strategy when we are over 40. This stimulation is usually combined with timed intrauterine insemination (if we're using these major and expensive drugs, we don't want to rely on natural sperm migration). There are three basic drug therapies.

Clomiphene Citrate (Clomid or Serophene)

Clomiphene citrate is the easiest and cheapest fertility medication we can prescribe. It works as an estrogen "pretender" and sits on the receptors in our hypothalamus and pituitary, masking any "real" estrogen in the vicinity. Our brain center is fooled into thinking there is no estrogen; it then puts out FSH to direct the follicles in the ovary to get going, develop, and produce needed estrogen. After 5 days of clomiphene citrate (started in the beginning of our cycle), there is a large amount of FSH, and the follicles have taken off. Once they've reached a critical size (which is measured with ultrasound), we can wait for spontaneous ovulation or we can give an injection of HCG (human chorionic gonadotropin), a hormone secreted by placental cells in early pregnancy and similar to the pituitary's LH (luteinizing hormone). The HCG injection, like our natural LH surge, stimulates the release of the egg within thirty-six hours. It's at this moment we "go for it," with either timed intercourse or, better yet, intrauterine insemination.

The advantages of clomiphene citrate are its low cost, low multiple-pregnancy rates (less than 7 percent), and ease of use. The disadvantages are that it is an anti-estrogen; it can thin the endometrial lining after several cycles of use, preventing implantation; it can also reduce cervical mucus production. Twenty percent of women with ovulatory problems don't even respond. We allow women in younger age groups to try clomiphene citrate for four to six cycles. When we're over 40, fewer attempts are warranted, and it may be appropriate to go for more aggressive types of ovarian stimulation without first failing with clomiphene.

Gonadotropin Therapy: Fertility Shots

Fertility shots consist of Pergonal, prepared from FSH and LH, or Metrodin (FSH alone). This is the ultimate "corporate takeover"; we're not waiting for our own brain center or pituitary to make these hormones. We're giving them in large amounts in order to hyperstimulate the ovaries so they'll produce multiple follicles and eggs. This form of therapy requires intensive surveillance by repeated ultrasounds to determine the number and size of follicles and blood tests to check estrogen levels. If we overshoot the mark (too many follicles), the result may be a multiple pregnancy (triplets or more), with a high risk of miscarriage, premature delivery, and babies with physical and mental problems. Even if we don't get pregnant, hyperstimulation can result in large ovarian cysts that may rupture, bleed, or cause fluid imbalance. I've seen women land in intensive care units from the complications of ovarian hyperstimulation.

Once the follicles reach the ideal size and estrogen levels are good, we give HCG, cause release of the eggs, and—thirty-six hours later—perform intrauterine insemination. This therapy is aggressive and expensive. For example, each ampule of Pergonal or Metrodin costs up to $40, and we can use two to four a day for 10 days or more. Ultrasounds cost hundreds of dollars each, and estrogen tests are at least $50. A typical monthly course of gonadotropin therapy can range from $1,000 to $3,000. Overall success rates are again dependent on the quality of our over-40-year-old eggs and range from 4 to 8 percent. (We are not counting the "pregnancy" rate, but the "having a live baby" rate.) The rate per cycle is even lower, about 1.4 to 2 percent.

ASSISTED REPRODUCTION

"Gathering" Eggs for Direct Fertilization

This is our brave new world of infertility. Once we have the eggs and the sperm, the combinations and permutations are amazing. We can harvest the eggs from our ovaries for any of the following procedures:

IN VITRO FERTILIZATION (IVF)

An "out-of-body" meeting with sperm, causing fertilization and growth of the subsequent embryo before it is reimplanted into our uterus. The ovaries are usually hyperstimulated to produce multiple eggs with fertility drugs. We can then remove these eggs by putting a needle through the numerous plump follicles and aspirating their fluid. This egg "search and capture" can be done with ultrasound guidance, so laparoscopic surgery is avoided.

GIFT (GAMETE INTRA-FALLOPIAN TRANSFER)

GIFT is direct "tubal meeting" of the egg and sperm. We place both in a Fallopian tube and allow them to fertilize in the most natural of environments, hoping that after several days of cell division and multiplication, the normal route will take the new embryo into the uterine cavity, where it will implant and grow. Again, the eggs are usually obtained after hyperstimulation with fertility drugs. They are retrieved and placed in the tube through laparoscopic surgery, so this does require a general anesthetic. It also requires that we have at least one normal Fallopian tube.

ZIFT (ZYGOTE INTRA-FALLOPIAN TRANSFER)

We can go one step further, combining in vitro and GIFT. The eggs are retrieved, fertilized outside the body, and allowed to begin to develop. Once the fertilized egg has developed for one to two days (we now call it a *zygote*) and looks good, we put it back into the tube, whence, in another one to two days, we expect it to find its way to the uterine cavity. This is what happens in a natural pregnancy, and even though the initial meeting was not held in the tube, the zygote knows the tube is just a temporary conduit to its new home, the uterus. As with GIFT, we usually hyperstimulate the eggs, and we need to perform laparoscopy to place the zygote into the tube.

OOCYTE (EGG) DONATION

We can mix and match with any of these procedures. If our eggs are absent (the ovaries have been surgically removed) or in poor condition (our FSH is high), or if we have had no success with our own eggs, we can use donor eggs of younger, healthy women. We carry and deliver a pregnancy that is 50 percent that of our partner from a genetic point of view, but our own genes are not involved. This allows us to be the biological but not genetic mother.

USING A SURROGATE

If we have had a hysterectomy, we can retrieve our eggs, fertilize them with our partner's sperm, and—using in vitro techniques—place the resulting embryo in a surrogate woman who has agreed (and usually has been paid) to allow the pregnancy to grow in her uterus for nine months. (Now we are no longer the biological mother but retain our place as the genetic mother.) This option has raised major legal and moral issues and is currently in the combined hands of lawyers, lawmakers, and fertility experts.

Assessing Assisted Reproduction

IN VITRO, GIFT, ZIFT, DONOR OOCYTES:
HOW FAR, HOW MUCH, UNTIL I HAVE THAT BABY?

All of these assisted reproduction techniques should be giving us a "take-home baby" rate of 20 to 30 percent per procedure. They do in 24-year-olds, but as we pass the 40-year mark, our rate decreases to below 5 percent. If our FSH level is above 25, the percentage is zero. Should we fail with the first attempt at assisted reproduction, the probability of success for each subsequent try probably drops one percentage point.

So how much does this really cost? A study published in the *New England Journal of Medicine* on in vitro fertilization revealed some astounding numbers. The charge for a single in vitro fertilization procedure averages $8,000. We have to take time off from work (lost income), we may have complications requiring hospitalization (cysts and infections), and we are more likely to have expensive multiple births (20 to 25 percent multiple births, 2 to 3 percent triplets or more). If we add in hospital charges for neonatal intensive care for these babies and assume 0.2 percent of us might have maternal complications and longer hospital stays, we arrive at the following numbers: For the "ideal couple" who are young, have no sperm problem, and undergo in vitro fertilization because of blocked tubes, the cost runs from $50,000 per delivery for the first cycle (yes, there are four zeros in this number) and $72,000 for the sixth cycle. For our group—couples in which the woman is over 40—the average cost per delivery is $94,000. If we combine this with male factor infertility, the cost rises to $160,000 for the first cycle and an incredible $800,000 for the sixth.

Failure-wise and cost-wise, we don't seem to do much better with GIFT or ZIFT. When performed in women under 40, both procedures are expected to give a pregnancy rate of close to 30 percent. Once we're over 40, this drops to less than 10 percent, and since roughly half of these pregnancies will be faulty and miscarry, we get a take-home-baby rate of 5 percent at the same exorbitant financial and emotional costs.

Unfortunately, we have to add in another consideration when we pursue assisted reproduction. All these high-tech procedures should be performed by very specialized fertility experts working in appropriately run facilities. Currently, there is little or no regulation of their advertising, claims, or techniques. We should be able to understand how they record their success rates—pregnancy rates don't count; take-home-baby rates do. What do they do with frozen sperm and embryos? What do their consent forms mean—to them and to the couples signing them? Our need to know should equal our need to procreate. Who said either would be easy?

DONOR OOCYTES: WE CAN BEAR BABIES AT ANY AGE; OUR ONLY IMPEDIMENT IS OUR EGGS

Our uterus doesn't age; if stimulated with the proper hormones, it can "work" and sustain a good pregnancy into our sixties. If we use donor eggs from younger women and perform in vitro fertilization, our take-home-baby rate per cycle ranges from 21 to 38 percent! Considering that one donor (whose eggs are usually stimulated with fertility drugs) can donate her eggs to two women, the cost per delivery can fall to about $24,000.

This new world of assisted fertility requires our own (not the physicians') bravery. We have to be realistic in facing the fact that we may have missed our chance to have our own genetic offspring. Most of us will pass through emotions of disbelief and denial, followed by frustration and anger—at ourselves for having failing eggs, and at the experts for failing to help us. We expect to be able to make things work as long as we study, work hard, and pay to get the best. At some point, we have to reach acceptance, not of remaining childless, but of remaining oocyte-less. Our best bet after 40 (especially if we have tried the other steps listed in this chapter) is to use donor eggs. If we're healthy and have an intact uterus and access to good sperm, we can conceive and deliver. If we're brave enough to undertake this venture, we will indeed open up our own new world—that of motherhood!

4

MIDLIFE PREGNANCY
A Risky Business?

The previous chapter dealt with the problems of getting pregnant. We were willing to put ourselves and our partners through the most complicated and expensive procedures. Is the development phase of pregnancy going to be as high-tech or as fraught with failures as the conceptual phase? What is at risk here—the pregnancy, our health, or the genes and well-being of our much-wanted progeny? First, let's consider the pregnancy and whether our age affects its viability. Then we'll consider other risks.

Miscarriage:
Why Can't We Make a Bad Pregnancy Good?

MISCARRIAGES AND AGE

We know that our eggs lose their viability with age. Their state of readiness (with the chromosome pairs already divided in half) becomes confused and, yes, defective. When they're fertilized by sperm, they may produce the wrong number of chromosomes. If a pair of chromosomes in the undeveloped egg fails to separate correctly when it develops during ovulation, the addition of the sperm's chromosomes results in the fertilized egg having three sets of the chromosome, not the correct two. This is called *trisomy*, and Down's syndrome is an example of this condition. In other instances, the pair doesn't divide, goes the "wrong way," and doesn't enter the genetic material of the pregnancy. The fertilized cells then contain the sperm's "lonely" single chromosome without its matching mate. The wrong number of chromosomes is found in close to 50 percent of our eggs after the age of 35 (we've checked this after they've been extracted for in vitro fertilization). These defective eggs either can't be fertilized (a major cause for our increasing infertility) or, if fertilized, can't develop into a normal pregnancy. The result of whatever manages to initially grow is an embryo with a genetic makeup that is usually incompatible with normal life, and miscarriage often follows.

We estimate that the majority of our miscarriages (called *spontaneous abortions*) occur because of abnormal chromosomes in the developing pregnancy. There is virtually nothing we can do to prevent this. We can't make a bad pregnancy (from a genetic point of view) good. Our risk of miscarriage rises to at least 50 percent by the age of 45. The only way we can decrease this inherent chromosomally caused risk is to use donor eggs (see previous chapter). We then approach a more normal miscarriage rate of between 15 and 30 percent, again depending on the age of the egg donor. The rate is never zero, even when we are in our twenties. The fertilization process of exchanging and sharing genetic information can and does go wrong at any age.

Other, nongenetic causes of miscarriage also increase with age. These include fibroid tumors, which can deform the uterine cavity, making implantation and growth of a fetus more difficult, and poor progesterone production, which causes inadequate endometrial growth in early pregnancy. Cervical incompetence (a condition in which the cervix lacks proper strength and closure) and subsequent loss of the pregnancy after 12 weeks increases in our age group. It's not that our cervix is old and tired, but because it may have sustained more trauma in our preceding twenty years—the result of abortion, miscarriage, or our mothers' exposure to DES. A weakened or shortened cervix can't stay shut against the pressure of an expanding pregnancy. As it opens, the amniotic sac surrounding the pregnancy breaks, the fluid is lost, and contractions ensue, causing abortion of the entire pregnancy.

There are also rare instances where we miscarry because our pregnancy is not immunologically protected. Our immune cells view a fetus as a foreign body (which, of course, it is) and, in certain conditions, set out to destroy it the way they would an infection. If we have certain antibodies called *anticardiolipid antibodies* (seen more often with immunological diseases such as *systemic lupus erythematosus*, or SLE), we are more likely to undergo this antipregnancy reaction and miscarry or have problems with an ongoing pregnancy.

We can do something about these nongenetic miscarriages. Uterine fibroids can be assessed by ultrasound or hysteroscopy. We can remove *submucosal fibroids* (those projecting into the endometrial cavity) with hysteroscopic resection. Large fibroids in the uterine wall may require major surgery and *myomectomy* (removal of the fibroids with subsequent reconstruction of the uterus). This procedure can cause scarring and subsequent infertility if the tubes become blocked, and it should only be undertaken as a last resort.

If our progesterone levels after conception are low, we can add this hormone in the form of natural progesterone suppositories. These should be given until the tenth week of pregnancy, when the placenta takes over from the ovary, producing all of the progesterone that the pregnancy could possibly need. Immunologic problems sometimes respond to steroid therapy. We've also tried aspirin and bed rest.

Miscarriage is a real tragedy at any age, but especially after 40, when our opportunities are finite and dwindling. It's like making the Olympic team, only to miss the bus on the way to the meet. We feel we have little or no time to make up for our loss. Many of my patients, when told that their pregnancy is "no good," feel they have done something wrong. They didn't eat right; they carried heavy packages; they exercised, or they didn't exercise . . . Guilt compounds their grief and mourning for the loss of an anticipated baby. We don't cause our own miscarriages, and physicians can offer only empathy, not pills, to "make it better." But if we want to finally deliver that healthy baby, we all have to start again, as soon as two months after the miscarriage has occurred.

CHECKING FOR A VIABLE PREGNANCY

Because of their high risk of miscarriage, many of my over-40 patients want reassurance that all is well as soon as they have a positive pregnancy test. (One of my patients called me two days after intrauterine insemination, demanding a test to immediately ensure that her pregnancy was normal!) Initially, we can check only in indirect ways. We can measure the level of HCG (human chorionic gonadotropin), which is produced by the developing placental cells. In early pregnancy, a daily doubling of this level is reassuring. After 6 weeks' gestation (we count from the first day of our last menstrual period) or 4 weeks from conception, a vaginal probe or transvaginal ultrasound can be performed. We should see a sac of fluid in the uterus (*gestational sac*) containing a very small embryo, and in that embryo we should now begin to see pulsations that represent its heartbeat. Early ultrasound will also demonstrate the number of pregnancies (remember, multiple pregnancies can occur in as many as 25 percent of women undergoing fertility assistance). Once we see that wonderful heartbeat, especially in a single pregnancy, our chance of miscarriage falls from 50 percent to less than 10 percent!

When the pregnancy is viable, what do we do and "worry about" next? Reproduction seems like a track-and-field meet. We have to jump over one hurdle after another to win or even finish the race. We've made it over the first one—the uterus is growing; ultrasound has shown a fetus with a heartbeat. The early pregnancy is okay, but what about the fetus? What about our own health? What about labor, delivery, and the baby?

The Fetus: Genetic Testing

We already know that reproductively, the saga of "missing" continues. If the chromosomes "miss" the right division and coupling, we may miss getting pregnant. Or, if we do, we're likely to miscarry. This natural safeguard is not foolproof. The risk of delivering a baby with a significant chromosomal abnormality is 0.26 percent at age 30, 0.56 percent at age 35, 1.5 percent at age 40, and 5.4 percent at age 45. For Down's syndrome, our risk increases from 0.3 percent at age 35 to 1 percent at 40, 3 percent at 45, and 9.1 percent at 49. There is an even higher rate of abnormal chromosomes if we test in the first two trimesters of pregnancy, but about one third of these pregnancies will be lost at later dates or are stillborn. There are two main tests that allow us to detect these chromosomal abnormalities. If any are found, we can decide whether to terminate the pregnancy or, if we choose to continue, be prepared to deal with pregnancy, birth, and newborn complications.

AMNIOCENTESIS

We perform this procedure between 15 and 20 weeks of pregnancy. At this stage, there is abundant amniotic fluid surrounding the fetus and there are large quantities of fetal cells in the fluid. An ultrasound will show us the fluid levels and also the position of the fetus. Using this as guidance, a needle is placed through the lower abdomen into the uterus and is directed to a fluid pocket. Between 20 and 40 cubic centimeters of amniotic fluid is aspirated. The cells in this fluid are separated and cultured. Since only a small percentage of amniotic cells are alive (many are just dead cells sloughed off the fetus's body), these have to be grown and allowed to multiply for about ten days. They are then stained, and their chromosomes are measured and counted.

This test also allows us to look at *alpha-fetoprotein (AFP)*, a major protein produced by the fetus in its gastrointestinal tract and liver. Some is excreted with urine, and fetal urine is one of the components of amniotic fluid. We know how much alpha-fetoprotein should be in the amniotic fluid in normal pregnancies between 13 and 20 weeks' gestation. Higher levels can indicate a defect in the fetus's body, allowing a greater outpouring of this protein. This occurs in conditions where the canal containing the developing spinal column and brain is partially or completely open *(neural tube defect)*, when the stomach wall is not closed *(ventral wall defect)*, or with certain gastrointestinal problems such as obstruction. Whenever we sample fluid for chromosomes, we also check levels of alpha-fetoprotein, so that we can diagnose these major malformations.

Advantages

This is our safest procedure. A large U.S. study showed that the incidence of fetal loss after amniocentesis was barely higher than the rate for nontested pregnancies (3.5 percent versus 3.2 percent). Overall, we have about a 0.5 percent rate of complications. These include fetal injury from the needle, leaking membranes from the needle puncture site (this may seal over after several days), and bacterial infections. The procedure is technically easy (just aim for the fluid pocket), and once the needle is in place, the initial, fleeting, cramplike pain is over. Most of my patients are so engrossed in the ultrasound picture that they forget to say "ouch" (however, one patient's husband fainted when he saw the needle!).

Disadvantages

It takes ten days to grow the cell cultures. We often don't get the results for two weeks, and those two weeks seem endless. In the interim, we begin to feel the fetus moving and kicking. Do we allow ourselves to embark on our odyssey of maternal attachment? Rarely, we are told that the cells didn't culture, we can't get a result, and we need to repeat the test. I feel that the greatest disadvantage of amniocentesis is the timing of the results. Telling a woman who is already 17 to 20 weeks pregnant that her fetus is not normal is horrendous. If she chooses to terminate the pregnancy, she must undergo a second-trimester abortion. This is a lot more difficult from a technical and, more important, from an emotional basis than terminating in the first trimester. To help push this time frame forward, we've developed the technique of early amniocentesis. This is performed between 9 and 14 weeks of gestation, uses less amniotic fluid, and may be an early alternative to CVS (see below). Complication rates (mostly ruptured membranes) are higher than for late amniocentesis but, in good hands, are similar to those of CVS.

CVS (CHORIONIC VILLAE SAMPLING)

CVS is performed between weeks 10 and 12 of pregnancy. Under ultrasound guidance (allowing us to see where the placental and fetal tissue is thickest), a small tube is either placed through the cervix or through a small puncture site in the lower abdomen. Ten to 25 milligrams of tissue are then aspirated. This tissue contains large amounts of fetal cells, which can be immediately stained; the chromosomes are then counted to check for Down's syndrome or other chromosomal disparities. Some of the cells are also cultured to ensure that our immediate chromosomal assessment is correct. We can also study the cells' enzymes and DNA to allow for genetic diagnosis of up to seventy hereditary disorders ranging from sickle-cell anemia, thalassemia, cystic fibrosis, muscular dystrophy, and Tay-Sachs disease to certain forms of mental retardation (including fragile X syndrome).

Advantages

With CVS, we've barely missed two periods and yet we can already determine the presence of a genetic problem. If the pregnancy is abnormal and we choose to terminate, we undergo a simple first-trimester abortion, which can easily be performed in a doctor's office. Conversely, and more happily, the minute we've heard that the pregnancy is genetically good, we can truly begin to rejoice in our condition. At this early date, we can even ascertain the sex of the fetus, which, down the line, is great for color coordination (and, of course, choosing names).

Risks and Disadvantages

The risk of fetal loss with CVS is at least twice that with amniocentesis, ranging from 1 percent to as high as 4 percent. Bleeding, spotting, and cramping can follow in 10 percent of procedures. Prenatal cellular genetic testing (if we get enough and the right cells) has a 99 percent accuracy rate for both CVS and amniocentesis. Rarely, however, our maternal cells are stained and cultured instead of fetal cells. This risk can be reduced by careful dissection of the tissue and microscopic identification of the "different-looking" fetal tissue. Since we get both fetal and placental tissue with CVS, we are more likely to get misleading results with this technique than with amniocentesis. If abnormal cells are present after cultures (in both CVS and amniocentesis), it may be that they divided incorrectly during the culture process. After all, this is not the normal way these cells were meant to grow. In these cases, the original cells in the fetus are fine, but we have to be sure. If, after CVS, we get chromosomal counts that are not uniform we have to repeat the count with a later amniocentesis.

The last small disadvantage of CVS is that it will not directly screen for neural tube defects. Since we cannot obtain fluid for alpha-fetoprotein with this procedure, we do the next best thing. We sample our own blood between 16 and 20 weeks of pregnancy. If abnormally high levels of alpha-fetoprotein are released by the fetus into the amniotic fluid, some is absorbed through the placenta into our bloodstream. The tests are sensitive enough to detect these levels, and if they are high, we can successfully diagnose 90 percent of fetuses with *anencephaly* (no developing brain) and 69 percent with other neural tube defects (including spina bifida). If we combine the blood tests with second-trimester ultrasound (looking at the brain and spine of the fetus at 18 to 20 weeks), we can ensure even higher rates of detection.

"Genetic" Ultrasound:
Another Test to Ensure Fetal Well-Being

This is not just a quick scan to check for heartbeat and size. A highly trained ultrasonographer should carefully image the second-trimester fetus at about 20 weeks. Its brain should be viewed (we can see its anatomy and rule out many developing abnormalities such as hydrocephalus), as should its heart (does it have four chambers?), major vessels leading to and from the heart, its abdomen, its limbs, and, of course, if we want, its sex organs. Major anatomic malformations (some of which may be incompatible with life) can be detected, allowing us once more to decide about continuing the pregnancy or to plan for corrective procedures while the fetus is in our uterus (such as draining excess fluid from the brain or kidneys). We will also be prepared to perform appropriate surgical procedures immediately after delivery. Once we are over 40, our risk of delivering babies with genetic malformations that are not due to known changes in chromosomes increases. We should use genetic ultrasound as an adjunct to CVS or amniocentesis.

Our Health in Pregnancy:
Are We Sacrificing the Former to Achieve the Latter?

We've been led to believe that the older we are, the more likely we will "get sick" (I'm never quite sure what that phrase means), have complications, and even die in our belated efforts to bear children. The statistics that are so grimly quoted may, however, be invalid for most of us who are healthy, well nourished, and well educated and obtain early prenatal care.

Maternal Death: The Ultimate Complication

Statistically speaking, by age 40 or older, we are 8.6 times more likely to die as a result of pregnancy and delivery than when we were 20 to 24 years old. This is taken from maternal death rates recorded between 1980 and 1985. These numbers included *all* women over 40, and when we examine them more carefully, we find that socioeconomic and demographic factors were probably more important than age itself. Race, poverty, education, marital status, the number of previous pregnancies and children to care for, and, most important, access to and quality of prenatal care were what counted. The death rate for poor, nonwhite women who fell into the "wrong" categories was 4.6 times higher than that of white "advantaged" women. So the 8.6 factor should not be used to scare us but rather to improve contraceptive choices and prenatal care for women who have been disenfranchised from reproductive health.

Although the numbers may be better than those quoted, we still run about a four times increased risk of mortality (this translates to about 50 maternal deaths for 100,000 live births). The major reasons for our maternal mortality are complications of high blood pressure (stroke and heart attack), pulmonary embolism (clots in the lungs), hemorrhage, and infection. As we get older, we're clearly more prone to high blood pressure. This can become worse during pregnancy. We are also more likely to develop gestational diabetes, which is associated with an increased incidence of high blood pressure, fetal complications, and need for cesarean section, or C-section. After 40, we undergo more emergency C-sections (see below) and operative deliveries, and these can put us at greater risk for pulmonary embolism, bleeding, and infection. Our higher C-section rate is definitely associated with a higher mortality rate, especially if our general health is already compromised.

Preexisting diseases usually worsen the older we get, and this can result in an increase in our death rate independent of pregnancy. However, pregnancy certainly doesn't help. These diseases include chronic heart ailments, kidney or liver disease, diabetes, high blood pressure, chronic infections, immune disorders, and cancers. If these conditions are not fatal in pregnancy, they could lead to a higher C-section rate for fetal or maternal problems. We see this again with high blood pressure, diabetes, heart disease, systemic lupus erythematosus, and addictions to cigarettes, alcohol, and illicit drugs.

If you have a chronic medical disorder, consult with prenatal specialists about your risks, and if you decide to "go ahead," make sure you're getting your care from a well-established team of high-risk obstetrical experts.

MEDICAL COMPLICATIONS DURING PREGNANCY

There is a huge span (and probability of prevention) between death and illness. It's a lot more valid to examine this latter problem, since it's the one with which we're most likely to deal. Again, we have to distinguish between those of us who are healthy and pregnant over 40 and those women who enter their pregnancy with preexisting or underlying medical problems.

It would appear that we're twice as likely to develop gestational diabetes after 40, especially if we're overweight (we're also more likely to develop diabetes without being pregnant). Eighty percent of women who develop gestational diabetes will in later years become diabetic. The stress of pregnancy brings this disease out before its predestined time. All pregnant women should undergo diabetes evaluation with a *glucose tolerance test* (50 grams of glucose in a sweet drink is consumed, and blood sugar levels are tested one hour later) at 24 to 26 weeks' gestation. If these levels are high, we then need a fasting and three-hour glucose tolerance test (using 100 milligrams of glucose). If this test is also abnormal, we must follow special diets to keep our overall blood sugar levels below 120 milligrams per deciliter. When diet doesn't do it, we have to add insulin. How will this inability to metabolize glucose affect our health during pregnancy? It could make us more prone to developing high blood pressure or pre-eclampsia, we tend to grow larger babies, and are more likely to require delivery before 40 weeks. These factors make our doctors more apt to deliver our babies by cesarean section. But with careful monitoring and good surgical technique, we should be fine. After we've completed our pregnancy, we have to be sure to be checked on a yearly basis for late-onset diabetes.

We're also more than twice as likely to develop pregnancy-induced high blood pressure than younger women, but again, that may be a matter of underlying (and often previously undiagnosed) hypertension or obesity (and we obviously know if we are overweight). Studies have shown that calcium supplementation can lower blood pressure and reduce hypertensive problems in pregnancy. So the least we should do is add calcium to our vitamins the minute we know we're pregnant (we actually should have been adding calcium via milk or with supplements since puberty!). We might require bed rest, hospitalization, and medication to lower our blood pressure, together with vigilant monitoring of our baby's well-being. There may be a higher rate of bleeding complications from separation of the placenta (this is called *abruptio placentae*). We certainly run a higher risk of C-section. However, bear in mind that 85 percent of women with chronic high blood pressure have uncomplicated pregnancies! A normal prepregnancy blood pressure is reassuring. If high blood pressure then develops in our over-40 pregnancy, it is usually much more manageable in the absence of underlying disease. In either case, the pregnancy will generally not contribute to a worsening of future hypertensive problems.

In short, if we're not overweight, if we eat right, and if we have no underlying high blood pressure or diabetes, chances are our health will remain unaffected even after 40, so our next concern should be the delivery itself.

Labor and Delivery: Can Our Over-40 Bodies Do It?

Who's at fault for the 30 to 65 percent rate of cesarean sections in our age group? Is it our over-40 bodies, our own anxieties, or those of our physicians?

Let's first consider our bodies. Is labor different as we age? The answer is "yes," but qualified with "sometimes." We tend to have longer labors and labor dysfunction; our contractions are not as efficient in pushing the baby down and dilating the cervix. We're more likely to require contraction stimulation with intravenous oxytocin (one common trade name is Pitocin), and to need the oxytocin twice as long as younger women, and at higher doses. It would appear that with age, our uterine muscles may stubbornly resist making a maximum effort.

Studies have shown that the uterine blood vessels that feed the placenta and the fetus are stiffer after age 40. More than eighty percent of the uterine arteries appear to contain "excess" collagen, which replaces normal smooth muscle in the vessel lining. This process prevents these vessels from expanding as well as they should in pregnancy in order to accommodate the huge blood flow. Stiffer vessels limit blood flow when it's needed most, during the stresses of contraction and labor. Our "reserve" is gone, and the baby reacts to this lower blood supply; its heartbeat may change, indicating fetal stress followed by fetal distress. When fetal distress occurs, we stop the cause—labor—and rescue the baby with an emergency C-section.

Because we may have experienced events that could scar our uterine lining—such as previous C-sections, abortions, or uterine surgery—we are more likely to have a "malplaced" placenta. Rather than implanting in the upper or middle part of the uterus, it settles in the lower portion and across the cervix. This is a *placenta previa;* it can cause significant bleeding in the last few months of pregnancy as it is pulled away from the dilating cervix. This condition requires cesarean section, since we would hemorrhage if we attempted a vaginal delivery through the placenta or around the separated edge. If bleeding occurs before the ninth month, we may end up with a premature infant, cesarean section, and considerable blood loss.

Women over 40 have waited a very long time to have their babies, so they tend to take very good care of themselves during their pregnancy. Eating by the book is fine, but we sometimes overdo it—we gain too much weight (more than 40 pounds) and get huge externally (us) and internally (our babies). We are also at higher risk for gestational diabetes and this, too, leads to big babies (a condition called *macrosomia*). Add this to a higher incidence of "lazy" labor, less pliable uterine arteries, and our normal-sized pelvis, and we won't deliver vaginally. Multiple pregnancies (and our rate is 25 percent with assisted reproduction) are often "taken" by C-section to protect the babies (who are at risk for growth retardation and who may need to be delivered early), as well as for anatomic reasons (delivering the second baby, especially if breech, can be more traumatic).

We then come to the psychological issues. Are we being sectioned because anxiety (ours and our physicians') has triumphed over medical indications? No baby is expendable, but if we've waited so long, possibly endured years of infertility therapy, cleared all our hurdles, and have the finish line in sight, we don't want to take any more chances. We may never have another pregnancy or "makeup" baby. We want our healthy baby out, and out *now*, and if it means being surgically aggressive, so be it. This may not be clinically justified, but it's difficult to always judge the psychological stresses that mold our clinical decisions.

Risks for the Object of It All: The Baby

As we get older, are we more likely to lose our babies (*perinatal mortality*) or have them born sick and in need of intensive care? A lot depends on our prepregnancy health—and on whether we're having a family all at once with a multiple pregnancy, whether we underwent genetic testing and terminated abnormal pregnancies, or whether we developed pregnancy complications. Overall, most studies do show a significant increase in perinatal mortality and morbidity after 40, but, again, these studies tend to lump all over-40 mothers together and don't always compensate for the factors I just listed.

PERINATAL MORTALITY

The principal factors causing this to increase after the age of 40 are high *parity* (having had a lot of previous deliveries), low socioeconomic status, poor prenatal care, and undetected genetic and congenital malformations (which also go together with poor or no prenatal care). Clearly some of these "poor-outcome" factors can be eliminated. Low birthweight resulting from growth retardation increases the risk of infant death. Conditions that limit blood and nutritional supply to the fetus are usually attributable to an underlying cause such as high blood pressure, poorly controlled diabetes, chronic illness, malnutrition, chronic infection, or smoking.

Prematurity is another cause of low birthweight and death. This is harder to predict but, again, if you have no uterine problems (fibroids, incompetent cervix, uterine scarring), multiple pregnancies, chronic vaginal infections, high blood pressure, or general poor health, you don't necessarily have to start bed rest at 26 weeks "just in case." Proper monitoring of uterine growth—an ultrasound at 20 weeks, followed by subsequent ultrasounds if size problems are suspected—should let you know if you are at risk and need more aggressive care, which includes bed rest, frequent fetal monitoring, and early delivery before the baby is compromised.

When we "crunch" the final numbers and control for our age-related frequency of multiple gestations, hypertensions, diabetes, abnormally placed placenta, and previous abortions, we still find that the risk of fetal death is 2.4 times greater than in the pregnancy outcomes of women under 30. The message from this statistic is that we need close surveillance. Most obstetricians recommend that we count fetal movements several times a day from 28 weeks and that we begin weekly fetal monitoring or nonstress testing at 32 weeks, and twice weekly at 36 weeks of pregnancy.

FETAL MORBIDITY: BABIES THAT CAN'T GO HOME WITH US

We've made huge strides in saving very small premature babies. Many that would once have died are now saved in high-tech intensive care units. The same factors that increase neonatal mortality in infants born to women over 40 will, of course, increase their morbidity. Once more, if we don't have risk factors for prematurity or growth retardation, our babies will probably do fine. The effect of maternal age on birthweight generally appears to be "ruled" by our medical complications (see above). There may be a small component of compromised, nonpliable uterine blood supply, which may contribute to a risk for delivery of a low-birth-weight infant independent of our health and social status.

If we've had an uncomplicated pregnancy, we can plan to take our baby home. Good fetal monitoring during labor with appropriate response to signs of fetal distress or prolonged nonproductive labor should allow a healthy baby *in utero* to continue to be healthy out of our body and in its intended environment—the crib at home.

Reducing Our Risks

There are a number of things that we can do to minimize our over-40 pregnancy risks. Before we even get pregnant, we should assess our health. If we are hypertensive or diabetic, or have other chronic medical problems, we may be heading for a complicated pregnancy requiring bed rest, hospitalization, and early operative delivery. Our babies may end up spending weeks or months in an incubator making up for time lost in our uterus. We should evaluate these risks and our motivation. If we want to proceed, we will need the best medical experts at the most advanced medical centers to provide our prenatal care.

Cigarette smoking is associated with high miscarriage rates, intrauterine growth retardation, premature separation of the placenta (*abruption*), premature rupture of the membranes, and premature delivery. A little smoking goes a long way; just ten cigarettes a day can poison your baby's environment and stunt its growth, resulting in underdevelopment and even sudden infant death. One study conducted in New York in the late 1980s showed that 26 percent of pregnant women between the ages of 35 and 44 smoked! Quit now! Will you ever have such a great reason?

Mild to moderate drinking increases our risk of miscarriage, fetal growth retardation, and fetal malformation. Alcohol is one of the most potent teratogens (a substance which causes abnormal fetal development). It can cause a group of developmental problems including stunted growth, mental retardation, and misshapen heart, limbs, and face. This cluster of developmental calamities has been termed *fetal alcohol syndrome*. It generally occurs if pregnant mothers drink heavily (six drinks a day), but portions of this syndrome may affect our offspring after moderate or even light alcohol consumption.

We have to clean up our diets before and during pregnancy. Nutritional deficits can affect our fetus's risk of congenital defects. If we add just 0.4 milligram (400 micrograms) of folic acid daily from the time we start trying to get pregnant, we may be able to reduce our risk of having a fetus with a neural tube defect by over half. Dark green vegetables, whole grain cereals, and legumes are excellent sources of folic acid. If we've had a previous pregnancy with neural tube defects, or there is a family history of this disorder, we should consume 4 milligrams of folic acid daily.

We need 1,500 to 2,000 milligrams of calcium a day to support our pregnancy and protect our bones. This is one of the few times in our adult lives that our bone-building cells can outnumber and outperform our bone-eating cells if given enough calcium. We can actually use this time to add to our bone density. Calcium may also decrease pregnancy-induced high blood pressure. If we supplement calcium we should stay away from some of the "natural source" calciums, which may contain high levels of lead (bone meal, dolomite, and oyster shell). Lead can severely affect a developing fetus. The refined and chelate forms of calcium may have less of this contaminant. Milk products are probably the safest way, in this regard, to get calcium during pregnancy.

We increase the volume of our blood by 50 percent during pregnancy. This dilutes our blood cells, and we usually need iron supplements to keep up.

Women with diabetes can reduce their risk of having babies with congenital anomalies such as heart defects by carefully controlling their glucose levels before they get pregnant and in early pregnancy.

Nutritional deficiencies need to be corrected, but excesses can also be a problem. Eating too much protein (no, you shouldn't live on steaks, eggs, and protein drinks) is associated with fetal growth retardation and places extra strain on our kidneys.

Recent surveys have raised concern over too much vitamin A. If a pregnant woman consumes more than 10,000 units of preformed vitamin A per day, she is estimated to have a 1 in 57 chance of delivering a baby with head and nervous system malformations. So check your vitamin supplements, because although beta-carotene is OK, excessive vitamin A is not!

If we want to procreate in our fifth decade, we should probably de-caffeinate. We know that pregnancy slows down the metabolism of caf-feine to half its usual pace, so whatever we drink stays with us for seven to ten hours. Caffeine passes through the placenta to the fetus, so we're supplying a very-long-term, steady dose. Caffeine has not been found to cause fetal malformations and, indeed, according to the National Insti-tutes of Health, three cups of coffee per day are not associated with a higher risk of abortion or fetal growth retardation. There have been studies, however, that have implicated three cups or more a day with stunting of growth, causing smaller-weight babies. Three studies have also shown a 1.7 percent increase in the risk of spontaneous abortion for each cup of coffee pregnant women consume per day. Once we've had our babies, we also need to be aware of the fact that the caffeine we drink passes through our breast milk. The quantities are small, but no one advises putting caffeine into baby formula, so why should we ruin an otherwise perfect food?

Obesity can cause us to have large, fat babies (who will subse-quently have a lifetime of weight control problems), pregnancy-induced high blood pressure, prematurity, and cesarean section. What we gain in pregnancy (aside from our kids) also affects our future risk of obesity. A study that followed 800 women through their pregnancies and postpar-tum years showed that those who, while pregnant, gained the weight recommended by the Institute of Medicine put on 5 pounds at the end of five years (See Table 4.1). If they gained more, they ended up 8 pounds heavier. If they gained less, they were only half a pound heavier than their prepregnancy weights. What happened between pregnancies was also prophetic. If they didn't lose their added weight or gained less than 10 pounds, they put on 7 to 9 pounds after their second baby was born. If they gained more than 10 pounds, they ended up with an extra 16 pounds. It appears that we need to lose our weight during the first six months after delivery. The longer it's on our bodies, the more likely it is to become permanent. If we're obese, we're also more prone to long-term health risks such as diabetes, high blood pressure, heart attack, and breast cancer. We're not having our children for someone else to raise because we can't!

Pregnancy is not a time to lose weight, but with properly adjusted eating in those of us who are overweight, we can limit our weight gain to

TABLE 4.1   **PREGNANCY WEIGHT GAIN RECOMMENDATIONS BY THE INSTITUTE OF MEDICINE**

Pregnancy Status	Recommended Total Gain*
Underweight: under 90% ideal body weight	28–40 lb.
Normal weight: 90–120% ideal body weight	25–35 lb.
Overweight: 120–135% ideal body weight	15–25 lb.
Obese: over 135% ideal body weight	15+ lb.

*Short women (under 62 inches) should strive for gains at the lower end of their range

between 16 and 24 pounds without compromising our baby's size or our own.

Most of us who have waited until our forties to start or complete our families have done so because of career, social, and economic choices. Hopefully we now have the maturity, finances, and family backing to allow us a new choice—that of good prepregnancy and prenatal care. We may be considered risky, elderly *gravidas* (pregnant women), but in the absence of poor health and our own neglect, and with the help of our doctors, we can pull this off and deliver healthy offspring.

....

Understanding Menopause

5

PERIMENOPAUSE
A Label or a Real Event?

"Peri" is one of those encompassing prefixes that we like to use in medical jargon. It means "around" or "near," so in this chapter we're discussing being "around" menopause or nearly menopausal. Very few life events (except sudden death from trauma) occur without prior physiologic changes—there is almost always a "peri."

If menopause is defined as the permanent cessation of our periods (we don't decide it's permanent for six months to a year), it follows that we are "peri" until we have reached this watershed (or tampon-shed). Doctors should be able to be more specific than that, especially since we are now capable of performing blood tests that give us the real hormonal scoop. But since most of us don't spend our mid- to late forties having frequent hormonal blood tests, we still define this transition by changes in our cycles and/or development of characteristic symptoms:

- Irregular cycles
- Hot flashes
- Mood changes

When and for How Long Do We Go Through This Transition to Menopause?

This simple and important question wasn't scientifically answered until 1987. The Massachusetts Women's Health Study followed 2,570 women, ages 44 to 55. They were considered perimenopausal if they had had cycle irregularity in at least two consecutive interviews (they were interviewed every nine months) and/or three to eleven months of no periods. They were postmenopausal if they had had no period for more than eleven months. On the basis of findings from this fairly large group of cooperative women, we now have the following important information:

1. The average age of natural menopause is 51.3 years.

2. The average age at the beginning of perimenopause is 47.5 years.

3. The average length of the perimenopausal transition is 3.8 years.

4. Ninety percent of women go through perimenopause (the remaining 10 percent abruptly cease menstruating and become menopausal).

5. Smokers go through menopause 1.8 years earlier than nonsmokers and have an earlier and shorter perimenopause.

6. Many symptoms increase in perimenopause and decrease in menopause.

Since few of us are "average," we should look at some of the variability in these numbers. It's rather unfortunate that the youngest women followed in this study were 44, since perimenopause can occur at earlier ages. Seventy-nine percent of women at 45 went through perimenopause in their five follow-up years, some at the very beginning. Conversely, 3 percent of 50- to 55-year-old women still hadn't gone through this transition during the same five years. It has also become clear that we can have hormonal variations and subsequent symptoms while still having regular periods. Do these count, and as we deal with them, can we be classified as perimenopausal?

Labeling the transition is probably less important than understanding what happens to us between our normal ovulatory cycles in our third and fourth decades and our total lack of cycles in the menopause. These changes are real, and the quality of our lives in our forties depends on our acknowledging them and considering our health-care choices to deal with or control them.

What Happens to Our Hormones During Perimenopause?

Our estrogen levels decrease progressively. It would make scientific sense, therefore, if we could determine that we're perimenopausal by simply testing our hormone levels. But blood tests are not always helpful, because the one consistent thing in perimenopause is inconsistent hormone levels. Initially the estrogen drop is subtle and remains in the "normal" lab range. This is particularly true if we're not exact in our timing of these tests (remember, estrogen will always be low in the early part of our cycle and will subsequently rise). As estrogen and inhibin levels decrease, FSH rises. If a particular cycle is a catastrophe and no follicle develops, we can have very low estrogen and high FSH values. They may even reach menopausal levels! But the next month, this high FSH may "awaken" residual "lazy" follicles and estrogen will be produced. FSH is then pushed down, and our lab values look normal.

One elevated FSH (greater than 30 milli–international units) does not menopause make and, conversely, a single normal FSH and estradiol does not negate perimenopause. We may need to perform these tests every two weeks for at least two months before we reach a hormonally based diagnosis of perimenopause or menopause. Even this may not be enough and, indeed, we may need to continue monitoring FSH levels.

Since hormonal tests are expensive (an FSH and estradiol measurement can cost $100), it may be wiser to look at our cycles and symptoms and use the blood tests when we need more exact information for therapy choices. For example, if I see a woman in her mid- to late forties who is having significant hormonal symptoms (hot flashes and mood changes) and no periods for several months except perhaps for spotting, I use FSH and estradiol tests to see if she is perimenopausal or menopausal. These tests might need to be repeated, but I use the current results to help us decide whether to treat her condition with low-dose birth control pills (in perimenopause) or hormone replacement therapy (in menopause).

This testing can also enable us to distinguish ovulatory problems that are not perimenopausal from those associated with this transition. Our "freak incidence" is high whenever we miss periods in our late thirties or early forties. Once we've confirmed that we are not pregnant, we want to make sure we're not perimenopausal (1 percent of women do become menopausal before the age of 40).

Anovulation (lack of ovulation) and missed periods can occur whenever stress, rapid weight loss, travel, medical conditions, or medical therapies affect our sensitive pituitary-ovarian balance. If we've missed periods and any of the above applies, an FSH and estradiol test is helpful. If the results are normal, we probably are (or, to be more exact, our follicles are) normal. We've stopped ovulating due to psychological or medical stresses. We can then either manage the underlying condition or simply bring on regular periods using progesterone or birth control pills.

Another gland can contribute to irregular cycles and perimenopausal symptoms—the thyroid. After childbearing, and as we pass into our fifth decade, we increase our risk of *hypothyroidism* (inadequate thyroid production). Low thyroid can make our cycles irregular, and can bring on the same hot flashes we associate with perimenopause and menopause. Before we start arbitrarily prescribing hormones, we'd better check and make sure we are giving the right ones. Those of us whose tests show low thyroid may have all our perimenopausal problems resolved (and gain control of our weight) with simple thyroid supplementation. Our perimenopause may be a "thyroid pause" that can easily be corrected.

Other Symptoms of Perimenopause

IRREGULAR CYCLES

Why do 90 percent of us have irregular cycles during this transition? Our store of ovarian follicles has been diminishing gradually throughout our lives, but the number drops precipitously in our early forties. On an individual basis, these follicles cease to perform as well as they did in the past, creating hormonal changes that may cause us to bleed early, late, longer, or not at all. If the follicles manage to do a decent job at every stage of our cycle, we continue to have regular periods. When they don't, though, we have irregular cycles, the official hallmark of "medically determined" perimenopause and the end result of our premenopausal ovarian changes. (See chapter 1 for a detailed account of our cycles.)

Some of the changes we might experience are:

Shorter Cycles

These are due to poor development of the follicle and "premature ejaculation of the egg," or to no ovulation with a feeble attempt at estrogen production, which falls once the follicle dies.

Longer or Missed Cycles

If no follicle dominates, estrogen levels may remain low for weeks, or even months. This is a *pseudomenopause* and is accompanied by lack of uterine lining buildup (so there's nothing to slough off) and missed periods. Chances are, we will also have significant menopausal symptoms during this period (or, to be accurate, lack of a period). But wait—we have a secret cache of follicles left, and finally (after much prodding from our overworked pituitary), it responds. Estrogen is once again produced, our symptoms diminish, our lining thickens, and then sheds, and we get a period.

A second scenario can also occur: A follicle develops and undergoes pseudo-ovulatory changes. There is no proper egg release, but progesterone is produced. This abnormal follicle forgets it's supposed to have a postovulatory two-week life span. It plods on, producing some estrogen and some progesterone. PMS symptoms occur and seem to last forever. Finally, it gasps and dies, and the uterine lining sloughs. A late period occurs, together with relief from PMS.

Intermittent Spotting and Bleeding

This is the result of irregular shedding of the lining of the uterus. Little bits and pieces break away (we bleed), there is a meager attempt at endometrial repair (bleeding stops), and then the process breaks down again. This bleeding is due to a disharmonious committee of unorganized follicles, instead of the usual dictatorial rule of a dominant egg with superior hormonal production. If we had similar problems in a factory production line, we would need to shut down (which eventually occurs with menopause) or propose a corporate takeover. This type of bleeding often signifies little or no progesterone production. The uterine lining is being subjected to unopposed estrogen and, with time, may get truly confused, develop abnormal glands, and finally become cancerous.

Prolonged or Heavy Bleeding

Lack of ovulation and production of unopposed estrogen can cause the uterine glands to become very full (*cystic*) and convoluted. The lining is built up over longer periods of time, and when it finally breaks down (either from a decrease in estrogen or because the existing estrogen couldn't keep up with its nourishment needs), the bleeding can be very heavy. Because the slough is uneven and some areas break down before others, the bleeding is prolonged. Since unopposed estrogen is the culprit, this symptom may signify cancer or precancerous changes.

Additionally, with age, we are more prone to uterine pathology such as adenomyosis, fibroids, and polyps, all of which can increase bleeding.

"I'M HAVING A BAD HORMONE DAY": OTHER SYMPTOMS

When our hormones vacillate, we may experience hot flashes and mood changes, and do so long before our periods change and "prove" we're perimenopausal. Both of these symptoms may begin in perimenopause and continue through menopause as well.

Hot Flashes

Hot flashes occur in over 50 percent of women going through perimenopause, and over 35 percent describe these flashes as "severe." This symptom alone prompts half of us to visit our doctor (one study showed that we're twice as likely to see a physician because of hot flashes than irregular periods!).

What is a hot flash? In the 1700s, it was described by the Germans as "commotion of the blood." Later, the French called it a "puff of heat." In the 1800s, it was believed to be analogous to the wayward maiden's blush, an emotional reaction to stress (or being wayward). Feminist writer Germaine Greer recently agreed with this Victorian assessment and recommended hydrotherapy!

The physiology and causes of hot flashes are not at all similar to those of the flush; they're more accurately akin to the breaking of a fever (definitely less romantic). The culprit, again, is falling estrogen, which most likely triggers a "storm" by causing the hypothalamus to increase production of hormones or proteins. Interestingly, this is the same area of the brain that produces GnRH, the hormone that controls FSH and LH. In the absence of estrogen, these hormones get overstimulated, and their outpouring affects our brain's temperature-regulating center, which sits near the hypothalamus. This "thermostat" is easily irritated, and in fact 10 percent of all women have hot flashes throughout their reproductive lives; some begin feeling them in their teens. As our estrogen drops, we may experience them just before or during our periods.

During one of these hypothalamic storms, the center is aroused, causing it to dispatch the erroneous message: "It's too hot in here. Let's cool this body down." Our natural cooling system kicks on: Our heart rate accelerates and our blood vessels dilate to rapidly move four to thirty times more blood to our body surface, where outside air cools it. We also perspire, and this fluid evaporation gives us a second outlet for the release of heat. These cooling events quickly accomplish their goal, decreasing our inner-core temperature by half a degree in a matter of minutes. The fickle thermostat now decides we're too cool and commands: "Let's heat this body up!" Suddenly our vessels constrict, we lose our flush, and we begin to shiver as our body attempts to generate heat.

My personal response to my first series of nighttime hypothalamic storms and hot flashes (which occurred when I was 46) was to brush away any aspect of my medical training and storm to my nearest department store for a thinner bed cover (thank goodness, there was a sale!). When my husband puzzled over the appearance of a new comforter that was, in his words, "skimpy," I assured him that this would prevent us from overheating in our sleep. Only when my hot flashes continued did I wake up—covered with sweat—and realize that my low estrogen and hypothalamic response were causing these hot flashes. The new comforter stayed.

It's important to note that we can't always blame perimenopause or menopause for this distressing symptom. Hot flashes can have a number of nonhormonal causes, which can even affect men (although they are rarely seen in public with a fan). Alcohol consumption may affect our inner temperature control and result in hot flashes. This is especially apparent in individuals who have low activity of an enzyme that helps break down alcohol. Individuals who flush easily with alcohol consumption are also more likely to become alcoholics (so if you flush when you drink, beware).

Rarely, a tumor in the bowel (*carcinoid*) produces a substance called serotonin, which can cause sudden development of hot flashes with no other hormonal explanation. A different tumor that grows in the adrenal gland (*pheochromocytoma*) may manifest itself through a combination of high blood pressure, excessive perspiration, and palpitations.

Finally, we have the dilemma of differentiating a hot flash from a panic attack. If the episodes of excessive perspiration and flushing are regularly accompanied by a racing heartbeat (even when resting), sensations of terror and anxiety, "crying jags," or fear that a heart attack is occurring or that death is imminent, the diagnosis of a panic attack is pretty evident. Women with mitral valve prolapse seem to be more likely to experience these attacks. Most doctors view this as a psychiatric problem and treat the attack (with some success) with a combination of psychotherapy, anti-anxiety medications, and drugs to control rapid heartbeat. Since we can be perimenopausal and have panic symptoms at the same time, it's reasonable to combine hormonal therapy with antipanic therapy when one treatment is not adequate.

Mood Changes

Perhaps we should reconsider what the acronym PMS stands for: not pre*menstrual* but pre*menopausal* syndrome! Our brain has receptors for estrogen, progesterone, and testosterone. Slow decreases in these hormones may cause less upset to our receptors than sporadic and radical vacillations. In other words, once we finally hit menopause, our central nervous system has had years to "get used to" lower levels and, indeed, despite the common belief that depression and mental illness increase in menopausal women, our scientific data show that just isn't true. Twenty percent of women (in contrast to 10 percent of men) will develop depression during their lifetime. Fifty percent of us have this occur between the ages of 20 and 50; the mean age is 40. During our perimenopause, we "out-depress" men by a ratio of 3, or even 4 to 1!

What symptoms commonly compose (or decompose) these depressive mood changes? The list is "depressingly" long:

- Irritability
- Tearfulness
- Excessive worry and anxiety
- Mood instability
- Food cravings and increased appetite
- Decreased energy
- Decreased libido
- Poor motivation
- Early-morning wakening
- Interrupted sleep
- Emotional detachment

Any of these sound familiar? I can pick out at least four that I have personally experienced, and my family would be happy to complete the list! I've had successful professional women sit in my office and challenge me to show them that they are not turning into heretofore unknown entities who have lost control. One patient described herself as an alien; she had alienated her family, her colleagues, and her actions from her feelings. Many psychologists and sociologists argue that what we're suffering from is midlife blahs, that because we realize we may not have attained our goals, our venerated youth is gone, and we're faced with the four Ds (demise of parents, divorce of spouses, deteriorating relationships with children, and drudgery at work), we are now decompensating. I don't see this as being applicable to either myself or the majority of my patients with premenopausal mood changes. It's too much of a coincidence that these symptoms "just happen" to accompany our changed cycles and, for over 80 percent of us, perimenopausal elevation of FSH.

We know that our hormones directly affect our neurotransmitters and may regulate mood, memory, appetite, and sleep. Low levels of estrogen are known to coincide with high levels of a substance called MAO (not the dead Chinese leader but the enzyme *monoamine oxidase*), which breaks down *catecholamines* and serotonin. (These are neurotransmitters that act as messengers in our brain and nervous system.) Their depletion is thought to be a significant factor in precipitating depressive episodes. Changes in our levels of estrogen, progesterone, and testosterone can increase or decrease the release of these substances transmitted between the nerve cells in our brain. We have little difficulty in accepting that our fluctuating hormones cause changes in our uterine response (and periods); why should we be reluctant to consider that our hormonally receptive nervous system is similarly affected?

Treating Perimenopausal Symptoms

STABILITY—IN HORMONAL FORM

Many of us feel we are losing control; our follicles are dwindling and inconsistent in their response to the "call of the pituitary," and our bodies respond in ways we neither appreciate nor care to accept. What are our options?

The Hormonal Takeover:
Use of Low-Dose Birth Control Pills

If our ovaries can't give us an even response, but instead taunt us with a roller-coaster ride of estrogen and progesterone production, we can simply shut them down while providing a steady, timed amount of these hormones. This is accomplished with low-dose birth control pills. The safety and use of these pills after 40 have been discussed in detail in chapter 2. Briefly, their effect on our perimenopausal symptoms and problems might include:

- Cessation of hot flashes
- Control of irregular bleeding
- Fewer mood, energy, and concentration changes caused by low estrogen; possible improvement of PMS
- Protection against endometrial cancer
- Decrease in risk of ovarian cancer
- Possible prevention of bone loss

- Lower incidence of fibroids, endometriosis, and ovarian cysts
- Decrease in arteriosclerotic heart disease
- Decrease in benign breast disease

Once we are on the Pill, we should have blessedly regular cycles. I have a patient who is currently 52, has been on the Pill for the last four years, and with each visit cautions me that I had better not tell her to stop taking it. She doesn't want to know if she is currently menopausal; she loves masking the possibility with this therapy. But she and I do need to know, so every six months I have her return at the end of her Pill-free week (or, if a patient uses 28-day packs, during the week of placebo pills) and I draw an FSH level. If it's over 50, menopause has probably occurred, and it's time to discontinue the birth control pills and consider hormone replacement therapy. Once we're menopausal, we don't need the stronger synthetic estrogen in the Pill. We now have nothing to suppress; it's time to just add what's missing and, if we choose to do this, we should use the natural, less potent estrogen of hormone replacement therapy. (My patient's last FSH was 20, and she is still taking her low-dose birth control pills.)

Hormonal Addition Rather Than Suppression: Use of Hormone Replacement Therapy (HRT)

HRT has been touted by the Europeans as being the "*haute* success" in the treatment of mood changes and PMS in perimenopausal women. They use nonoral estrogen either as an implant (which is not commercially available here) or as a patch. They recommend the use of the larger patch (0.1 milligram) or even a double patch to be changed twice weekly with the addition of progesterone for 10 days each month to protect the uterine lining. They warn that during the first month of therapy, there may be a transient increase in symptoms, but that by the end of the third month, symptom levels should be reduced by 50 percent.

This form of cyclical hormonal therapy may not suppress our own ovarian function. Remember, the estrogen in HRT is one fourth as potent as that in birth control pills. As a result, our follicles' ups and downs continue. When they are "up" and produce normal amounts of estrogen, the addition of the estrogen in the patch may be too much, leaving us feeling overdosed with breast tenderness and bloating. When our natural estrogen levels fall, our endometrium can respond, and we may bleed despite HRT. We now have to deal with a symptom that can signal cancer.

Finally, there seems to be a higher risk of breast cancer in some women using HRT in the European studies when compared to American women. It's possible that extensive and high-dose use of estrogen in the perimenopause is a factor. This therapy will need at least another decade of analysis before doctors can give the reassurance they would like as they prescribe estrogen for perimenopausal symptoms.

Progestins to Control Irregular Bleeding

This works quite well. We're simply providing the missing progesterone (in synthetic form it's termed *progestin*) at the right time for the right number of days when our own ovulations are faulty. Most physicians prescribe medroxyprogesterone acetate (Provera or Cycrin), 5 or 10 milligrams for 10 to 12 days at the end of each cycle, or norethindrone acetate (Norlutate), 5 milligrams. This builds up the uterine lining, which will then slough and bleed once we stop taking the pills. We need to self-produce estrogen for the initial endometrial development. If none is present, the progestin won't work. I sometimes use this as a "trial of menopause." If several cycles of progestin do not stimulate bleeding (with a normal uterus), we no longer have estrogen on board, and chances are we have crossed the transition to menopause.

In addition to cycling our bleeding, progestins protect our endometrium from unopposed estrogen and the risk of endometrial cancer. I have patients who bleed every four to five months, have minimal perimenopausal symptoms, and who delight in the absence of regular periods. I become the "spoiler." I counsel them to take a progestin at least every other month—which, of course, causes bleeding. But, more important, they aren't left to their unopposed estrogen and future risk of endometrial cancer.

The progestins and I are "spoilers" in other ways. We may increase PMS. In an effort to keep my patients happier (with their medications and me), I switch those who bloat and get depressed on synthetic progestin to natural progesterone. Between 200 and 300 milligrams a day for 10 to 12 days should give them adequate protection and bleeding control.

NONHORMONAL THERAPIES:
THERE MUST BE A "NATURAL" WAY TO CONTROL THESE
SYMPTOMS

The majority of us will go through this transition without major depression, out-of-body and -control experiences, and certainly without psychoses. We're sleeping well and are only minimally annoyed by our hot flashes. Our menstrual irregularities are not causing us to hemorrhage, bleed continuously, or become anemic. We have normal weight, good health, no genetic history of ovarian cancer, and are using adequate contraception. We don't feel the need to replace, add, or otherwise "fiddle" with our hormones. What can we or should we do during perimenopause?

1. Know what's happening and why. This diminishes anxiety and stress, which, in themselves, contribute to our symptoms.

2. Avoid hot flash stimulators—alcohol, caffeine, spicy food, stress, overheated rooms, thick comforters, and clothes that can't be layered.

3. Eat to prepare for the next half of our lives. Make sure we're getting at least 1,500 milligrams of calcium a day so that we protect our bone density. Our diet should have plenty of grains, fruits, and vegetables and be low in fat.

4. Exercise. This can decrease stress and raise endorphin levels and our sense of well-being. Studies have shown that hot flashes are half as common in physically active women as in those who are sedentary.

5. Herbs such as dong quai and black cohosh may diminish PMS symptoms and hot flashes (see chapter 8).

6. Increase our intake of natural dietary estrogens such as soybean products. Japanese women consume these at the expense of fat and meat and seem to have significantly fewer perimenopausal symptoms than we do.

7. Vitamin E and evening primrose oil (see chapter 8) may help to reduce PMS symptoms and hot flashes (many researchers feel this is a placebo effect).

8. An over-the-counter hormonal replenishing gel (Pro-Gest) made from wild Mexican yams *may* help reduce symptoms. This gel has not, unfortunately, been put through scientifically controlled studies that look at its efficacy (see chapter 8).

9. Stop smoking! Smoking lowers our estrogen levels and causes an earlier perimenopause and menopause by as much as two years.

Perimenopause: The Staging Ground for the Next Half of Our Lives

Because 90 percent of us have irregular cycles and hormonal symptoms, we've been reminded that our ovaries are "a-changing," and we should start doing the same. Who knows? We could read a book (hopefully, this one), consult a doctor (and we all know how many years we've gone without a checkup), and get appropriate present and future woman-care information. Perimenopause is a dress rehearsal for menopause. We're all going to be present at the live performance, no matter how young we are. Better be ready.

6

MENOPAUSE
The Most Misunderstood
Transition of Our Lives

"**M**"-words have been used to define many of the important periods (literally and figuratively) of our lives. Menarche is our first period. We then have monthly menses (periods) which can be interrupted by pregnancies (yes, a "P"-word that occurred for most of us after marriage). As a result of most of these pregnancies (some miscarried), we became mothers. We matured. After another "P" transition (perimenopause), we reached the penultimate "M" status—menopause. The word is self-defining—a "pause" of our menses (periods). It signifies the end result of an ongoing endocrinologic transition.

Our society has imbued this transition with so much negative symbolism that I sometimes feel like a mother trying to rescue her child from a cult. Quiet reasoning and understanding may help, but anger and raised voices crying "What have they done to us?!" are also in order.

The Final Period: When and Why

We define menopause as our last menstrual period but, obviously, we can't know it's the last one until we haven't had any more, usually for six to twelve months. This is a retrospective diagnosis, a sort of "look back and remember when."

WHEN

The average age of menopause is 51, meaning that it usually occurs between 47 and 53. Although we're far from scientific in predicting when the event will transpire, we have found that certain factors in our heredity or past behavior can affect the timing of our last period and onset of menopause.

Early Menopause

1. Smoking. This can "hurry up" ovarian failure by two years!

2. A family history of early menopause (mother or older sisters).

3. Previous chemotherapy or radiotherapy; this can destroy ovarian function, especially in women over the age of 35.

4. Living at altitudes above 10,000 feet. This is an empiric finding. It's not clear why, but menopause can occur one to two years earlier than expected.

5. No term pregnancies; a history of short menstrual cycles (incessant ovulation may contribute to more rapid loss of oocytes).

6. An early perimenopause (see previous chapter); if this started in our late thirties or early forties, menopause will probably occur within the next four years.

Late Menopause

1. Family history of late menopause (mother and sisters).

2. Early menarche (first period before age 11). Some studies indicate that this is associated with late menopause; others have shown a correlation with early menopause!

Premature Menopause (Before Age 40)

This may not be "normal," but it happens to 1 percent of women before the age of 40. Many will be told they are "too young to be menopausal" and will be dismissed and inappropriately treated with possibly devastating results on their present and future health. Here are some of the causes:

DAMAGE TO THE OVARIES

Our ovaries are most vulnerable in their developmental stage, and we have the greatest number of oocytes when we are five months postconception in our mother's uterus. If our mothers had viral infections, it's possible that our ovaries could be affected, so that we were born with a depleted number of oocytes. We had enough to go through puberty, and we may also have had enough to get pregnant (although menopause in our twenties won't have given most of us enough time). But at some point before the age of 40, we run out of oocytes and we can't develop follicles capable of responding to our pituitary commands.

Ovarian damage can, of course, be caused surgically, the ultimate damage being the removal of both ovaries (*bilateral oophorectomy*). If only one ovary is removed and the other compromised (by such surgical procedures as cyst removal or hysterectomy with damage to blood vessels supplying the ovary), a slow dwindling of the remaining follicles will result in menopause occurring months or years after the procedure, but much earlier than the expected time.

The vulnerable oocytes in our ovaries can also by prematurely destroyed by radiation or chemotherapy that is used to treat malignancies of childhood and early adulthood. The good news, however, is that the younger a woman at the time of therapy, the less likely she is to have permanent destruction of her ovarian function.

Rarely, the ovaries and their follicles are attacked by our own antibodies. We really don't know what causes this autoimmune process, but it can destroy our ability to ovulate and produce hormones. This process can be accompanied by additional derangements in our immune system causing us to reject other major organs, especially the thyroid.

GENETIC CAUSES

Some families have a genetic premature menopause. This condition is linked to one of the X chromosomes, which we inherit from our mother (XX) and our father (XY). One parent may contribute a defective X chromosome, which reduces the genetic determination of the initial number of oocytes that develop in the ovaries.

The greatest prematurity of menopause is what I call "menonever"—never developing a period (*primary amenorrhea*) and never producing ovarian estrogen because the ovaries didn't develop. The medical term is *ovarian dysgenesis* (a dysfunction in the genesis of ovaries), and it can occur sporadically (translation: we don't know why) or as a result of an abnormality of one of our X chromosomes. If our normal female chromosome complement has two Xs and, by mistake, we didn't get one of the Xs during fertilization, we end up with XO; this is called *Turner's syndrome*. The second X chromosome is needed to develop our ovaries (but not our vagina or uterus). If even a part of that second X is missing, our ovarian development is deficient. Conversely, if we get too many Xs (*trisomy X*, or triple X), the opposite occurs and our ovaries are given incomplete signals for development, which may result in premature menopause.

WHY

For 90 percent of us, our dwindling oocyte numbers have already given notice during perimenopause. Remember, we went from 7 million oocytes at the fifth month of gestation to 1 or 2 million at birth and "only" 400,000 at puberty. We hit the few hundred to few thousand mark when we reach menopause. We don't hit zero at menopause, but the few hundred to few thousand follicles left are so functionally inept that estrogen production declines steeply to miniscule levels. These are insufficient to give us periods or, more important, to satisfy the estrogen receptors in our target organs—the brain, heart, blood vessels, bones, genital tract, bladder, and skin.

If we approach the diagnosis of menopause prospectively (not all of us want to wait a whole year to figure out we've had our last period), we need to look at our hormonal levels. Our estrogen will remain low (estradiol levels below 30 picograms/milliliter), and our FSH (trying for the rest of our lives to get those ovaries to work) stays high at levels that are greater than 50 milli-international units. Several menopausal readings with ongoing symptoms and lack of periods are about as confirmatory as we can get without waiting that defining year.

Although our ovarian production of estrogen has failed in menopause, it doesn't mean we become totally "estrogen-less." We produce several forms of estrogen, both from the ovaries and peripheral organs, and there is a shift in this production. During our reproductive years, our ovaries were our major source of estrogen. The strongest estrogen, estradiol, was produced at higher levels than the weaker estrogen, estrone. The concentration of estrone falls after menopause, but remains higher than estradiol (in other words, the relationship reverses). We also have a change in male hormone production. When we were younger, our ovaries produced two types of male hormone, a small amount of the "potent" male hormone, *testosterone,* and a larger amount of the weak hormone, *androstenedione.* This balance, too, shifts with menopause, and we get much less androstenedione. Because our menopausal ovaries continue to produce some of the more potent testosterone, our total ovarian male hormone production falls only 30 to 50 percent, whereas ovarian estrogen decreases by at least 90 percent. Once we're menopausal, we still have an additional source of estrogen; it's produced from male hormone in our peripheral tissues, including our fat, muscle, and skin. This conversion is performed more effectively once we're menopausal. We're compensating—our outer-body estrogen production is making up for our inner body's (ovarian) failure.

The more fat we have, and the older we are, the more we convert testosterone to estrogen. So postmenopausal obese women have more estrogen than those of us who remain thin. "Fat-made" estrogen can literally insulate us from some of our menopausal symptoms, as well as long-term development of diseases related to estrogen depletion (see sections on osteoporosis and Alzheimer's). That doesn't mean that fat is an overall health advantage. This same estrogen producer increases our risk of endometrial cancer, breast cancer, ovarian cancer, and heart disease. (See part III.) The battle of the bulge should still be fought!

The Wherefore: Physical Signs and Symptoms of Menopause

HOT FLASHES

I have always been puzzled about the term "sign" (often used synonymously with "symptom" in medical terminology). I imagine a large poster proclaiming, with appropriate graphics, that a disease or condition is contained herein. In the case of menopause, we do bear (and bare for) the trademark sign, hot flashes. Our flushing, perspiring, fanning, and subsequent shivering publicly advertise our status of estrogen depletion. Up to 93 percent of us have "signed on."

The prevalence of hot flashes is highest in our first two years of menopause, ranging from 58 to 93 percent. They are reported to occur more in women in Western than in non-Western cultures, and Japanese women are supposedly least affected. This has been attributed to their diet, which contains a large amount of plant estrogens, or *phytoestrogens*, and their culture, which emphasizes willpower while deemphasizing physical complaints.

Hot flashes can vary in frequency from hourly to once a day. A third of menopausal women with flashes report having more than ten a day. Intensity is a subjective issue to scientists; it is probably less so for those of us who have to change clothes and sheets or repeatedly shower. In one study, 26 percent of menopausal women with hot flashes reported that this symptom was severe (the same high rating was applied by 47.4 percent of women undergoing surgical menopause and 36.8 percent of premenopausal women who experienced this symptom). Almost half of us perceive a forewarning or "aura" prior to flashing. We may feel a sense of anxiety, a reddening of our skin, a change in heart rate, or a sensation of heat. During the hot flash, we also share some common feelings (just because we're red and sweating like pigs doesn't mean we become emotionally passive). These include irritation, annoyance ("Why can't I control this?"), frustration ("Enough already!"), and sometimes a sense of panic, suffocation, or, rarely, suicidal thoughts. When these damn things recur during the day, they are physically and emotionally draining (and I'm not just referring to water loss).

It's a struggle to maintain a cool composure and command of our work situations while losing our personal temperature control. Initially, when I began to sweat in the operating room, my colleagues thought I had encountered a surgical dilemma. I quickly learned to comment how well "the case" was going and how hot the lights were, then request that the temperature be lowered. This helped me reestablish my psychological control. Turning red and perspiring during business discussions is another control disaster. This response has so often been connected to deceit, uncertainty, or stress (we would fail lie detector tests during our flashes), that our sincerity, skill, and intelligence are suddenly put to question. We can also lose control of the quality of our personal relationships if we reject close encounters and intimacy because we don't want our partner's body heat to raise our own. Unfortunately, this symptom not only creates social and emotional havoc when we're awake, it continues to disrupt our bodies' temperature control while we sleep.

In order to have what we so glibly term "a good night's sleep," we have to put our brains to rest by cycling through various brain-wave patterns. These culminate with our dreams, or REM sleep (this is an acronym for "rapid eye movement," which occurs together with some pretty revealing fantasies during our dreams). If we interrupt the progression of these stages, we "fog" our mind. Menopausal hot flashes may awaken us several times during the night as we find ourselves drenched in sweat, throwing off bedcovers, and opening windows, but hot flashes have also been shown to occur throughout the night (documented by changes in our heart rate, skin temperature, and brain pattern) without causing conscious awakening. These insidious flashes will also disrupt our brain waves' peace. Sleep deprivation can lead to fatigue, irritability, decreased energy, and depression, a type of jet lag without the reward of arriving at a new destination.

How long should we expect these flashes to continue? Studies have shown that the majority of us (about 60 to 65 percent) can expect to experience flushes for one to seven years, about 25 percent for seven to ten years, and 10 to 15 percent for more than eleven years. Women in their seventies and eighties certainly do report having hot flashes (I know my mother does). Our numbers may be skewed because few studies of this and other menopausal symptoms include "older" women (as if the effects of estrogen deprivation disappear after our late sixties!).

Can we predict who among us will be dealing with severe or prolonged hot flashes? Only to a small and perhaps not very scientific extent. We know that surgical removal of the ovaries, especially in women who are not near their natural menopause, will result in significant flashes for 80 to 90 percent of them. One of my patients (who had surgery for an early cancer) was sopping wet twenty-four hours postoperatively. The staff thought she had a severe infection and suggested intravenous antibiotics. She was given estrogen and her "fever" rapidly resolved.

Women who go through their natural menopause before age 52 have an increased probability of having hot flashes. Also, thin women, especially if they smoked during perimenopause (both factors reduce estrogen) seem to be destined to be more frequent consumers of electric and handheld fans.

We can't "will" our hypothalamus to behave, but we can diminish factors such as stress, heat, alcohol, spicy food, and caffeine, all of which have been show to aid and abet our internal temperature reactivity. Nor do we have to continue to perspire, flush, and lose sleep. Fortunately, there is help. Estrogen replacement therapy is a true "cure" (see chapter 7). Hot flashes usually subside within four to six weeks and will be gone for as long as we continue therapy. (The flashes can recur if we stop hormonal therapy.) If we can't or won't use estrogen, we might not get complete relief, but we can get help (see chapter 8).

VULVAR AND VAGINAL SYMPTOMS

Understanding the Symptoms

The lower part of our genital tract needs estrogen. Once it has lost this hormone, it undergoes what I term "starvation involution." The first "to go" is vaginal fluid secretion. The vagina doesn't maintain its usual moisture and fails to lubricate properly during sexual arousal and intercourse. This "dry zone" is due to diminished blood flow to the vaginal walls, fewer cells lining the walls, less mucus produced by the cervix, and less fluid coming down from the uterine cavity. The vaginal walls also change. In a process called atrophy, they become thinner, less elastic, and pale. The stretchy wrinkles that previously allowed the walls to expand for expulsion of babies (and entrance of the penis that helped contribute to the making of these babies) smooth out and disappear. The thin, less distensible surface is now easily traumatized by sexual intercourse and can bleed. If we're not sexually active, scar tissue can form between touching surfaces.

These extreme changes won't occur overnight once we're menopausal and will occur even less if we use those nights to have regular intercourse. Decreased lubrication can develop early in perimenopause as soon as we have diminished estrogen levels. Discomfort with intercourse (*dyspareunia*) can also occur at this time and is unfortunately common. It is estimated that this is the second most frequent complaint (after hot flashes) instigating visits to the gynecologist. One study has shown that without hormonal therapy, 30 percent of us will have dyspareunia. Once it hurts to have intercourse, we are less likely to want to engage in sex (who wants to hurt?), and because we anticipate pain, our sexual desire may decrease. With reduced blood flow to the vagina, we experience less engorgement during sexual arousal. This can affect our normal stimulatory process and orgasm. Finally, our sexual response can be affected by one more regional factor: the tone of our muscles surrounding the vagina. If we can't squeeze them, we lose important participation and pleasure (ours and our partner's).

Vaginal atrophy is not just a sexual problem; it's a very real medical problem. With loss of estrogen, the vaginal pH changes from a normally acidic low to a higher, more alkaline pH. This less acidic environment discourages the growth of one of our most important organisms, lactobacillus, which acts as a bacterial guard against abnormal flora. Once these "bad guys" overgrow (notice, I gave them a male personification), they can cause discharge, irritation, and can rise up into the urethral opening of the bladder, creating urinary tract infections.

Our vulva and genital skin can be just as estrogen-sensitive as the inner vagina. It, too, can atrophy, losing its collagen and fat. The hood over the clitoris can retract, leaving this part of our anatomy exposed and more likely to be irritated by pressure from sitting and friction from underwear. Wiping, inserting creams or tampons, as well as the friction of intercourse, can cause swelling and pain in the clitoral area. The thinning of the vulvar skin, combined with an irritating vaginal discharge, can lead to terrible itching. It's not ladylike to scratch, but during the night, when the itching seems worse, many ladies do, with resultant abrasions to the skin and infection.

Prevention and Treatment of Vulvar and Vaginal Atrophy

The preceding description is not a pretty one and fits into a concept of menopausal "withering womanliness." We have to neither wither nor lose our genital competence. There are a number of options:

ESTROGEN THERAPY

This treatment offers us the greatest success. If started early in menopause, it will prevent all of these atrophic changes. Systemic estrogen replacement therapy (as either pills or patches) should give us estrogen levels that are adequate to maintain healthy vulvar skin, vaginal wall thickness, blood supply, fluid production, and muscle tone. Estrogen can also be supplied "on target" with estrogen creams that are inserted into the vagina.

REGULAR INTERCOURSE OR MASTURBATION

How's this for a doctor's prescription! When we're sexually active, we keep our vaginal pH down and discourage growth of abnormal bacteria. Regular use tones our surrounding muscles, and we end up with no pain and more gain.

VAGINAL MOISTURIZERS AND LUBRICANTS

We spend a fortune throughout our lives moisturizing the skin everyone sees. There are thousands of products available, all advertised by gorgeous 20-year-olds. Very few products have been developed for our inner moisture needs, and it is certainly more difficult to promote them. Replense and Gyne-Moistrin are vaginal moisturizers that can be helpful if used on a regular basis. Nonirritating creams (without alcohol or scent) can help the vulvar skin. I occasionally see good results with simple A&D ointment. We should use lubricants just before we have intercourse. We oil mechanical parts that rub (like the engines of our cars); we just need to do the same to prevent our own inner friction. Use the lubricant like a massage oil; rub it on your partner and have him rub it on your vulvar and clitoral area. It helps to achieve a tactile intimacy and prevents irritation. There are several products on the market with such wonderful names as Moist Again, Lubrin, and Astroglide. Vaseline is not a good lubricant; it can dry and cake. K-Y Jelly has been used for years, but I prefer a liquid to a gel. My personal favorite is Astroglide (although the name prompts some weird associations). Most of these lubricants are conveniently displayed next to condoms in the drugstore, so you don't even have to ask for them by name.

VAGINAL DOUCHES

The vagina is a self-cleansing organ, and there is no medical need to douche. We know, however, that a high pH is associated with overgrowth of the wrong bacteria; it can be beneficial to lower the pH and encourage acidity. For those of us who suffer from chronic discharge, vinegar douching may help, though it should not be used more than twice a week.

KEGEL EXERCISES

These are designed to improve the tone of the muscle around the vagina and opening of the bladder. Put your finger in your vagina and squeeze; feel which muscles you're using. Then (after removing your finger), contract ten seconds, relax ten seconds. Repeat this fifteen times and try to do this exercise three times a day. Try to work up to a "rep" of twenty-five squeezes at one time. Make sure you're not using your abdominal, leg, or buttock muscles. Check by placing your hand on your abdomen; if it moves during the exercise, you're cheating. Reisolate (with your finger) your pelvic floor muscles and try again. It's an "invisible" exercise, and you can perform it while driving, sitting at your desk, or when you go to the bathroom (the same muscles should stop the stream of urination).

VULVAR AND VAGINAL HYGIENE

1. Don't use bath oils or bubble baths; they can increase vaginal pH and result in more infections.

2. Empty your bladder before and after intercourse; this flushes out any urethral invasion by bacteria.

3. Wear underwear that is comfortable and that allows moisture to be absorbed away from the vulvar skin (look for the cotton or "wicking" fibers found in breathable underwear).

4. Use gentle, nondeodorant soaps in the vulvar area.

5. If you are prone to irritation, stay out of hot tubs, Jacuzzis, and chlorinated swimming pools.

6. Get out of wet bathing suits or damp exercise clothes as soon as possible.

BLADDER SYMPTOMS

Our bladder and bladder opening (urethra) originated from the same tissue as the vagina during our embryonic development. When we lose our estrogen, our lower urinary tract, like the vagina, loses elasticity, support, and some degree of function. The long-term consequences of estrogen deprivation are covered in chapter 5, but urinary problems can appear in the early stages of menopause.

Stress Incontinence

One study has shown that 56 percent of premenopausal women have this symptom, and it decreases to about 41 percent six years after menopause.

Frequency

"Didn't I just go to the bathroom?" This seems to increase minimally after menopause and in the same study quoted above, was found to rise from a 28 percent prevalence during perimenopause to a rate of 33 percent six years after menopause.

Voiding at Night (Nocturia)

This does not seem to be a result of estrogen depletion, but the normal pooling of blood in our lower body during the day. Once we finally lie down at night and our legs go up, the fluid is reabsorbed into our bloodstream, processed by our kidneys, and excreted into our bladder, where it collects. After a while, the bladder "protests" this nocturnal stretching and contracts. We feel we have to leave our cozy beds and pay a nocturnal visit (or two) to the bathroom. This also occurs in men (we are all more prone to collect fluid as we age). I am always amused when I bump into my husband as we both grope our way through our dark bedroom to the bathroom at 3:00 A.M.!

Urgency

"I have to go, and I have to go now!!!" It is not clear that this is estrogen-related. Fifty percent of premenopausal women complain of some degree of urgency, and this number remains fairly constant in menopause.

Bladder Infections

These cause a combination of the above symptoms—urgency, frequency, and burning on urination. Change in the vaginal pH and thinning of the vaginal mucus increase our bladder infection rate during menopause.

SKIN CHANGES: OUR COSTLY BATTLE OF THE WRINKLE

The cosmetic companies, facialists, and plastic surgeons love menopause! Estrogen depletion affords them a reason to go about correcting our skin's loss of moisture and suppleness along with the resulting sagging, bagging, and wrinkling.

We know that collagen is good stuff. Our skin, bones, and cartilage are all composed, in large part, of collagen. Indeed, it constitutes about one third of our total body mass. Forty percent of our collagen is found in the layers of our skin, where it's responsible for resilience and tone. We have peak quantity of skin collagen between the ages of 20 and 40. Sun damage can decrease the formation of certain types of collagen by as much as 50 percent, and smoking can also adversely affect collagen. After 40, there is an age-related collagen loss, but this becomes significantly accelerated (a run on wrinkles) after menopause. Menopause throws three strikes against our skin: collagen depletion, fluid loss, and decrease in total skin thickness. The decline in collagen content occurs at a more rapid rate in the first few years of menopause, up to 30 percent in five years, and declining to a rate of 2.1 percent per year over a period of ten years. Our skin thickness and moisture seem to follow our collagen loss. Our skin often becomes dry and flaky and bruises easily; a "reptilian" conversion that one prominent skin cream commercial implies we can prevent (as we see a 25-year-old model putting cream on her perfect skin while an alligator slithers by).

Our eyes might be the mirror of our souls, but our skin gives away the secrets of our bones. They share their collagen dependence on estrogen. If we have a tendency to lose collagen in one, the same will occur in the other. Pale, fine-skinned white women (especially if they are thin) who suffer significant skin loss changes in menopause are undergoing similar bone loss with the development of osteoporosis. Our dermatologic concerns mirror our bone concerns; both are valid. The saying "Vanity, thy name is woman" might correctly be switched to "Vanity, thy name is collagen."

So what we need is a collagen maintenance program. We won't get it in creams, facials, or plastic surgery; we will with estrogen. Replacement of this hormone increases the production of collagen, its water-binding qualities (moisture), and skin thickness. It's been shown that for women with low skin collagen content, estrogen may initially increase collagen content within six months and later prevent continued loss. For those of us with thicker, darker skin, estrogen will be prophylactic. No collagen buildup occurs (we don't need it), but we won't continue inexorably toward the estrogen-deprived "pruning" of our skin.

WEIGHT GAIN: DOES PAUSE OF MENSES MEAN PAUSE OF WEIGHT CONTROL?

We have a greater positive caloric balance than men. Positive balances are great for the weight of our checking accounts but impact negatively on our body weight. If we take in more calories than we burn, we gain weight. Our basal metabolic rate, or calories that we expend without doing anything, is 116 calories a day less than that of men. Men also have a higher sleeping metabolic rate; they burn more calories than we do even when they're asleep by 208 calories a day. As we enter our middle years, it becomes more difficult to fight our lowered metabolism. During our perimenopause, we tend to gain 0.8 kilograms (about 2 pounds) a year. Most of this is deposited in our hips, buttocks, and thighs. We may take a size 10 top, but we need a 12 or 14 bottom. This is called *gluteal*, or *gynecoid*, obesity. This weight gain does not appear related to loss of estrogen.

After menopause, there is a shift in our fat distribution and body composition. Our lean body mass decreases, the fat mass increases, and there is a shift in where it goes, from our hips to our abdomen. This is male-pattern, or *androgenic*, obesity; we carry our fat "like a man." This in and of itself is a known risk factor for atherosclerosis, coronary artery disease, and heart attack (see chapters 9 and 10). The question is whether we also gain weight above and beyond our tendency to do so in perimenopause. Some studies show no correlation between estrogen depletion and weight. Others, unfortunately, do. A survey of nearly 500 women in the early postmenopause showed that 64 percent reported gaining weight regardless of whether their menopause was natural or surgical. Those who gained did so in proportion to their premenopausal weight status. If they were not obese, they averaged 10 to 15 pounds, and if they were already "weight-challenged," they upped the scales by 21 to 23 pounds! Another study of a similar size (number of women, not pounds) that did not rely on patient reports, but actually weighed the subjects in 1984 and 1987, found that those who were 42 to 50 years of age at the start of the study gained an average of 5 pounds. Twenty percent gained 10 pounds or more, and only 3 percent lost 10 or more pounds. There was no difference in weight between those who became menopausal during these three years and those who did not. To date, the studies have been inconclusive, but few of us want to just sit around waiting for fat distribution or redistribution to occur—with either age or menopause!

Psychological Symptoms of Menopause

MENOPAUSE, MOOD, MIND, AND WHAT ELSE . . . OH YES—MEMORY!

Early psychoanalysts felt that menopause had a significant negative influence on our mental health, that the emotionally charged symbolism of menopause was what depressed us. Life at this time was described as "pale and purposeless." Even psychotherapy wouldn't help, and "resignation without compensation" was the only solution. To add gender insult (am I being hostile here?), it was felt that this was a bad time for our mental health because we were more prone to penis envy! (Apparently, it had been mitigated in our reproductive years because our periods reminded us of our ability to have babies.) Freud felt that we mourned our reproductive loss and that this caused a state of melancholy. More recently psychologists have told us that this period stresses our fears of growing old and loss of femininity, factors which contribute to our loss of self-esteem.

Depression: Myths and Facts

Before we address these theories like mature, intelligent adults (who have not lost their ability to analyze despite the negative expectations of these psychoanalysts), let's examine whether depression actually increases in menopause. An overwhelming number of studies point to the fact that it does not! If we look at the number of women treated or hospitalized for psychiatric disorders, we find that their number drops in the decade following menopause. If anything, we psychiatrically peak in our perimenopausal years and return to "inner peace" after we have dealt with the turmoil of our fluctuating hormones.

What *does* happen is that if a woman over 50 develops significant anxiety or depression, she has been conditioned to believe it's, of course, "your menopause, my dear." Her first stop (after, perhaps, some consultation with friends or family, who reinforce the menopause theory) is to see her gynecologist or primary care physician. We get skewed statistics if we look at the complaints of women attending menopause clinics. About 50 percent are clinically depressed, but it is this psychological problem that got them there in the first place; "there" was the wrong place. They should have been consulting psychotherapists.

It's easier for us to blame menopause than to admit to having a depressive illness. To distinguish clinical depression from mood disorders, we have to assess what the symptoms do to our lives. A woman with severe depression will have decreased interest or pleasure in most of her activities. She may have significant weight loss or weight gain, either be unable to sleep or sleep too much. She may feel restless or barely be able to move. She has daily fatigue, feels worthless, or may have excessive or inappropriate guilt, as well as difficulty concentrating, indecisiveness, and recurrent thoughts of death. These obviously interfere with her daily activities. Women with moderate depression have only some of these symptoms and are unable to complete all of their activities, but can perform some. Those of us with mild depression have a few symptoms and feel that it requires extra effort to do what we need to do to get through our day, but we manage.

More significant depression in menopause may occur in two instances: in women who have undergone surgical menopause and subsequent sudden loss of estrogen and male hormone (the latter is partially conserved in natural menopause), and in women with a history of depression and psychiatric illnesses, whose previous vulnerability to mental illness seems to increase in menopause. Many of these women have bio-logical factors causing their depression, including a deficiency in neuro-transmitting substances such as norepinephrine and serotonin, which relay messages between brain cells in the hypothalamus and in an area called the limbic system. Estrogen may influence the production and re-ceptor sensitivity of these transmitters. When the transmitting fuel is down, low estrogen may be an additional stress, and the symptoms of true depressive illness can get worse.

Most of us feel fine, and studies done on the general population of women in their fifties show no change from the 8 to 10 percent preva-lence of depression that affects the female population during its repro-ductive years. Menopause does not cause "mental pause."

If physicians don't ask us the right questions or listen to what we're really telling them, they reinforce the "It's all due to menopause" belief. We all—doctors and patients alike—need to get the full picture. Are we dealing with dying parents (80 percent of all 50-year-olds have a living mother or father, and 25 percent of us have to take time off from work without pay to care for them)? Do we have adolescent children whose remarks or behavior make us feel old and ineffectual, or a spouse who's sick, either mentally or physically? Are we going through a divorce? Do we have work and economic worries? Surely these depression factors are not caused by menopause. During other periods of our lives, they are considered ample reasons for depression and anxiety, and, of course, they continue to be.

We've achieved a victory of sorts. Even the psychoanalysts agree: We do not become poor, purposeless, depressed souls once we're menopausal. But that doesn't mean we can't undergo some changes in our mood or feeling of well-being if our estrogen levels fall. We may experience these in perimenopause, but symptoms often continue through our first few years of menopause. These include:

Insomnia

The frequency of this symptom doubles from our premenopausal days (or nights), and about 40 percent of us don't get a good night's sleep. The most common reason is interruption of our REM sleep by hot flashes. Estrogen deprivation may also increase wakefulness without any loss of temperature control.

Fatigue and Low Energy

This is usually associated with the insomnia caused by hot flashes.

Irritability and Nervousness

This appears to be more prevalent in perimenopause but can continue to occur, another domino effect of hot flashes and poor sleep.

Decreased Libido

Decreased libido (see chapter 16) may be due to vaginal atrophy and painful intercourse. Lowered estrogen and male hormones may also affect our sexual brain centers.

Nonclinical Depression

Not a newfound clinical depression, but a general sense of fatigue, low energy, and lack of cheerfulness. Again, this is often associated with hot flashes and insomnia.

Memory: Short-term, Long-term . . . Did I Already Cover This?

Does it seem that we are more likely to forget where we put the keys or our glasses, or even where we left a family member? Yet we remember the names of those older-looking people we meet at our high school or college reunions! Scientists have tried to take this subjective forgetfulness and apply objective tests to see if our cognitive functions—which include memory, acuity, and ability to learn—are affected by estrogen depletion. Menopausal women have been tested to measure their memory, eye-hand coordination, reflexes, and the ability to learn new information and apply it to a problem. It seems that we do undergo some loss of short-term memory, but our long-term memory is unchanged. When 48-year-old women who underwent hysterectomy and removal of both ovaries were randomized and given either estrogen or a placebo for three months, those on estrogen had higher scores on tests of immediate verbal memory, even in comparison to their preoperative scores. In contrast, the women who received placebos showed no change in their scores but had lower scores in their ability to learn new material. We need larger studies and long-term follow-up before we can attach an estrogen quotient to our mental acuity.

DO WE NEED HELP?
HORMONES, ANTIDEPRESSANTS, AND PSYCHOTHERAPY

Since menopause has little impact on our mental health, most of us will not need any "therapy" except perhaps understanding that "menopause is okay" and "we're okay."

If we are depressed or have other psychological symptoms, will estrogen help? Is this our "feel better" panacea? The answer is an equivocal "maybe," for some of us (how's that for medical certainty!). If we are dealing with the fallout (or fall-apart) from hot flashes, estrogen will help. If depression is mild, merely a mood change that can be colored blue, then estrogen might help. When psychologically healthy women underwent removal of their uterus and ovaries and were given estrogen for three months, their depression scores were significantly better than those of women given a placebo. When these same "content" women were taken off the estrogen and switched to placebo, their scores got worse. They subjectively felt down and sad. Estrogen increases the rate of destruction of the MAO enzyme in our brain. The lower our MAO enzyme levels, the better we probably feel, since MAO breaks down serotonin. So, indirectly, estrogen can help keep our brain serotonin levels up.

If our depression is significant and not correlated with hot flashes or insomnia, then we have to consider that we're dealing with a psychiatric disorder. Hormone replacement therapy won't provide the fix. Psychotherapy and other pharmacologic approaches might. Clinical depression is often caused by a chemical imbalance and low levels of certain neurotransmitters. To change these levels, we can prescribe the new antidepressant drugs that inhibit serotonin uptake (or re-uptake) by the neurons in the brain. The names of these drugs (Prozac, Zoloft, and Paxil) have become synonymous, rightly or wrongly, with a new sense of American "well-being."

The effect of these drugs on appropriate patients (and I stress the word *appropriate*) is elating. Between 50 and 65 percent experience marked improvement or complete remission of their depressive symptoms. I recently saw a patient whom I had referred for psychotherapy.

She was on Prozac and felt wonderful. While touting what it had done for her, she stopped mid-sentence, looked at me, and asked, "Have you tried it yet?" I laughed and promptly went to the bathroom to see if I looked like I needed a major psychotherapeutic drug. I, like most women, feel fine. There are days we might react to stressful events and feel down, but this is not clinical depression. These medications are not supposed to be used for instant gratification or the elimination of mood changes that affect all of us in our daily lives. No, I haven't "tried" Prozac—yet . . .

Another class of medications termed *cyclic antidepressants* is widely prescribed. These are divided into *tricyclic* (which means they have three chemical rings) and *heterocyclic* medications (which have more rings in their chemical configuration). They all work by affecting the uptake or levels of neurotransmitting substances. The tricyclics include Elavil, Anafranil, Norpramin, Torfranil, and Sinequan. The heterocyclics currently marketed are Wellbutrin, Desyrel, Asendin, and Ludiomil. These alleviate symptoms such as loss of appetite, decreased perception of pleasure, loss of energy, slowness, suicidal thoughts, and feelings of hopelessness, helplessness, and excessive guilt. A third class of antidepressants are the MAO inhibitors. (Remember, MAO is the enzyme in the brain that breaks down the neurotransmitter serotonin.) This group includes Marplan, Nardil, and Parnate. They are more likely to be used in women with symptoms of increased appetite, excessive sleepiness, high levels of anxiety, and phobic or obsessive-compulsive behavior.

All of these medications have side effects. The cyclics can cause weight gain, drowsiness, lowered blood pressure when standing, and irregular heartbeat. The MAO inhibitors can cause insomnia and agitation, lowered blood pressure when standing, and weight gain. The new "in" serotonin re-uptake inhibitors are supposed to have fewer serious side effects, but they can cause agitation, insomnia, and gastrointestinal problems (mostly diarrhea).

Medical therapy can cause medical problems. Psychotherapy will certainly have fewer medical side effects and has been found to benefit 45 to 60 percent of women with mild to moderate depression. Some degree of psychotherapy is always indicated, if only to ascertain which of us will benefit from medication and, if so, what type. A combination of both therapies is warranted if we get an inadequate response from one. This should benefit 50 to 60 percent of women with severe and recurrent depression. There is one more combination of therapies that helps the symptoms of this disorder—adding estrogen to antidepressant therapy. There is evidence that it potentiates the effect of some antidepressants, allowing us to use lower doses and have fewer side effects.

Our Reality Pause

Let's look at menopause with a new sense of educated reality. How does this hormonal transition affect our lives? First, the negatives:

- We usually develop hot flashes, and these can cause sleep disturbances.
- Problems may result from atrophic changes in the vaginal area.
- Mild psychological symptoms may develop; most are due to poor sleep.
- Dryness and thinning of our skin can occur.
- If we gain weight, it moves from our hips to our waists.
- Sex drive may change, but this is partially due to our vaginal symptoms.

Next, the positives:

- We are freed from contraceptive worries.
- PMS is over.
- We don't have periods, cramps, or heavy bleeding.
- Our menopausal symptoms gave us the impetus to see our doctor and read books so that we can choose to go through the most important health transition of our lives, passing from the "fix it, it's broken" mentality to the "I can prevent its breaking" state of mind.
- We have choices and remedies for just about every symptom listed under the negatives, so once we have dealt with them (and subtracted them from our list), we are left with our positives.

Menopause is the completion of a life cycle that started before we were born. It does not constitute a stop, but is actually the start of the next phase of our lives. We need to know a lot more than why we don't have periods. Our knowledge of long-term issues—the effect of estrogen depletion on our hearts, bones, and brains—and our unique female diseases and medical problems are far more important. These will determine the quality of the next thirty to forty years of our lives.

7

TAKING HORMONES
The Good, the Bad, and the Questionable

To take or not to take—that is the question. Twenty million of us will have to make this decision over the next two decades as we enter menopause and change our concerns from birth control to hormone control. The question continues even after we pass through this transition. Women in their sixties through eighties who stopped taking or never took hormone therapy are still welcome to participate in this mass dilemma. Few medical therapies have so great a potential to affect our "well-being," our "unwell-being" (development of disease), and our ultimate mortality. Hundreds of studies have been conducted on estrogen and progesterone. They have been analyzed, statistized, glorified, and criticized. The bad news (side effects and possibility of cancer) hits the public media before the ink in the medical journal dries: ESTROGEN LINKED WITH CANCER! The good news (as in life) gets less coverage and less attention: ESTROGEN MAY DECREASE ALZHEIMER'S DISEASE (note when it's good, there is always a modifying "may"). Let's look at the facts.

ERT and HRT: An Introduction to the Risks and Benefits of Hormone Therapy

Since the term "hormone therapy" implies use of estrogen and progesterone, and each has its benefits and problems, it is necessary to begin by dividing our information into two categories: *estrogen replacement therapy (ERT)* and *hormone replacement therapy* (estrogen plus progesterone, or HRT). (Later, we'll also look at male hormone—androgen—therapy and DHEA.)

ESTROGEN REPLACEMENT THERAPY: ERT

Benefits of ERT

As we've noted, good news always seems to get less attention than bad news. To offset this tendency, let's begin with the benefits of ERT.

REVERSING MENOPAUSAL SYMPTOMS

Menopausal estrogen deprivation does not go unnoticed by our body or our mind. None of the common menopausal symptoms—hot flashes, disrupted sleep patterns, vaginal dryness, inability to concentrate, unreliable short-term memory—threatens our lives, but each can seriously compromise the quality of our lives. After all, health is more than just the absence of disease. Estrogen therapy reverses the symptoms caused by estrogen loss. These hormone pills or patches deliver relief almost immediately. The flushes and sweats stop, our sleep patterns improve, intercourse doesn't hurt, and our mental well-being improves: we feel like "well beings."

Therapy for these symptoms can be started at the onset of menopause, either after periods have stopped for several months (and symptoms have appeared), or if periods are very irregular and several blood tests show that FSH levels are high and estrogen or estradiol levels are low. Since our hormones are still working during the perimenopause, albeit with starts and stops, we are better off treating hot flashes, sleep disturbances, and vaginal dryness during this transition with low-dose birth control pills, which suppress the misbehaving ovaries. Estrogen replacement therapy, unlike birth control pills, does not suppress the ovaries. The estrogen used in hormonal replacement is only a quarter as potent as the estrogen in the birth control pill. We don't need much once our ovaries quit; and, fortunately, the small amount that effectively controls our symptoms also controls the onset of significant disease.

Many of our menopausal symptoms subside with time, as our bodies and brains adapt to their estrogen-poor environment. After two to five years, a significant number of women report that they are "over meno-pause." Unfortunately, though, some of us never get over the symptoms: we continue to experience them for the next third of our lives. A very reasonable approach to the hormone question is to address the "here and now" of menopause. If we enter this transition and feel rotten, we can start therapy. Once we feel better, we can reevaluate. Our decision to stay on estrogen will depend on our risk for certain diseases such as heart attack, osteoporosis, and breast cancer. Medical research will continue, and new and improved data will help us chart our next five-year to thirty-year plan.

PREVENTING OSTEOPOROSIS AND HEART DISEASE

The National Center for Chronic Disease Prevention and Health Pro-motion and Epidemiology Office of the Centers for Disease Control and Prevention (amazing how government agencies have such long titles) recently published a decision analysis on the long-term risks and benefits of estrogen replacement. Although we are reduced to numbers, the num-bers are gratifying. If 10,000 women were to take estrogen for twenty-five years, they would have a 48 percent decrease in fatal coronary heart dis-ease events (otherwise known as heart attacks). This would translate to "only" 567 cases (or more correctly, women). Deaths from hip fractures would be reduced by 49 percent (seventy-five women), while deaths from breast cancer would increase by 21 percent (thirty-nine women), and deaths from endometrial cancer would rise by 207 percent (twenty-nine women). On balance, ERT would prevent 574 deaths, and women would gain 3,951 quality-adjusted life years compared to women not using estrogen. What the CDC group did was analyze numbers from hundreds of studies and try to translate our lives and deaths into some sort of cost-benefit analysis. We come out ahead with estrogen, but it be-hooves us to look at each issue more closely and understand what this hormone does.

Osteoporosis: Estrogen "Bones Up"   There is no question that os-teoporosis is one of our most devastating diseases (see chapter 11). The good news is that estrogen can protect us against osteoporosis by encour-aging new bone formation and halting the normal 2 to 3 percent annual bone loss that occurs in the first five to ten years after menopause. Cal-cium and exercise alone just won't do this.

We know how much estrogen is needed to maximize bone sparing: 0.625 milligram of conjugated estrogen or the equivalent, raising our estradiol blood levels above 50 picograms/milliliter. A smaller amount, 0.3 milligram, may also work if we "enable it" with 1,500 milligrams of calcium. Some of us who are at high risk (about 15 percent) need even more than the 0.625-milligram dosage for protection. If there is any question, bone density scans should be performed to make sure we are getting our maximum estrogen benefit. Estrogen protects our bones only as long as we take it. Once we stop, early menopausal bone loss restarts at the rate of 2 to 3 percent a year. We lose our estrogen advantage after five years. As far as our bones are concerned, "ever-use" of estrogen is not enough; we need "forever-use."

Estrogen works even if osteoporosis is already present. As late as our seventies, it will stop progression of the disease and help to rebuild lost bone. Our fracture rates decrease dramatically, and bone pain associated with this disease is lessened. Those of us who first begin using estrogen at age 65 are predicted to have a 14 to 19 percent higher bone density than those who never use it, and we'll reduce our fracture risk by 57 to 69 percent. It may never be too late to support our bones with estrogen.

Cardiovascular Benefits: Estrogen Each Day Can Keep Heart Attacks Away   Since 1970, more than thirty-two large epidemiologic studies have been conducted on this subject. They consistently show that estrogen has an extraordinary benefit on our hearts. It decreases our risk of fatal heart attack, our number-one killer, by at least 50 percent (see chapter 9). If a similar claim could be made for a drug affecting men's risk of heart attack, that medication would be found in almost every medicine cabinet in America. Estrogen does not affect the hearts of men (there is a song somewhere in that statement); they don't have the right hormone receptors. We do.

Estrogen's wide-ranging beneficial effects on our cardiovascular system are detailed in chapters 9 and 10. Essentially, we estimate that 25 percent of estrogen's protective qualities result from lowering total cholesterol and lipids, increasing the good HDL cholesterol, and lowering the bad LDL cholesterol. The greater part of estrogen's benefits derive from its positive effects on virtually every component of our cardiovascular system—our blood, our vessels, even our heart itself.

What Dosage, How Long?

We have a harder time determining "smallest working dose" for heart disease than for osteoporosis, since we can't correlate estrogen dosage to artery "cleanliness" or heart muscle "pumping power." The dose of estrogen used in most studies demonstrating cardiac protection was equivalent to 0.625 to 1.25 milligrams of oral conjugated estrogen daily. Abstracting from this, we recommend 0.625 milligram as the low-est effective dose (this is also the dose doctors suggest to prevent osteo-porosis).

How long should we take estrogen? It stands to reason that as long as we take it, the better its current influence on our lipids and hearts. Studies support this. They show that women using estrogen for fifteen or more years have at least a 50 percent decrease in cardiac risk, whereas if they use it for less than three years, the number drops to 10 to 30 per-cent. In a seven-year study of over 8,000 women (average age 73) living in Leisure World, California, long-term use of estrogen gave even more encouraging results. Women who were taking estrogen and had used it for more than fifteen years had a 40 percent reduction in their overall mortality from *all causes* compared to women of the same age who never used estrogen. Women with a history of using estrogen in the past had a 20 percent lower all-cause mortality than lifetime nonusers. The longer they stayed on estrogen and the more recent its use, the better their mor-tality rates. Another recent study, of 454 women (average age this time was 77), gave similar results, with a 46 percent reduction in the rate of death from all causes with long-term use of estrogen.

If We Already Have Heart Disease or, Worse Yet, a Heart Attack, Is It Too Late for Estrogen?

No! On the contrary, some studies have shown that the protective effect of estrogen is stronger in women who already have coronary heart disease. In one study, over a thousand women with more than 70 percent stricture of their coronary vessels (severe coronary artery disease) were followed for ten years. Estrogen users had an 84 percent reduction in their risk of recurrent disease; 97 percent were alive after ten years. It is never too late (for our hearts) to start estrogen. Many physicians feel that if a woman has a heart attack, she should go from intensive care to hormonal care.

ERT AND OUR UROGENITAL TRACT:
TONE, SUPPORT, AND THE RIGHT BACTERIA

The loss of estrogen results in several vaginal and bladder problems.

Vaginal and Bladder Infections The estrogen-deprived lining no longer supports our normal vaginal flora or bacterial ecosystem. The pH changes (it goes up), and the wrong bacteria take over, causing vaginal irritation and infection. These can also spread to the bladder.

After we have our children, our pelvic support system is stretched (as we all know!). But with lack of estrogen, we add insult to injury: Relaxation takes over, the bladder may prolapse or sink down into the vagina (cystocele), and the urethra or bladder opening protrudes and becomes more exposed. In addition, the smooth muscle of the bladder does not contract as well. It has lost estrogen "tone." These combined factors often cause us to be unable to empty our bladders completely when we try to void (necessitating a repeat visit to the restroom after a very short time). The leftover stagnant urine can easily become infected as abnormal bacteria ascend from the vagina through the exposed urethra.

Estrogen therapy will promote the maintenance or development of thickened, healthy vaginal cells. It restores the normal vaginal pH, increases vaginal blood flow and fluid, decreases vulvar and vaginal pain and irritation, and improves vaginal lubrication during intercourse. Our bacterial ecosystem is restored, and we are less likely to get vaginal and bladder infections. Bladder tone can improve, and estrogen may prevent continued loss of pelvic support.

Incontinence Estrogen deficiency is probably not the main cause of our involuntary loss of urine after menopause, but it doesn't help. When we lose estrogen, we lose collagen supporting the urethra and bladder neck. If the angle between the urethra and bladder is lost and the sphincter muscle is weakened, we are more likely to become incontinent. Without estrogen, the lining of the urethra thins, and there is poor closure (those atrophic cells just can't pull their act or, more appropriately, their "opening" together). Urine "dribbling" may become an involuntary flow if we cough, sneeze, or lift. This is called "stress incontinence." Abdominal stress or pressure produces it, but the word "stress" really describes our own emotional reaction to this grievous problem. We also tend to develop more urinary urgency (just thinking about a toilet makes us want to go NOW!). This is urge incontinence and is caused by involuntary contractions of the bladder muscle.

Estrogen will improve the atrophic tissue in and around our urethra. It can lead to an improved urethral seal and better resistance, and lessen our symptoms of urgency and frequency. Forty to 70 percent of women with atrophic urogenital tissues and incontinence show some improvement with estrogen therapy. We should certainly try this before we even begin to consider corrective surgery.

Pelvic Prolapse Our stretched ligaments fall short (or long) of their support duties as we get older, especially if we have lost our estrogen. The uterus may descend and prolapse into the vagina so that the cervix, which is normally at the top of the vagina, is pushed into the opening or even protrudes out (*uterine prolapse*). This pulls the other organs down (if the uterus falls, so go the bladder and rectum). Bladder prolapse or cystocele pushes the vaginal roof downward. Rectal prolapse, or *rectocele*, causes bulging of the vaginal floor upward. This is anatomically incorrect but, more important, is physiologically and psychologically distressing. Our misplaced pelvic organs contribute to our problems of voiding and incontinence, as well as our ability to have bowel movements. We may feel constant pulling, pressure, or pelvic discomfort. It is hard to sit or stand. We can't or are too embarrassed to have intercourse.

Estrogen won't put our pelvic organs back into their right places, but estrogen deprivation may promote and hasten their descent.

Local Estrogen: Creams Work

Most women do not want to spend the last third of their lives worrying about the bottom third of their pelvises. ERT will prevent or reverse vaginal atrophy. The effect on our bacteria, infection rate, bladder symptoms, and support will follow. We can supply estrogen to our urogenital tracts with pills or patches, but sometimes this is not enough, especially if atrophy has caused decreased vascularity or blood supply. We may be better off applying estrogen vaginal creams directly to our target. We'll need nightly applications of the cream (2 grams) for one to two weeks to begin to build up the lining. Once our symptoms are improved, we can cut down the dose to 1 to 2 grams twice weekly for "urogenic maintenance." The good news is that for those of us who can't or won't use systemic estrogen (pills or the patch), use of the estrogen creams alone provides protection from vaginal atrophy. The effect of these creams is generally local; there is more absorption initially when the vaginal lining is very thin. Topically applied estrogen will not protect our hearts or bones, but our vaginas and bladders can be maintained in the estrogen style to which they have been accustomed.

Estrogen and Our Brain

Estrogen helps keep our brain cells or neurons "in touch." It promotes the production of an enzyme, *acetyltransferase*, which is needed to synthesize acetylcholine. This substance "hot-wires" our memory and thought processes by allowing messages to bound from one neuron to the next. Estrogen also appears to make neurons more sensitive to nerve growth factor, which (you guessed it) stimulates growth of our neurons and their network of connecting fibers. The denser the mesh of these fibers, the better their ability to carry out our thinking and memory.

Even men need estrogen for their brain (or brainy) functions. Theirs is obtained by converting the male hormone testosterone to estrogen within the brain. In this respect, they're lucky, since their supply of testosterone remains fairly stable until they reach their eighties.

By the time we reach 80, 40 percent of us will have problems with our brain cell connections. The mass of neuron-connecting fibers becomes tangled, and abnormal protein plaque is deposited. The levels of acetyltransferase decline, and we lose our ability to retain and retrieve information. This defines Alzheimer's disease, which currently affects 3 million women and whose victims will double in number over the next decade.

Some of us are more at risk than others. There is a gene that increases susceptibility, especially if the disease occurs before age 65. It codes for a certain lipoprotein (apolipoprotein E), which has been implicated in this brain degeneration process. Future medicine and counseling may include a check for this gene so that we can fight back preventively. One of the therapies could be estrogen.

We don't think that estrogen deprivation is the primary reason that our neurons miscommunicate, but by either decreasing the fiber mesh or limiting the protection of an important enzyme, the lack of this hormone may increase our vulnerability to predisposing factors for Alzheimer's disease. A recent California study of 2,400 women found that those who had been on estrogen therapy were 40 percent less likely to have Alzheimer's than those who had not taken this hormone. Other studies have suggested that ERT can improve memory function and decrease the rate of memory loss in women who already have mild to moderate Alzheimer's disease. We know that after menopause, fat tissue can produce estrogen. Those of us who are chubby may be unhappy with our dress size, but we make more estrogen than svelte or skinny women, and thin women are known to be at increased risk for Alzheimer's! Estrogen's positive actions on our cardiovascular function may also increase the blood flow to our brains. This, too, may limit our development of Alzheimer's.

We can also lose our mental function (and our lives) from stroke. Estrogen probably has the same beneficial effects on the vessels in our brain as on our coronary vessels. The National Health and Nutrition Examination Survey showed that the relative risk for stroke for women who *ever* received ERT or HRT as compared with those who were never treated was 0.69 (or 31 percent less), and that of fatal stroke was a low 0.37. This mimics the reduction we get from estrogen on coronary artery disease.

In deciding whether we want estrogen replacement, we have considered our hearts and our bones. We should also be concerned about our minds.

Estrogen May Prevent Cancer: Rectal-Colon Cancer

A recent study from the University of Wisconsin showed that the incidence of rectal and colon cancer was reduced by 46 percent in women who were currently or recently using HRT and by 30 percent if they had ever used it. This was a large survey and included over 600 women with cancer and 1,600 "controls." Estrogen and progesterone have been found to reduce the secretion of bile acids. Since these acids "irritate" the bowel and may increase our risk of rectal-colon cancer, their reduction may be cancer-sparing. This large-bowel cancer is our third most common malignancy after the age of fifty. Reducing it by more than 40 percent has major health implications, yet it has not received 1 percent of the media attention focused on the possibility that estrogen may promote other cancers.

Cosmetic Effects of Estrogen:
We Won't Die of Wrinkled Skin,
but We Can "Smooth" Our Menopausal Transition

Do we have a built-in wrinkle rate, and is there something (other than plastic surgery) we can do about it? The collagen content and thickness of our skin determine its smoothness and tone. Estrogen therapy can prevent this collagen loss and even increase skin collagen content from 3 to 5 percent in just twelve months. A Spanish study showed that the patch might be more effective than pills for this skin protection.

Most of us have earned our wrinkles. We can't mature with taut, endlessly even (and boring) skin, but few of us want to resemble prunes. Estrogen won't give us the perfect skin of a 20-year-old model, but it will make a cosmetic difference that is welcome.

Risks Associated with ERT

If ERT could help us achieve good hearts, healthy bones, well-functioning bladders, enjoyable sex, and wrinkle-free skin without side effects or risks, we would not be struggling with our individual hormone decisions. Like any medical therapy, estrogen can cause adverse effects, especially if it is improperly prescribed or not sufficiently monitored. There is no free lunch or, for that matter, free health (and I'm not referring to government-supported universal health care).

Our chief concern is, of course, cancer. Can estrogen cause cancer? The answer is yes if we're talking about endometrial cancer. It's equivocal if we consider breast cancer.

ENDOMETRIAL CANCER

Unopposed estrogen (without added progesterone) leads to unopposed stimulation of the uterine lining. This causes atypical overgrowth or hyperplasia and eventually endometrial cancer. Depending on the dose of estrogen and duration of its use, it can cause a 5- to 8-fold increase in the risk of this cancer.

Progesterone in fairly small doses will oppose the estrogen effect on the endometrium and effectively prevent development of endometrial cancer. The FDA Advisory Committee recommends that women who have intact uteri (intact means we've not had a hysterectomy) receive progesterone in addition to estrogen. This is HRT rather than ERT and brings forth a whole slew of other issues.

BREAST CANCER

This is the greatest concern about and barrier to widespread use of ERT. We can be told we are ten times more likely to die of heart attack than breast cancer, that we are at risk for hip fracture and even dementia, and we are not convinced. These are distant, poorly visualized events of old age. Breast cancer is a fear today. We have added confusion to this fear with a plethora of conflicting scientific data. This supposedly objective and, unfortunately, frequently subjective seesaw has caused a major "better not use this stuff" attitude in many doctors and women. Recent analyses of all of the data are somewhat reassuring but remain, at best, confusing. A major analysis of twenty-three studies showed no increased breast cancer risk. In analyses of other studies, if an increased relative risk was found, it appeared to occur only after fifteen years and varied from 1.1 to 1.5, depending whose data and analyses we "follow." The recently published Nurses' Health Study found a 28 to 32 percent increase in risk for breast cancer (or relative risk of 1.28 to 1.32) in women who took estrogen for five years or more (and were still taking it), but a University of Washington study published one month later found no increase in breast cancer in women who took estrogen for as long as twenty years! Another study designed to confront our estrogen fears was carried out by the American Cancer Society. Researchers followed more than 400,000 women from 1982 to 1992 and in March of 1996 reported that taking estrogen pills for up to ten years did not increase the risk of dying from breast cancer.

The higher doses of estrogen (equivalent to 1.25 milligrams of conjugated estrogen) may have a greater impact on this risk, so obviously we want to use as low a dose as possible. The cancers that do develop while we take estrogen seem to be less invasive and have a more favorable prognosis when compared to the cancers in age-matched women who are not taking estrogen.

We want a firm scientific conclusion, but alas, we don't have one. We are not sure there is an increased risk in breast cancer, but if it develops, it appears to be more contained, and it takes a long time to show up. Many epidemiologists consider this risk "modest." The term "modest" may be inconsequential to those of us who ultimately have to deal with a diagnosis of breast cancer. So once more, we are on our own to individually consider the possibility of this cancer. If we are already at risk because of family history, we might not want to add that 0.3 to 0.5 to our odds unless our symptoms or risk of other diseases, such as coronary heart disease, osteoporosis, or even Alzheimer's, are significant.

HORMONES AND GALLSTONE FORMATION:
CAUGHT BETWEEN A STONE AND A HARD PLACE?

Use of estrogen replacement with or without progesterone is associated with a two-fold risk of developing gallbladder stones composed of cholesterol. Estrogen acts like a cholesterol traffic cop; it concentrates and diverts cholesterol in our liver into bile for excretion. This is how our body gets rid of noxious substances. The bile collects in a distendable sac, our gallbladder, and then flows into our intestines and, finally, out with our stool. The higher the cholesterol content of the bile, the greater the chance of it forming stones. This effect is estrogen dose– and potency–related; 1.25 milligrams of conjugated estrogen (a fairly high dose of Premarin) raises the cholesterol level of bile by 18 percent, while the 50 micrograms of ethinyl estradiol found in the "higher"-dose birth control pills raises it 50 percent.

Some of us are at risk for gallstones because we have exposed ourselves to conditions that increase either our cholesterol intake and production or our estrogen levels. Diet, weight (obese women also produce more estrogen), and multiple pregnancies (when our estrogen levels rise by a factor of 100), as well as age, affect our stone production. So the "three F's" apply—fat, forty, and fecundity (multiple pregnancies). Estrogen therapy may add to this risk (a sort of improvised fourth "F," as in "forever" estrogenized). With the advent of *laparoscopic cholecystectomy* (removal of the diseased gallbladder through a small incision using laparoscopy techniques), gallstones need not require major abdominal surgery with long-term hospitalization and recovery. This form of gallbladder disease should, however, not be dismissed, especially in women with the "three F's" against them. The use of the estrogen patch rather than pills might decrease this hormone's effect on the liver and diminish this small but significant risk.

Hormone Replacement Therapy: HRT

What Is HRT?

Progesterone compounds are either synthetic, and called progestins, or natural, in which case we're allowed to use the word "progesterone." Because we all know the latter term, I'll use my author's prerogative and refer to all progestins as progesterone in this chapter. In my discussion of therapy, I'll separate them and go back to "official" terminology.

If we have a uterus, take estrogen, and don't want to risk a 5- to 8-fold increased risk of endometrial cancer, we have to pay a price; that price is progesterone. It complicates our routines, our symptoms, and our compliance, and has skewed (or "screwed") our research data. Progesterone can cause vaginal bleeding. It's often prescribed cyclically (10 to 14 days each month) in an attempt to copy our premenopausal cycles. Most women will bleed when they stop their progesterone; some even have cramps. There is a point when we just don't want to deal with this. Our anticipated goal of a period-free life after menopause has been radically changed by our need to take progesterone. Continuous-dose therapy (taking very low doses of progesterone every day with estrogen and not cycling off) may be the answer to this problem.

Progesterone can also cause PMS-like effects. Since we still don't know what causes PMS, it's hard to pinpoint why progesterone does this, but for some women, the 10 to 14 days they must take this hormone for uterine protection are uncomfortable, if not miserable. They may develop bloating, breast tenderness, mood changes, depression, and headaches. There are ways to deal with these side effects, but they require our willingness and that of our doctors to switch and change the progesterone, the dosage, and the mode of cycling until we find our right individual HRT therapy plan.

What Happens to the Benefits of Estrogen When We Add Progesterone?

If progesterone prevents unwanted estrogenic effects at one site (the endometrium), is it an equal opportunity spoiler? Will it prevent the positive estrogenic effects at other sites (our hearts and bones)?

HRT AND OSTEOPOROSIS

Progesterone appears, like estrogen, to promote new bone formation, so adding it to estrogen does not diminish our bone protection; it may even enhance it.

HRT AND CARDIOVASCULAR DISEASE

There has been much debate among physicians, chemists, physiologists, and, of course, the makers of progestational compounds as to whether the addition of this hormone will attenuate or eliminate the cardiac protective effect of ERT. Much of the concern has been based on the assumption that the estrogenic benefits to our lipids (raising HDL and lowering LDL) would be blocked by synthetic progesterones. It appears that this "blockage" is only a small one and our lowered LDLs are not affected. Natural progesterone seems to have less of this blocking effect than the synthetic form. But synthetic progesterone lowers our triglycerides. Considering that new data have correlated high triglyceride levels in women with risk of heart attack, its decrease should protect us and is welcomed. We know that 75 percent of estrogen's cardiac protection is connected to its effect not on our lipids but on our vessels, our blood, and our heart. It would appear that these additional sources of coronary benefit are not adversely affected by any form of progesterone. By adding this hormone, we are not giving up our estrogen-enhanced cardiac futures.

So we now have all the theories, but what actually happens to us? It would have been very helpful if our researchers had followed women who took estrogen and progesterone for fifteen years and compared them to women using ERT only. These studies are only now under way.

HRT AND BREAST CANCER

We're concerned here, because our data are really poor. We know that before menopause, when we have our natural progesterone production the last two weeks of our cycles, our breast cells are affected, and *mitosis,* or cell division, increases (our breasts also tend to feel tender and full). But the progesterone eventually matures these breast cells, and they stop dividing. Once they've completed their growth and know their "purpose," they are less likely to mutate. Some researchers feel that progesterone may close the open-window effect of estrogen and actually protect our breasts, especially if it's given in a continuous dose.

What will progesterone do if we use it in conjunction with estrogen during HRT? The few studies that have looked at breast cancer and HRT conflict. Two older studies showed an increased risk for breast cancer; a third showed a decrease. To further confuse us, two opposing U.S. studies were released just a month apart in 1995. The first caused a media-sponsored hormonal blowout. This was the Nurses' Study, which followed over 120,000 women with questionnaires from 1976 to 1992. By 1990 close to 70,000 were postmenopausal. They documented 1,935 cases of new breast cancer among these women. Those taking estrogen plus progesterone for five years or more had a 40 percent increase in their risk of breast cancer versus a 30 percent increase if they took estrogen alone. This difference was not considered statistically significant, but it certainly suggested that the addition of progesterone to estrogen therapy does not reduce the risk of breast cancer among postmenopausal women. The second study, published in the *Journal of the American Medical Association*, gave hormonal reassurance and subsequently received far less media attention. Five hundred women between the ages of 50 and 64 who had newly diagnosed breast cancer were compared to a similar group of healthy women. There was no statistical link found between any hormone use (estrogen alone or estrogen and progesterone) and breast cancer. Actually, the women who had used hormones for eight years or longer had a lower risk! To date, the FDA Advisory Committee has given up, stating "[We] do not feel that the data is adequate to answer the question of whether or not progesterone alters any breast cancer risk that might be induced by ERT." We'll probably need at least another ten years before we can adequately address this concern.

"YOU SHOULD NOT TAKE HORMONES": MISCONCEPTIONS OF THE PAST AND PRESENT

We—doctors and patients—have all confused apples and oranges in our hormone market. I know I've said this before, but it bears repeating: The hormones in birth control pills and those used for hormone replacement therapy are totally different. First, the estrogen in birth control pills is synthetic while natural estrogens are used in ERT. The estrogen in the birth control pills of the 1960s and 1970s was ten to twenty times more potent than today's ERT, and even the new low-dose birth control pills are four times more potent. Old studies on high-dose birth control pills demonstrated an increased risk of blood clot formation, heart attack, and stroke, especially in women over 35 who smoked. High-dose birth control pills were found to affect glucose levels and diabetes and, on occasion, induced high blood pressure. By democratically declaring all estrogens equal, we concocted an inaccurate stew of contraindications to ERT. Women with a history of clots, pulmonary embolism, high blood pressure, diabetes, heart disease, heart attack, and stroke, as well as those who were obese or smoked, or were just "too old," were invariably told, "You should not take hormones!" These women were left to cope with, and often prematurely die from, these serious health problems.

It's time to look at each of these so-called contraindications in the light of current lower dosages, regimens, and years of experience and realize that, indeed, they may be *indications* for the use of ERT.

Coronary Heart Disease and Previous Heart Attack

Estrogen seems more effective in preventing a heart attack if we are already sick and have coronary heart disease. It decreases the risk of heart attack by 84 percent (versus 50 percent for those of us who start out with apparently healthy vessels and hearts). If we've had a near miss and survived a heart attack, we have been forewarned. To become forearmed, we have to consider estrogen "cardiac therapy."

Stroke

This is our third leading cause of death (see chapter 10). Recent large studies show that our risk of mortality from stroke is reduced by 30 to 50 percent if we use estrogen replacement therapy. The pathways of estrogen protection are probably very similar to those of heart protection. Looking at a national study of nearly 2,000 menopausal women followed for up to sixteen years, it's been shown that postmenopausal estrogen use resulted in a 31 percent reduction in the incidence of stroke and a 63 percent reduction in death caused by stroke. More regionally, 9,000 menopausal women living in Leisure World, California, were studied and, again, women on ERT were shown to decrease their risk of stroke by 47 percent. A Swedish study of 23,000 menopausal women followed for an average of 5.8 years showed that estrogen decreased their risk of stroke by 30 percent and their risk of certain types of brain hemorrhages and clots by as much as 50 percent. Many of these women also took progesterone (HRT), and it did not seem to counteract the protective effect of estrogen on the incidence of stroke.

If we are at risk for stroke (family history, high blood pressure, diabetes, arteriosclerosis, or previous stroke), we should put estrogen onto our "good" list. Although the dilemma of hormone therapy can cause us to experience a collective headache, estrogen might prevent the most devastating headache, stroke.

A History of Abnormal Clots

Any woman who has had *thrombophlebitis* (clots in the deep veins of her legs) or, worse yet, a potentially fatal *pulmonary embolism* (clots that travel to the major vessels of the lungs and block them) is scared. When the event occurs, she has to be hospitalized, given intravenous *anticoagulants* (blood thinners), and then take anticoagulant pills for months. I speak from personal experience, because I developed thrombophlebitis during my residency in obstetrics and gynecology. I remember that I was then told (in my twenties) that I should *never* take hormones!

There has been no clinical evidence that either ERT or HRT increases our risk of abnormal clots, thrombophlebitis, or pulmonary embolism. There have been some changes documented in clotting factors in the lab, but these do not seem to translate into actual events in our bodies. A history of previous clot problems (such as mine), even if they occurred with birth control pills, does not mean we can't use ERT when we are menopausal. The drug companies and textbooks have been slow to accept this and often state that previous thrombophlebitis or pulmonary embolism is, indeed, a contraindication to ERT. For drug companies, this is a continuation of what I term "butt-protecting" disclaimers.

Diabetes

There is nothing "sweet" about this disease, which causes an elevation in our blood sugars. If you're diabetic, your risk of coronary heart disease and heart attack is five times greater than that of a woman who does not suffer from this disease. Diabetic women are at even higher risk for heart attack than diabetic men (our lipoproteins become much worse than theirs under the same diabetic conditions). Obtaining estrogen protection against heart attack is more than welcome! Contrary to belief, estrogen will not adversely affect blood sugar levels or diabetic control. Indeed, glucose metabolism may be improved with ERT, and we often see better blood glucose control and a decreased need for insulin. One study showed a significant decrease in the frequency of diabetes in post-menopausal women treated with ERT.

We already expend so much effort in achieving insulin control in diabetes; we should be adding hormone control.

High Blood Pressure (Hypertension)

This is a silent killer and one of our major risk factors for heart attack and stroke (see chapters 9 and 10). The prevailing belief among both doctors and women (and, again, the disclaimers produced by the drug companies) is that estrogen therapy predisposes women to an increase in blood pressure. Wrong. Again, we have confused birth control pills with ERT. In truth, the predisposing culprit is our age and perhaps the daily stresses of the world we live in. Most women who take estrogen actually have a decline in blood pressure (remember, it relaxes the vessels and promotes dilation). A small percentage of women may experience what we call an idiopathic increase in blood pressure (that means it is an individual, unexpected, or unexplained reaction, or we're just too "idiotic" to understand why it occurs). Our bodies don't always behave according to accepted plans and theories. If we do develop high blood pressure while using estrogen, we don't always have to cease and desist. Simply changing from oral estrogen to the patch may take care of the problem.

When we consider that estrogen lowers the risk of heart attack and stroke, which are exactly the feared results of high blood pressure, this disease becomes an indication for estrogen use. ERT may help stop this prevalent, silent killer from decimating our ranks.

Smoking

If the threat of lung cancer doesn't scare us away from inhaling poisonous smoke, the specters of heart attack and stroke should. Apparently, some of us don't scare easily enough, so we must ask, What does estrogen have to offer those of us whom cigarette companies describe as "mature women who smoke"? Perceptions range from estrogen is a "no-no" for smokers to estrogen "fixes" everything. We've been concerned about the use of birth control pills in women who smoke. High-dose oral contraceptives can increase certain clotting factors in our blood. Smoking promotes this effect, and a clot, or thrombus, can form in an otherwise normal coronary artery, causing heart attack. This does not occur with the estrogens used for ERT. On the contrary, we know that, if anything, the "natural" estrogens decrease platelet adhesiveness and clot formation. On the other hand, ERT will not compensate for our smoking abuse. The levels of active estrogen with ERT appear to be lower in women who smoke than those who don't. Smoking may increase liver breakdown of estrogen. Smokers also have an increase in the production of certain adrenal hormones that oppose estrogen's effect. Smoking also decreases some of the beneficial effects of estrogen on our lipids and continues to hasten our rate of osteoporosis despite the reparative effect of estrogen.

Because estrogen replacement is less effective in women who smoke, the hormone levels in their blood should be checked. They may need higher doses (especially with the patch) to effectively reach the 50 to 60 picograms/milliliter level that is our therapeutic goal. ERT will not cancel the more than 5-fold increased risk of heart attack or 2-fold risk of stroke, but it may diminish it. Smoking is not a contraindication to ERT, but if we care enough about the quality and duration of our lives to take estrogen, we should care enough to quit smoking.

Obesity

Many women feel that estrogen will make them fat. Physicians frequently feel that fat women don't need estrogen. Let's look at the term "overweight" or, yes, the other awful words, "fat" and "obese," and make sure we are all on common ground (or common body mass). Wearing a size 12 dress instead of an 8 does not constitute obesity. We're *medically* overweight if we are 20 percent heavier than our ideal body weight, and this figure is based on our age and our build —not the models in *Vogue*. Is estrogen therapy responsible for the thickening around our waists (or, to put it bluntly, the total loss of this part of our anatomy) and our endless struggle with extra pounds from our late forties through our fifties? Considering that only 20 to 30 percent of "eligible" women are currently using ERT, we would then expect the other 70 to 80 percent to have better luck with their figures and weight. *Not!* Women on estrogen therapy weigh less than women who don't take hormones. There may be a small weight gain in some women with initiation of ERT, but it levels off.

Some studies indicate that ERT may indeed reverse some of our general postmenopausal increase in fat stores while also increasing muscle mass. There is additional good news: Estrogen helps prevent deposition of fat cells in our midbody areas. This male-pattern obesity is correlated with increased levels of insulin and triglycerides and subsequent atherosclerosis, leading to heart attack. Estrogen helps keep our bodies and hearts "feminine."

If we are already "weight-challenged," should we not take estrogen? This would eliminate a lot of us. Unfortunately, 33 percent of white women and 60 percent of African-American women in their forties are overweight, and this increases to 50 percent for whites and stays at 60 percent for African Americans in their fifties. We know that fat cells make weak estrogen. Logically, enough fat should produce enough estrogen. Obese women do have a lower incidence of stroke and Alzheimer's. But those benefits are dramatically overshadowed by weight-related increases in diabetes and heart attack. In other words, "fat" estrogen does not offset the adverse impact of fat. Estrogen replacement will not worsen our weight challenge. It can help redistribute our fat, and it will afford protection from heart attack.

We add one more protective component with HRT: The combination of obesity and menopause is a simple arithmetic equation. It equals increased "unopposed" estrogen. This equates with increased risk of endometrial cancer. The progesterone of HRT offsets this risk. If we're overweight and on HRT, we are less likely to develop endometrial cancer than obese women who have erroneously (and meanly) been told that they are "too fat" to need or warrant estrogen therapy.

"Too Old"

Another fallacy regarding ERT! Firstly, what does "too old" mean? My 17-year-old thinks that my generation and I are too old for many things, including conversation (with her), ecological responsibility, and sex! If we are too young to get old, when are we old? Many of the ailments to which age predisposes us are exactly those that are diminished with ERT: coronary heart disease (CHD), osteoporosis, stroke, and Alzheimer's. We have definitive evidence that even with advanced CHD and osteoporosis, estrogen promotes some reversal and affords protection from their progression (see part III). The older we get, the greater the chances of our continuing on, but we want to gain quality of years, not just quantity.

Although we may decide that our daughters and granddaughters are right on one issue—that we're too old to share their obsession with rap—we can make informed (and more harmonious) choices about hormone replacement therapy—at any age.

Benign Fibroid Tumors of the Uterus

At least 20 percent of women over the age of 35 have these benign uterine tumors. We know that during our reproductive years, our own estrogen stimulated these tumors to grow. Why some of us have fibroid-growing estrogen receptors and develop these benign tumors, while others don't, is a mystery. It's not that we produce more estrogen (our hormone levels are the same as those of tumor-free women). There appears to be an age-related increase in receptor sensitivity and fibroid development as well as a familial and ethnic tendency (African-American women are more susceptible to fibroid growth). When we deprive these receptors of estrogen, the fibroids shrink. This can occur with natural or surgical menopause, as well as with the use of certain drugs that prevent estrogen production by the ovaries (GnRH agonists).

So it stands to reason that if we take ERT or HRT, we would expect fibroid growth. With few exceptions, however, this does not seem to be common with the dosages we use. Perhaps with time, the receptor count or sensitivity of the fibroids diminishes. Estrogen replacement therapy will not usually cause sudden growth or development of fibroids.

There is, however, a silent, nonpalpable (meaning we don't feel it during pelvic exams) fibroid that can create an HRT-related problem—bleeding. If a fibroid grows into the endometrial cavity, its presence may remain undetected without ultrasound. When we take HRT, especially in a cyclical fashion, and the endometrium sloughs, this tumor may cause heavy or prolonged bleeding. Abnormal bleeding on HRT should be checked with a vaginal ultrasound. If a mass or thickening in the endometrium is found, hysteroscopy will allow us to determine if the bleeding culprit is a submucosal fibroid (and, of course, also rule out cancer). We then have two choices: Stop hormone therapy or remove the darn thing with hysteroscopic resection.

We can live with our fibroids unless they are very large or cause bleeding. These benign tumors won't kill us or affect our vitality. However, coronary heart disease, osteoporosis, stroke, and Alzheimer's will. Women on hormone therapy need annual exams. If we have uterine fibroids, they should be monitored, but their silent presence need not bolster the argument against estrogen therapy.

TRUE CONFESSIONS:
WHEN ESTROGEN SHOULD NOT BE USED

Let's not fool ourselves: Estrogen is not an over-the-counter product that should be popped (pills) or slapped on (the patch) by all. When do we "just say no" to estrogen?

Breast Cancer

Recent (less than five years ago) breast cancer, especially if it contained estrogen receptors, is currently believed to be a contraindication to estrogen replacement therapy. As physicians, we're afraid to prescribe it and, as breast cancer victims, terrified to use it. If estrogen is a tumor promoter (rather than originator), we want to make sure we harbor no residual tumor cells to promote. So traditionally we don't take estrogen and instead look for acceptable alternatives to help us through our symptoms and help prevent coronary heart disease and osteoporosis.

Tamoxifen is in many ways an excellent alternative to estrogen for women who have had breast cancer. Its primary benefit is, of course, the reduction of recurrent breast cancer by at least 25 to 35 percent when taken for up to five years. Tamoxifen also affords some major secondary gains by improving our lipoprotein profiles (it lowers cholesterol and LDLs) and diminishing calcium loss from our spine. It doesn't help hot flashes (and, indeed, it can make them worse), vaginal dryness, or bladder and skin changes. As yet, we don't know what happens to our incidence of stroke or Alzheimer's after we've completed tamoxifen therapy. Like unopposed estrogen, it stimulates the glands of the endometrium and can increase the risk of endometrial cancer. Those of us who have a uterus and take tamoxifen should be monitored with yearly ultrasounds or endometrial samplings.

"JUST SAY NO"—THE SEQUEL

Does "no" mean "never" for women with a history of breast cancer? As with so many of our medical rules, we've learned to stop being so arbitrary. Or maybe just less sure of ourselves—we doctors are slowly coming down from our pedestals (and some of us need motorized cranes to facilitate this descent!). There have been no studies that actually show an increased risk of breast cancer recurrence or reduced survival rates after use of ERT. On the other hand, we don't have studies with enough breast cancer patients or sufficient years of follow-up to reassure us.

There is one fact that might warrant consideration of ERT for women with breast cancer: Taking estrogen while we develop breast cancer does not appear to make the outcome of the disease worse. In fact, the prognosis of women who took ERT before diagnosis is better than that of women who never took estrogen. Additionally, women who are diagnosed within a year of taking ERT have a longer survival rate than women who have not taken estrogen for more than a year before diagnosis.

With or without ERT, 10 percent of women with small tumors, "good" types of cancer cells, and negative nodes will have breast cancer recurrence. Those with large tumors, "bad" types of cells, and positive nodes will have more than a 50 percent recurrence rate. One half of us with breast cancer fall between these groups, with an average recurrence rate of 30 percent in ten years. We have to understand this if we want to reconsider ERT. It's possible that if we get a "natural" or inevitable recurrence, estrogen could make it grow. Because tamoxifen reduces recurrent breast cancer, some cancer specialists advocate its use together with estrogen in post–breast cancer patients who wish to continue ERT. As patients and physicians, we're becoming less arbitrary. There is no black-and-white (except on mammograms); we have to look at multiple factors. The reasons to consider use of ERT after breast cancer might include:

1. Having a distressing time with quality-of-life symptoms (hot flashes, sleep deprivation, mood changes, memory loss) that we can't seem to alleviate with alternative therapies.

2. Having a high risk for coronary heart disease. There is no triumph over breast cancer, if in the ensuing years we die prematurely of heart attack!

3. Developing significant osteoporosis (but remember, there are some excellent nonestrogenic therapies).

4. Any of the above (this is beginning to resemble the SATs, but health has its own tests) and surviving breast cancer for a number of years (many M.D.s quote five years; it seems to have special medical connotations). An additional factor might be knowledge that the original cancer was small and did not have estrogen receptors.

5. No recurrence for more than ten years (no matter what the original tumor "showed").

6. A cancer specialist (*oncologist*) or gynecologist who is sympathetic to a woman's desire to take estrogen (especially if reason number one is a factor) and willing to take an unknown medical-legal risk. This may be the dumbest criterion, but let's remember, someone has to write that prescription!

The American College of Obstetricians and Gynecologists Committee on Gynecologic Practices has stated:

> No woman can be guaranteed protection from recurrence [of breast cancer]. The short-term and potential long-term benefits of ERT are well recognized. . . . In postmenopausal women with previously treated breast cancer, consideration of ERT is an option, but must be viewed with caution.

In other words, we're sailing through uncharted waters without official maps. Women who have had breast cancer will have to get out their compasses and chart their own courses until substantial studies give us definitive guidelines.

Previous Endometrial Cancer

With regard to earlier endometrial cancer, we might ask, "Even if estrogen may have caused this, can we forgive and forget after we've been treated?"

We should not take ERT, or even HRT, if we have undiagnosed abnormal bleeding. I recently took care of a woman who had bled two out of three weeks for months while perimenopausal. She was given cyclical hormones to correct this bleeding and, although her symptoms diminished, she still complained of intermittent spotting. She reported this as a discharge (actually, it was "old" brown blood; slow bleeding and exposure to oxygen turn the blood a rusty brown). Vaginal cultures were done (the doctors heard the word "discharge" and didn't pay attention to color distinctions), and she was informed that she had no infection and basically was dismissed. This woman was overweight, had never had children, and had a history of irregular periods. She *looked* like she was at risk for endometrial cancer. When she finally saw me, she was convinced that all of her problems would be solved by increasing her estrogen and changing her progesterone. Instead, she got scanned and underwent a hysteroscopy. We found that she had endometrial cancer. Luckily, it was still at an early stage, and a hysterectomy (together with removal of her tubes, ovaries, and some pelvic lymph nodes, which showed no tumor spread) cured her. Can this woman and others like her take estrogen in the future?

Most oncologists would suggest she take Megace (a high-potency progesterone) for several years after the initial cancer surgery. The medical reasoning is that if any cancer cells (or "almost"-cancer cells) escaped the knife, they would succumb to a bombardment with strong progesterone. Megace also diminishes hot flashes and helps prevent osteoporosis.

One statistic says that women who take estrogen and develop endometrial cancer and are treated live longer than women who have never taken estrogen and do not develop this type of cancer. If we expect to do so well, despite this cancer, and continue on with our lives, should we not provide protection from coronary heart disease and osteoporosis, as well as improve quality of life?

Again, this is an individual patient-physician decision. I and many others do prescribe estrogen as early as three to five years postsurgery. This is, however, one of the few exceptions to our rule of "no uterus, no need for progesterone." I give continuous HRT (estrogen and progesterone) as a safeguard with the thought that progesterone will prevent any "uncertain" cells remaining "somewhere" from being influenced by unopposed estrogen. "Uncertain" and "somewhere" may not sound very scientific and probably descends into the realm of superstition (progesterone wards off endometrial cancer ghosts). But who says we should forgo safe betting in our choices of ongoing care?

Unwanted Symptoms with ERT: Weren't We Supposed to Feel Better, Not Worse?

I wish every patient for whom I prescribed estrogen had all the "expected" benefits (hers and mine) and no adverse reactions. I've had women ask my exchange to beep me during non-office hours (I guess as a kind of retribution) to tell me how awful they felt on estrogen. Their complaints vary from nausea, bloating, and breast tenderness to increase in breast size (and by now, most of us don't equate large breasts with either femininity or attractiveness—they're just more to support with larger bras!). With time, some of these initial reactions diminish, but for some women just a week of nausea or bloating is enough for them to stop therapy. Women who tend to have chronic headaches may get worse with ERT or HRT (although many of my patients relate that their headaches improve after taking estrogen). These "bad-head" days may be related to cyclical therapy, when we stop or start the estrogen and/or progesterone, causing hormone levels to change. If we eliminate the cycling and take the same dose of hormones daily (continuous dose), the problem may be eliminated. We've also found that the patch may be associated with fewer headaches and less nausea.

Remember, there are half a dozen types of estrogens on the market. If unpleasant symptoms develop with one form, it is worth switching and trying another before we give up. Some of our symptoms might also improve if we change bad health habits. Caffeine increases breast tenderness; high salt intake increases water retention; overeating and underexercising make us fat. So let's make sure of where the real culprit lies before we "beep" our doctors or abruptly throw away our hormones.

Ways and Means of Hormone Therapy

NATURAL ESTROGEN: WHICH IS BEST, BETTER, OR JUST OK?

There are over half a dozen types of estrogen to choose from (see Table 7.1). They are all considered natural estrogens. Once in our body, they are put through the same changes that occur to the estrogens we produce

TABLE 7.1 PREPARATIONS CONTAINING ESTROGEN

Product	Pharmaceutical Company	Type of Estrogen	Type and Dosage	Price (one-month supply at large chain pharmacy) for lowest-dose tablet
Premarin	Wyeth-Ayerst	Conjugated equine (horse) estrogens ~ 45% estrone sulfate; ~ 55% equine estrogens	*Oral:* 0.3, 0.625, 0.9, 1.25, and 2.5 mg tablets *Vaginal cream:* 1 g contains 0.625 mg	$13.96
Estratab	Solvay	Esterified estrogens ~ 85% estrone sulfate; ~ 15% equine estrogens	*Oral:* 0.625, 1.25, and 2.5 mg tablets *Vaginal cream:* 1 g contains 0.625 mg	$17.95
Menest	SmithKline Beecham	Esterified estrogens	*Oral:* 0.3, 0.625, 1.25, and 2.5 mg tablets	$9.95
Estrace	Mead Johnson	Micronized estradiol	*Oral:* 0.5, 1, and 2 mg tablets *Vaginal cream:* 1 g contains 0.2 mg estradiol	$14.95
Ogen	Abbott	Estropipate (piperazine estrone sulfate)	*Oral:* 0.75 mg estropipate in 0.625 mg; 0.625, 1.25, 2.5, and 5 mg tablets	$24.95
Ortho-Est	Ortho	Estropipate (same as Ogen)	*Oral:* 0.625 and 1.25 mg tablets	$17.95
Estraderm	Ciba	Estradiol	*Patch:* 0.05 and 0.1 mg	$27.95 (0.05 mg)
Climara	Berlex	Estradiol	*Patch:* 0.05 and 0.1 mg	$29.95 (0.05 mg)
Vivelle	Ciba	Estradiol	*Patch:* 0.0375, 0.05, 0.075, and 0.1 mg	$27.95 (0.05 mg)

in our ovaries. If we ingest estrogens as tablets, they are absorbed by our intestinal tract and go to the liver, where they are broken down and reconfigured to less potent estrogens called *estrone* and *estriol*. Some estrogen is attached to a sulfate, while other forms are oxidized and become *catecholestrogens*, which work in our central nervous system. It is these reworked estrogens that are released to our blood and can then enter our target cells. The difference between natural estrogen, which we use for ERT, and synthetic estrogen in birth control pills (such as ethinyl estradiol) is not how they are made (using animals or a lab), but how they are handled by our liver. The natural estrogens are extensively broken down. The synthetic estrogens are not; they are degraded very slowly in the liver and other tissues, and this causes them to have a much higher estrogen potency. If a natural estrogen is given by a nonoral route (absorbed through our skin or mucous membranes), its first pathway will not traverse the liver. It misses what we call "first-pass" metabolism, but once in our blood, it does eventually get taken up by the liver and put through the same reconfiguration that occurs with ovarian estrogens or the oral tablets.

Types of Estrogens

In an ideal pharmacologic world, we could issue expert and consumer reports rating the various estrogen products. We do this for cars— their cost, fuel efficiency, safety features, and overall performance. What about applying these criteria to our hormone medications? Every woman is unique, so there may be no true rating. Knowledge of each product, however, might help us and our doctors to individualize our therapy.

PREMARIN (TABLETS)

This is our "oldest" estrogen and has been on the market for fifty-two years. Most of the American studies on the long-term effects of estrogen on our hearts, bones, brains, and mortality have been conducted with this product.

Premarin is a mixture of estrogens obtained from what the pharmaceutical company (Wyeth-Ayerst Laboratories) refers to as a "natural" source (at this point, most of us think of springs). It is extracted from the urine of pregnant mares, which, if you think about it, is very "natural."

When mammals are pregnant, they produce huge amounts of estrogen and the runoff is "peed off" in the urine. There are quite a few estrogen compounds made by these mares; these include estrone (which we also produce and excrete in our urine), equilin, and 17-alpha-hydroequilin (horse estrogens—the word *equine* means *horse*), together with smaller amounts of other forms of estrogens.

Premarin is the most prescribed estrogen in this country. Physicians feel comfortable using it because it has been around so long. Recently the pharmaceutical company scientists have demonstrated some tamoxifen-like "anti–breast cancer" properties in the horse estrogen components of Premarin. They have also found that horse estrogens may be more potent than human estrogens in improving our lipoproteins (lowering and breaking down LDL and increasing HDL). So although some of us may not philosophically want to accept a kinship, or even a working relationship, with pregnant mares, their estrogen has been shown to be effective for women. Premarin is a reliable contender in the estrogen (I have to do this) horse race.

ESTRACE (TABLETS)

This, too, is a "natural" estrogen. Here, the "natural" means its active estrogen component, estradiol, is "naturally occurring" and it's identical to that produced by our ovaries before menopause. The estradiol in Estrace is derived from plant sources. It's micronized (chopped up into tiny pieces) to allow for better absorption. Once it enters our gastrointestinal tract, it is metabolized in our liver and converted to estrone. It is this estrogen that circulates and affects our organs. This is a relatively "pure" estrogen (the term "relative" is used, because colors, lactose, starch, and talc have been added as, by the way, they are to the other estrogen preparations). Patients and physicians may prefer this preparation because it mimics the ovarian function of women rather than that of horses. There has been some concern, however, over a Scandinavian study of over 23,000 women which showed an increased incidence of breast cancer (up to 1.7 relative risk after nine years) in women using estradiol. In all fairness, this study has been criticized because the women took fairly high doses (2 milligrams of estradiol) and just 1 in every 30 women were sent questionnaires. So whether this study should increase our concern about estradiol depends on which researcher we listen to. This is a good estrogen and has been shown to have all of the desired positive effects on our hearts and bones. If it "feels right," it will probably be right for women needing estrogen replacement therapy.

OGEN AND ORTHO-EST

These are essentially the same product put out by different pharmaceutical companies. The estrogen is prepared from purified crystalline estrone, the estrogen produced in our body after we metabolize the other types of estrogen therapies (Premarin and Estrace). So this pill supplies the "estrogen end product." This formulation is a little weaker than the "same dose" of Premarin or Estrace. It takes a dose between the 0.625-milligram and 1.25-milligram tablets to raise our blood levels of estradiol and estrone to the same degree as 0.625 milligram of Premarin or 1 milligram of Estrace. This lower estrogen effect could be beneficial if we're trying to diminish symptoms. If the dose is clinically too low (for example, we have persistent hot flashes), it can always be increased.

ESTRADERM PATCH

This looks like a large oval, "see-through" Band-Aid and is applied to unexposed skin (lower abdomen, buttocks, or thighs) and changed twice a week. It releases 17 beta-estradiol (the same component as in Estrace) in a continuous fashion, so theoretically we don't get the peaks and troughs of hormone levels that can be associated with our ingestion of estrogen tablets. The patch comes in two sizes: small (10 centimeters square), which is designed to deliver 50 micrograms of estradiol a day (the 0.05-milligram patch); and large (20 centimeters square), which, you guessed it, gives double the dose (the 0.1-milligram patch). We get maximum serum levels of estradiol and estrone in two to eight hours and, with long-term use, we get estradiol levels that are similar to the equivalent 0.625-milligram Premarin tablet and 1-milligram Estrace tablet (for the small patch) and 1.25 milligrams and 2 milligrams of the oral estrogens for the large patch.

Sounds great, but unfortunately our skin doesn't always absorb and transmit the way we plan. Fifteen to 20 percent of women develop local irritation (large ugly red blotches or welts on the skin under the patch). Changing the area helps (the skin on our thighs or buttocks seems to be less sensitive than that on our abdomen), but at least 2 percent of women have to stop using this system because of irritation. Aside from differences in sensitivity, we have differences in skin thickness and penetrability, so the amount of estradiol absorbed can vary by as much as 20 percent from woman to woman. If we're in hot climates and perspire, we are literally washing away some of the estrogen (also, the patches don't stick). It's probably a good idea to check our blood estradiol level to see how much is being absorbed. We want the level to be 50 picograms/milliliter or more. This will ensure we are "doing" or "absorbing" it right.

CLIMARA PATCH

This newly released patch (in 1995) releases 17 beta-estradiol slowly and steadily so it has to be changed just once a week. The hormone is incorporated into the adhesive and, unlike the Estraderm patch, there is no central "bubble," or reservoir, that contains the active ingredient. The patch is thin and translucent, lies flat, and, according to its manufacturers, has superior stickiness. It maintains a slightly steadier, but lower, level of hormone in our blood compared to Estraderm; on the average, the larger 1.0-milligram Climera patch maintains serum estradiol levels at 70 picograms/milliliter, and the smaller 0.05-milligram patch gives levels of approximately 35 picograms/milliliter. This latter dose (like that absorbed with the smaller Estraderm patch) may not be quite enough to protect some women from osteoporosis.

Climara, like Estraderm, causes some of us to develop skin irritation and welts. The company reports that 9 percent of women developed significant irritation, which caused "only" (their word) 6.8 percent to discontinue therapy.

VIVELLE PATCH

This was released in 1996 by Ciba Pharmaceuticals, the makers of the Estraderm patch. It's their answer to the Climara patch; there is no bubble and estradiol is incorporated into the adhesive. Vivelle comes in four strengths: 0.0375, 0.05, 0.075, and 0.1 milligram. This larger variety permits dosing flexibility, although in the past I've had my patients cut the Climara patch to get these same "in-between" doses.

Using the Patch Versus Taking the Pill

There are some differences between the patch and pill that we should know about, and these are due to lack of "first-pass" metabolism by the liver. If we don't eat the estrogen, it doesn't get absorbed by our gut and passed directly to our liver. The estradiol enters our circulation without passing "go," but—to continue our Monopoly analogy—the game continues and, eventually, the player (estradiol) goes around the board again and gets to pass "go" (the liver). There, instead of collecting $200, it is metabolized. Estradiol's later "liver entry" means it has less effect on the liver's function, and the liver has a smaller effect on it. So while oral estrogen (tablets) stimulates production of certain liver proteins (some of which bind up estrogen and make it less active), as well as certain clotting factors, the patch does not. We know that oral estrogen gives us better living through better lipoproteins. It raises HDL and lowers LDL. Much of this is done in the liver, and there was concern that we would lose this effect with the patch. But later is better than never, and after three to six months of estrogen patch use, we do find that our HDLs go up and LDLs go down. Another piece of good news: The patch has no effect on our triglycerides, whereas oral estrogen may cause them to increase in some women.

Now that we are transport experts (of estrogen), we can take some of the hocus-pocus away from the "why-am-I-on-the-Pill-while-my-friend-is-on-the-patch" controversy.

THE PATCH: WHY YOU WOULD CONSIDER USING IT

1. The pill caused nausea.

2. Your triglycerides are abnormally high.

3. You have variations in your hormone levels with pills, and this causes ups and downs in symptoms like hot flashes (levels can drop fourteen to eighteen hours after ingestion of estrogen tablets).

4. You have a history of migraines or your headaches worsen with oral estrogen.

5. You have had or are at risk for gallbladder disease.

6. You have a history of abnormal clots or a disease, such as lupus, that can change clotting factors. Although clinically, the pills are not associated with increased risk of clots, clotting factors are altered. This does not appear to occur with the patch, so the purists, hematologists, and lawyers might be happier if you use the patch under these circumstances.

7. You smoke. Oral estrogen causes release of certain liver proteins, and nicotine releases abnormal liver proteins. When the two combine they may cause increased clotting.

8. Your blood pressure increases with oral estrogen. This may be due to elevation of a substance called renin. There is no increase in renin with use of the patch.

The Pill: Why You Might Prefer This

1. You live in a hot climate, and the patch won't stick.

2. You developed skin reactions to the patch.

3. Your lipoproteins are awful, and you want to get started improving them as quickly as possible with ERT.

4. You are at high risk for coronary heart disease or osteoporosis, and there is a question whether you are absorbing the estrogen in the patch in levels that are needed to prevent these diseases (repeated estradiol levels are not 50 picograms or greater).

5. You don't want to show a "badge of honor" to menopause; you are self-conscious about seeing or having the patch seen.

6. You have to take your progesterone as a pill (currently, it's not available in a patch), so it's easier to just pop two pills at once.

Estrogen Creams

VAGINAL CREAMS

How much of the estrogen cream that we prescribe for "local" vaginal effect is actually absorbed? One gram of Premarin or Estratab cream contains 0.625 milligram of estrogen. The absorption of this cream results in blood levels that are approximately one half to one quarter of those obtained with a 0.625-milligram tablet taken orally. Estrace (estradiol cream) is weaker; 1 gram has only 0.1 milligram estrogen, producing even lower blood levels. It's interesting to note that micronized estradiol can be suspended in saline (salt water) and douched into the vagina. With this medium (liquid rather than cream), the absorption is four times greater. Micronized estradiol in tablet form (we're now taking our pills vaginally rather than orally!) is also well absorbed, and researchers are working on a vaginal ring which gives continuous estrogen release.

If we want the effect of the cream to be as local as possible, we should decrease the dose to just 1 gram twice weekly. This should be enough to keep our vaginal tissue healthy without estrogenizing the rest of us.

SKIN CREAMS

Estradiol Cream   Many European women rub on (or, more euphemistically, massage in) their estrogen. They are using an alcohol-based gel of estradiol. They apply it to their arms, shoulders, or abdomens. It dries in two to five minutes and leaves no sticky residue or odor (sounds like an ad for furniture polish!). The skin stores the estradiol and acts as a continuous "time releaser" for the estrogen. The doses and blood levels of estrogen are similar to those of the estrogen patch. It sounds great; the gel eliminates the skin reactions we may develop to the adhesive on the patch, and there is no need to constantly wear a visible "badge" of menopause. This product is not currently available from a pharmaceutical company in the United States, but if we want to "rub it in," we can get a similar gel from specialized "hormone-formulating" companies in Madison, Wisconsin.

Tri-Estrogen-Progesterone Cream   This cream is made from extracts of wild Mexican yam (the barbasco plant) and soybeans. Presently, we have to consider it as an "alternative" therapy. It certainly has not had the controlled studies or scientific scrutiny that we have given "established" estrogen therapy. The chief component of this cream is estriol, which is only 25 percent as strong as conjugated estrogen. We metabolize estrogen into estriol and secrete it in our urine. Women from ethnic groups with a low incidence of breast cancer have higher urinary excretion of estriol than women with a high incidence of breast cancer. It may just mean that they are clearing and peeing off their estrogen more efficiently, but some researchers are looking to see if estriol itself is an anticancer estrogen. Once more, we've got the questions (and hopes), but the data are not sufficient. There are claims that the progesterone in this cream (again, from plant sources) has been shown to stop the progression of osteoporosis. Again, we need numbers and studies. The cream can be applied in small amounts (one quarter of a teaspoon) twice daily to the wrist, chest, face, abdomen, back, shoulder, neck, or throat. I have had some patients tell me that it improved the skin of their face and neck when applied to these areas, but this is truly anecdotal and cannot be considered scientific evidence.

THE PROGESTERONES: SEARCHING FOR THE SPOONFUL OF SUGAR TO HELP THIS MEDICINE GO DOWN

If we have to take progesterone (meaning our uterus is intact), which will be the kindest and gentlest, as well as effective? Progesterones can cause side effects we would rather live without, such as bloating, breast tenderness, irritability, and depression (our old PMS symptoms!). Like estrogen, there are several different formulations of progesterone (see Table 7.2).

Provera and Cycrin
(Medroxyprogesterone Acetate, or MPA)

This is the oldest and most commonly used form of synthetic progesterone or progestin for hormone replacement therapy. It is the progestin being used in the HRT program of the Women's Health Initiative. It's a synthetic hormone in which chemical groups have been added to progesterone to improve its absorption and stability. Once we take MPA,

TABLE 7.2 PREPARATIONS CONTAINING PROGESTERONE

Product	Pharmaceutical Company	Type of Progesterone	Dosage	Price (one-month supply at large chain pharmacy)
Provera	Upjohn	Medroxy-progesterone acetate	2.5 mg 5 mg 10 mg	30 tabs (continuous therapy): $16.95 10 tabs (cyclical therapy): $10.95 10 tabs (cyclical therapy): $12.95
Cycrin	Wyeth-Ayerst	Medroxy-progesterone acetate	2.5 mg 5 mg 10 mg	30 tabs: $10.95 10 tabs: $8.95 10 tabs: $8.95
Generic medroxyprogesterone acetate		Medroxy-progesterone acetate	2.5 mg 5 mg 10 mg	30 tabs: $11.95 10 tabs: $7.95 10 tabs: $7.95
Aygestin	Wyeth-Ayerst	Norethindrone acetate	5 mg 2.5 mg (break 5 mg tablet in half)	10 tabs (cyclical therapy): $22.69 10 tabs (cyclical therapy): $11.35
Micronor	Ortho	Norethindrone	0.35 mg	30 tabs (continuous therapy): $31.69
Natural micronized progesterone	HealthPharmacies, Women's International Pharmacy (both in Wisconsin), and other pharmacies willing to compound this formulation	Progesterone	100 mg 200 mg	60 cents per 100 mg capsule (continuous; take 1 to 2 capsules a day) 75 cents per 200 mg capsule (cyclical; take 1 200 mg capsule; may add 1 100 mg capsule)

the progesterone levels in our blood peak in one to four hours and fall after twenty-four hours. The tablets are available in 2.5-, 5-, and 10-milligram doses. If given continuously, the lowest dose, 2.5 milligrams, is used (5 and 10 milligrams are used for cyclical therapy). Since there is a concern that progestins may attenuate some of estrogen's protective effects on our lipids and coronary heart disease, we should aim for the smallest dosage that we know protects the endometrium. Five milligrams is currently recommended for cyclical therapy, but some investigators are going down to 2.5 milligrams. I reserve the 10-milligram dose for patients who have breakthrough bleeding. When progesterone problems such as bloating and mood changes occur, I find that they do so on MPA. I often start my patients on this product, but if they report these symptoms, I "boutique" their progesterone therapy and try another form.

Aygestin (Norethindrone Acetate)

This progesterone is synthetic and is made by adding and subtracting chemical groups to testosterone (it is amazing what adding an ethinyl group here and taking away a methyl group there can do). The male hormone properties of this substance are virtually eliminated, and a "proper" progestin is formed which can be absorbed and is stable. This pill, like MPA, gives us a progesterone level that peaks in one to two hours after ingestion and falls in twenty-four hours. Aygestin comes in just one strength, 5 milligrams, which is roughly equivalent in its progestational activity to 10 milligrams of Provera or Cycrin. The tablet is scored so it can be broken in half (2.5 milligrams) to use as an effective dose for cyclical HRT. I find that for some of my patients, Aygestin may cause fewer side effects than MPA (this may just be a placebo response because we've changed the pill, and both the patient and I want it to work). I wish I had more objective data on these subjective progesterone "responses."

Micronor (norethindrone), the "Mini-Pill"

This synthetic progesterone is similar to Aygestin but has an acetate attached to it (frankly, in our state of chemistry knowledge, we don't care as long as it's absorbed and works). It's also a much smaller dose, 0.35 milligram, compared to 5 milligrams in Aygestin. It is used as a progesterone-only birth control pill, hence the description "mini."

This low dosage can effectively be used with estrogen for continuous-dose HRT. In other words, we take our estrogen daily and our mini-progesterone pill daily. Micronor is very conveniently packaged in a pack so we can see if we've missed a pill. Because of its low dose, there seems to be less breast tenderness and fluid retention, and the best news is that we get rapid reduction in breakthrough bleeding (90 percent of us will become pad- and tampon-free after nine months of use). This is a fairly new way to provide progesterone, and since it is so low-dose, we should be followed with endometrial monitoring.

Natural Micronized Progesterone

Natural progesterone is not absorbed well and becomes inactivated when ingested (our stomach enzymes and liver really do a number on foods and medications). This gastric attack has been overcome by mi-cronizing the progesterone into miniscule pieces and putting them into oil. This process also protects the medication from liver breakdown. The progesterone is "pure" and has no relationship to male hormone. It is not currently available as a brand-name drug, but is a product of what I term "Mom and Pop" companies and pharmacies. I have my patients order it from a pharmacy in Wisconsin, but several of our local companies tell me they can formulate the product. It is fairly expensive (I guess this is the ultimate "boutiquing" of progesterone), ranging in price from 60¢ to $1.00 for a 100-milligram capsule. These capsules give rapid and sus-tained blood levels of progesterone similar to those of Provera and Aygestin but, in some women, are associated with less fluid retention, breast tenderness, and depression. I prescribe it for my patients who have "failed" the synthetic progestins (or whom the progestins have failed), or for women who have a premenopausal history of severe PMS. The results have been gratifying, and many of these women who have threatened progesterone or total ERT strike are able to remain on hormone therapy without side effects.

New data from the PEPI Trial (what a great acronym for a menopausal study; it stands for Postmenopausal Estrogen/Progesterone Interventions) have shown that micronized progesterone does not di-minish the effect of estrogen in raising HDL, whereas the synthetic progestins have a mild lowering effect. Since HDL levels may be an im-portant factor for heart attack, we might want to consider this when choosing a progestin if we have low HDLs or are at cardiac risk. The progesterone comes in 25-, 50-, 100-, and 200-milligram capsules. For cyclical therapy, we take 100 milligrams in the morning and 200 milligrams at night, or just 200 milligrams at night (this progesterone can cause sleepiness, so I prescribe the major dose before bedtime). For continuous therapy I prescribe 100 to 200 milligrams nightly. It should be noted that the same company that makes micronized progesterone has come out with a capsule that combines 0.35 milligram of micronized estradiol (similar to Estrace) and 100 milligrams of micronized progesterone. If we take two to three capsules daily, a good continuous dose of both estrogen and progesterone is maintained, and we can get away from the Chinese food–ordering technique; two pills from Bottle A and one pill from Bottle B.

Megace (Megestrol Acetate)

This is a synthetic, high-dosage, high-potency progestin. It is used to treat recurrent or metastatic cancer of the breast and endometrium. It comes in 20- and 40-milligram tablets. Twenty milligrams of Megace taken twice a day have been found to decrease menopausal hot flashes substantially. For women who cannot take estrogen or who are on tamoxifen for post–breast cancer therapy, this strong progestin might make life "cooler." Another positive attribute is that Megace appears to increase bone mineralization and can provide us some protection against osteoporosis. On the negative side is our concern over possible long-term effects on our lipids and risk of cardiovascular disease. Another drug with my so-oft-stated caveat: We'll have to wait, study, and see.

MALE HORMONES (ANDROGENS): "WHY CAN'T A WOMAN BE MORE LIKE A MAN?"

Understanding Androgens

We can dismiss Professor Higgins's silly query, but Eliza Doolittle did produce male hormones, as do all of us. Sexual inferences aside, male hormone is the source of our estrogen production. (Or we could turn the concept around and state that estrogen is a male hormone that has completed its destined conversion.) We make two types of male hormone in our ovaries: testosterone (the stronger) and androstenedione (the weaker). Our follicles that develop during monthly ovulation convert both of these androgens to estrogen. Our adrenal glands also produce androstenedione, as well as DHEA (believe me, unless you are taking a biochemistry exam, you don't need to cope with these names). These relatively weak androgens enter our circulation and get transported to our ovaries, where they, too, can be converted by the follicles to estrogens. Male hormone, especially androstenedione, is also converted in other parts of our body to estrogen. This is called *peripheral conversion* and occurs in our fat (hence, the fatter we are, the more estrogen we make) as well as our muscle, skin, kidneys, and brain (our brainy conversion of androgen to estrogen may allow us to escape a destiny of becoming "more like a man").

From puberty to menopause, the follicles of our ovaries make male hormone and convert it to estrogen (mostly estradiol). This accounts for 60 percent of our circulating estrogen. The other 40 percent comes from peripheral conversion of male hormone. When we exhaust our supply of follicles and become menopausal, the ovary loses its ability to directly convert androgen to estrogen, but it still makes male hormone in its nonfollicular tissue, or *stroma*. So with menopause, we lose 80 to 90 percent of our estrogen, but only about 50 percent of our male hormone.

We know what to expect with the loss of estrogen (see the chapters on menopause and estrogen, and about half of this book!), but what does a fall in male hormone do to us physically and psychologically? Do we miss it? (This rhetorical question is not raised in order to generate a gender debate; we've already established that androgens are our "natural" product.) The "miss it" question is complicated. Yes, we have less male hormone, but we have dropped our estrogen levels to a greater extent. For some of us, the ratio of male to female hormones may be more important than their actual individual levels. So many of us in our fifties through our eighties will go through our lives without a thought or feeling of male hormone deprivation. But some of us may be more sensitive, or "male hormone–challenged." Loss of libido, lack of energy, mood changes, nervousness, insomnia, and decreased sense of well-being have all been listed as possible symptoms of androgen deficiency. Studies have shown that, compared to women receiving estrogen alone, women who receive male hormone with estrogen have a greater improvement in their psychologic and psychosomatic symptoms. They have more sexual fantasies, more sex (if a partner is available), and a generally high level of sexual satisfaction. Many women report (or test) that their energy levels are improved and they feel a general improvement in the quality of their lives. On a physical basis, male hormone appears to help rebuild depleted bone, especially in the vertebrae. The higher our androgen level, the less likely we'll develop spinal crush fractures.

As usual in medicine, there are also negative reports. Male hormone, especially in high doses, can lower HDL (our good cholesterol) and might diminish some of estrogen's protection against coronary artery disease. But triglycerides are also lowered, and this is considered beneficial. We have no long-term studies of estrogen plus male hormone (plus progesterone, if needed) on our incidence of heart attack.

We also have to consider cosmetic issues. We tend to grow more facial hair as we get older (we all notice the extra time spent plucking our chins with tweezers). This may be due to a change in our natural androgen-to-estrogen ratio. If we add more male hormone, will we grow beards? Twenty percent of women who take preparations of estrogen and testosterone develop mild *hirsutism* (hair growth). This is both dose-dependent and reversible. It can also be treated with a drug called spironolactone, which decreases our skin sensitivity to male hormone. I only mention this in passing; I can already hear the cries of "overmedication." Giving one drug in order to allow us to use another could be considered overly aggressive, but we may like how we feel and aggressively want to continue using male hormones; that doesn't mean we have to accept facial hair.

Should I Take Male Hormones?

Just because we live in a male-dominated society (which, we hope, is changing) doesn't mean we should all supplement ourselves with male hormones. Their use should be considered in the following situations.

1. Significant symptoms that began with menopause and do not "appropriately" improve on adequate doses of estrogen replacement: hot flashes, depression, irritability, mood changes, and loss of energy. The last problem should be attacked with male hormone only after appropriate efforts have been made to rule out other causes of low energy such as anemia, low thyroid, chronic diseases, or difficult, overdemanding lives.

2. Loss of libido that does not improve with estrogen replacement and does not appear to be related to other psychosocial problems.

3. Women who undergo surgical removal of both their ovaries before their "natural" menopause. This is a sudden, massive shock to our hormonal system—we're losing both our estrogen and most of our male hormones. Our symptoms are generally severe and often difficult to resolve unless we add androgens.

4. Severe breast tenderness on estrogen replacement therapy. Our breast tissue gradually becomes desensitized as we lose our estrogen in menopause. When we replace this estrogen with ERT, we sometimes develop significant breast pain (we can't even be hugged). Male hormone works to decrease this pain.

5. Significant vertebral osteoporosis. Adding male hormone to estrogen may be helpful in decreasing our risk or recurrence of crush fractures of the vertebrae.

Types of Male Hormones

If we decide to use male hormones, they come in various preparations (see Table 7.3). We can get them together with estrogen, in which case, we will take that tablet exactly the same way we would take estrogen, either day 1 through 25 or daily, depending on the type of therapy we have chosen.

Taking male hormone in no way protects the uterine lining and does not substitute for progesterone. So if we must use HRT, we also have to make choices about the type of progesterone and the way we wish to cycle or not cycle with this medication. For those of us who use the patch or take an estrogen that does *not* come with male hormone, a separate pill is necessary. Methyltestosterone tablets are 10 milligrams. I have my patients begin with just a quarter of a tablet and ask them to let it dissolve in the inner lining of their cheek (subbuccal administration) or under their tongue (sublingual). This low dose should not cause acne or facial hair and, if not swallowed, does not pass through the digestive tract, so there are no adverse effects on our lipids. If necessary, the dose can be raised to one half of a tablet (5 milligrams) to get the desired androgen effect. Adding male hormone in this fashion becomes complicated because some of us will be taking three different hormone pills at

TABLE 7.3   PREPARATIONS CONTAINING MALE HORMONES

Product	Pharmaceutical Company	Active Ingredients (per tablet)	Price (for 30 days)
Estrogen-Androgen			
Estratest H.S. (half-strength)	Solvay	Esterified estrogens, 0.625 mg Methyltestosterone, 1.25 mg	$26.95
Estratest	Solvay	Esterified estrogens, 1.25 mg Methyltestosterone, 2.5 mg	$31.95
Premarin with methyltestosterone	Wyeth-Ayerst	Conjugated estrogens, 0.625 mg Methyltestosterone, 5 mg	$32.95
Premarin with methyltestosterone	Wyeth-Ayerst	Conjugated estrogens, 1.25 mg Methyltestosterone, 10 mg	$50.95
Androgen Only			
Android-10	ICN	Methyltestosterone, 10 mg	$53.95
Methyltestosterone (generic)		Methyltestosterone, 10 mg	$8.95

various times and end up having to be mathematicians in order to decide which to take when and for how long, and by what route.

A new androgen patch has just been introduced for the treatment of "low-testosterone" men. If we could just get a few studies that would test the absorption and subsequent androgen levels from this patch in women, we would have a new non-oral route available to us. (This would make the following couple conversation possible: "Honey, I just ran out of my patches; can I borrow one of yours?")

Male hormone can also be given as a long-acting shot (DEPO-testosterone), and this can make our medication life easier. As an injection it bypasses our digestive system and liver. I have a patient in her fifties who began having back problems several years ago. She's always been delightfully thin and petite, so we knew she was small-boned to begin with. She had also been given high doses of thyroid for many years. Sure enough, bone-density studies demonstrated that she had severe osteoporosis and was developing crush fractures in her back. Since testosterone helps treat this condition, she currently takes daily estrogen and progesterone and comes in once a month for a shot of DEPO-testosterone. She is better (on her scans), but also feels better with less pain and a great libido!

DHEA: ANOTHER HORMONE WE HAVE TO WORRY ABOUT

When I first wrote this chapter on hormones, I planned to review the basics—estrogen, progesterone, and testosterone. But there is an additional hormone that has recently come under scrutiny with regard to our process of aging. As often happens during the nascent period of hormone research, this new kid on the block has been lauded as the substance of youth by some and scorned by others. The latter group feels that this is a form of male hormone inappropriate for women, turning Mother Nature into Father Nature.

This controversial hormone is *dihydroepiandrosterone* (just remember DHEA). It's the most abundantly produced product of our adrenal gland, which also makes the hormone cortisol. Only a small amount of DHEA is allowed to roam free in our blood. Most is bonded to a sulfate molecule so it becomes (you guessed it) dihydroepiandrosterone sulfate, or DHEAS. Our serum concentration of DHEAS is 300 to 500 times higher than that of DHEA. This steroid is a weak male hormone and can be converted to the more potent testosterone, but it also has an independent role and should not be looked upon as a mere intermediary on its way to becoming something more important and malelike.

We are born with very high levels of DHEA(S) (please note, this is the correct abbreviation for both forms of DHEA). These levels decrease until puberty and then rise again in our late twenties, our era of DHEA(S) supremacy. Henceforth, we begin our trek of DHEA(S) loss, not with a bang (menopause has no effect on its depletion), but with a whimper, until the level declines by 80 percent in our seventies and, indeed, continues to fall in our eighties and nineties.

Scientists have found that giving DHEA(S) to experimental animals causes some amazing effects. It prevents diabetes in genetically programmed diabetic and obese mice. It increases the tissue sensitivity to insulin of aged but otherwise normal rats. (Remember, they and we tend to become insulin-insensitive with age, and the resultant increasing levels of insulin cause fat tissue to be deposited in our bodies.) Weight gain of younger animals is slowed, even if they are overfed. DHEA(S) increases the life span of these rodents (just what the world needs—longer-living rats and mice); but what if it can do the same for humans? It restrains rodents' immune system from self-attack, increases the immunity of fighter cells, and inhibits the development of breast cancer in these animals. It also helps other cells resist mutation caused by cancer-causing substances.

The question is whether these rodent studies are relevant to us. Only minute amounts of DHEA(S) are naturally produced in the adrenals of animals other than humans and nonhuman primates. We're the only species capable of synthesizing and secreting large amounts of this steroid. Does that mean we'll miss it more than rodents as we age and produce less? There are conflicting reports (as usual) as to what dwindling DHEA(S) levels do to our health and well-being. Some studies have shown that Alzheimer's victims have a 50 percent decrease of DHEA(S) levels in their blood.

Low levels of DHEA(S) in men have been correlated with their risk of developing and dying of coronary disease. These DHEA(S)-less men appear to have a diminished overall survival. This connection has not been found in women. Indeed, those with the highest natural levels of DHEA(S) seem to have the highest mortality because of cardiovascular disease.

Since there is a sexual difference in both the levels of this hormone (they are higher in men) and disease propensities (also higher in men), there might be similar differences to the response of DHEA(S) when it is used as an anti-aging drug. Indeed, initial studies seem to support this hypothesis. Men treated with a high dose (1,600 milligrams) of DHEA(S) showed improvement in their lipid profiles. When women received the same amount, they went into male hormone "shock" and resembled "sick" (heart-wise) men. They became resistant to insulin, their insulin levels increased, and this in turn caused their HDL levels to drop. Since insulin stimulates male-pattern obesity, it is not good for our hearts or our weight. These adverse effects occurred with high or pharmacologic doses of DHEA(S). What happens if we simply give lower replacement doses that are just enough to bring our levels of DHEA(S) to where they were in our twenties and thirties? Thirteen men and seventeen women, ages 40 to 70, were tested in a "proper" placebo-controlled crossover trial with nightly doses of 50 milligrams of DHEA(S). The serum levels of this hormone were "restored" to those found in young adults in just two weeks. The women had a 2-fold increase in their male hormone levels, but their HDLs declined only slightly. There was no change in their insulin sensitivity or body fat. The exciting aspect of this study was that both the men and women had a remarkable increase in their perceived physical and psychological well-being. They found that they had increased energy, better sleep, and improved mood, and were more relaxed and better able to handle stressful events. They did not report a change in their libido. These positive changes occurred in 84 percent of the women and 67 percent of the men. Both sexes were also found to have an increase in certain growth factors that could potentially spare age-related destruction of their proteins and cells.

Another study using this low dose of DHEA(S) (50 milligrams) in 11 postmenopausal women showed they had a 2-fold increase in the destructive activity of their natural killer cells. One study of 11 women is hardly sufficient to let us reach any decision, yet we know that age is accompanied by a loss of our immune competence and, as a result, we have an increase in our rate of cancer. If, indeed, DHEA(S) can help reverse this, its impact would be major.

Since the dose of 50 milligrams works but seems to double our male hormone levels, a dose of 25 milligrams may be more appropriate. We await adequate test results. Until there are controlled long-term studies on large groups of women, we need to contain our age-old excitement about age containment. It's far too early to proclaim this hormone our steroid of youth.

Hormone Replacement Regimens: Modes, Styles, and Comfort

Like fashion, hormone replacement has tremendous variation and goes in and out of "style." Physicians have become designers, and their styles of therapy (reported in the "trade" magazines and then picked up by everything from your local paper to *Vanity Fair*) go in and out of vogue. My advice is to go for the comfort factor (even if it looks like a housedress) and the understanding factor (we shouldn't need graduate training to matriculate into menopause). Unless we know why our hormones are prescribed, understand how to take them, and anticipate the unexpected (especially bleeding), we will continue our abysmal track record of noncompliance. A study of 2,500 women who were given prescriptions for HRT and followed for five years revealed that 20 to 30 percent of them never filled their prescriptions. Twenty percent discontinued therapy after nine months, and 10 percent took their hormones intermittently (these women must really have expected a little hormone to go a long way!). We are a lot more consistent in operating and servicing our home appliances than our hormones and bodies!

Here are the current "accepted" regimens and a few we're still working on. There is no general "best," but there should be one that meets the needs, schedule, and comfort level of each of us.

CYCLICAL HORMONE THERAPY

Schedule

Estrogen is taken days 1 through 25; progesterone is added for the last 10 to 14 days (either days 16 to 25, days 14 to 25, or days 12 to 25). We stop both for the next 5 days and then restart the estrogen. The easiest way to remember this is to follow the monthly calendar. Begin the estrogen on the first of the month and continue for the next 25 days. Start the progesterone on the 12th, 14th, or 16th of the month, again continuing until the 25th; then you stop both and begin the whole cycle again on the first of the next month. Now, this won't always work out exactly. On 31-day months, we are off our hormones for 6 days, and in February we are off only 3, or in a leap year, 4 days, but nothing bad will happen if we vary our number of hormone-free days. The progesterone I prescribe varies according to the patient. The doses are fairly standard: 5 to 10 milligrams of Provera or MPA, 2 to 5 milligrams of Aygestin, or 200 to 300 milligrams of micronized progesterone.

Medical Reasoning for This Regimen

We are trying to copy our previous natural cycles. Remember, when we ovulated, we put out estrogen from the time of our period for about 14 days. We then released an egg, and our ovaries produced estrogen and progesterone for two weeks. In the absence of a pregnancy, the level of both hormones abruptly fell; the endometrium was no longer hormonally supported, so it sloughed and we got our period. We have looked to this rhythmic ebb and flow of estrogen and progesterone as our model for cyclical hormonal therapy.

Positive Aspects of Cyclical HRT

We "feel" we haven't changed. We usually have our periods once a month and, for many of us, this seems natural and reassuring. If progesterone can diminish estrogen's positive effect on our lipoproteins or we don't like the way we feel on any progesterone (synthetic or natural), we are limiting the number of days of this hormone to less than half our cycle.

Negative Aspects of Cyclical HRT

We usually bleed when we cycle off. After we have gotten rid of our periods, we often resent the hassle of dealing with them again. Since so many of us use the 25th of the month to cycle off, I always imagine a run on tampons by women over 50 around the 26th or 27th of each month. I wonder if the marketing mavens or those stocking the drugstore shelves have caught on!

Our five days off all hormones may cause us to briefly restart our menopausal symptoms (hot flashes, interrupted sleep patterns, and even mood changes). Those of us who are prone to headaches may find that cycling our hormones triggers the onset of this miserable problem. If we haven't found the right progesterone, our 10 to 12 days "on" may become a monthly odyssey into PMS.

Comments

This is the most effective way of beginning HRT in early menopause. The shorter the time between our last menstrual period (normal or otherwise) and beginning HRT for menopause, the more our bodies seem to want to follow the "old routine." Cyclical hormone therapy in the first few years of menopause generally causes less breakthrough or abnormal bleeding than continuous-dose therapy. With years of use, we tend to have lighter periods and, indeed, they often disappear on cyclical therapy. Sometimes they never appear, and I have had patients call me to complain that something was wrong; they didn't bleed. We never mind not bleeding; our only concern is bleeding off schedule.

Further, a recent study has suggested that taking cyclical hormones for one cycle every three months may suffice to protect our endometrium. A higher dose of Provera was used (10 milligrams), and there were reports of heavier "periods" and some unscheduled bleeding. Despite this, the women preferred taking the estrogen just four times yearly by a ratio of 4 to 1. I would be willing to use this on patients who prefer life with minimal progesterone but would certainly want to follow them carefully with yearly ultrasounds and/or endometrial samplings.

Tips for Using Cyclical HRT

It can take three or four months until you bleed when you're supposed to and your body falls into sync. If you continue to have abnormal bleeding (during the estrogen-only part of your cycle, or when you begin the first few days of progesterone), something may be wrong, and you should notify your doctor. If after one or two months you still have hot flashes, you and your doctor can try "upping" the dose of estrogen. If hot flashes begin twelve to fourteen hours after you take your estrogen tablets, dividing the dose between morning and evening may prevent its wearing off. You can also use the estrogen patch for cyclical therapy; stick it on twice a week from days 1 to 25. Just take it off for the 5 days at the end of the cycle.

CONTINUOUS ESTROGEN WITH CYCLICAL PROGESTERONE THERAPY

Schedule

We take the estrogen every day; we never cycle off. We need progesterone for 10 to 14 days each month. (I usually tell my patients just to add the progesterone from the 1st to the 12th each month.)

Medical Reasoning Behind This Regimen

This is "almost" copying our premenopausal cycles, except we are trying to "make it better." Since so many women hate their 5 days off hormones because they become symptomatic during this hormonal hiatus, we have tried to eliminate all estrogen-deprivation "trauma."

Positive Aspects

It's a little easier to remember just to start and stop the progesterone. Our periods may be lighter or even disappear. We don't necessarily need to stop the estrogen to protect the lining of the uterus; the 10 to 14 days of progesterone seem to suffice in counteracting the estrogen's effects on the endometrial glands.

Negative Aspects

Some women feel a "relief" when they cycle off of estrogen and progesterone. They experience a loss of water weight and bloating, as well as breast sensitivity, on their 5 days off.

Comments

Wyeth-Ayerst Laboratories has packaged a product called Premphase that supplies a daily dose of 0.625 milligrams of Premarin and 14 days of Cycrin, 5 milligrams, on a card that allows us to punch out the pills at the "right" time for this type of HRT.

Tips

Again, it can take three to four months before your body gets used to this type of semicycling. After that time, you should bleed *only* when you cycle off your progesterone. If you bleed at other times, notify your doctor.

CONTINUOUS HORMONES

Schedule

We take estrogen and progesterone daily.

Medical Rationale for Continuous Hormonal Therapy

We want to protect the lining of the uterus from unopposed estrogen. What better way to do this than with daily progesterone opposition? With time, the lining "gives up"—it becomes thin, the glands become puny, and we achieve our goal of a nonactive endometrium. If the lining is atrophied, it won't slough, and we won't bleed. We return to a menopause that truly is a "pause" of our menses or periods.

Positive Aspects

Not having to deal with a period is probably the chief advantage of this therapy. A constant level of estrogen and progesterone means our bodies don't have to cope with hormonal changes each month. This may reduce menstrual or hormonal headaches, bloating, PMS, and cyclical PMS-like symptoms. The amount of progesterone we use is half the dose we use in cyclical therapy. So if we are sensitive to progesterone, the smaller dose may cause fewer side effects. On the other hand, we don't know which is, in the long run, better for our lipids, hearts, or breasts, some days of higher progesterone, or all days of lower progesterone—no studies are yet available.

Negative Aspects

Between 30 and 40 percent of us will have breakthrough bleeding, especially the first four months of therapy. The closer we are to our natural menopause, the greater our chance for this type of bleeding. It's one thing to deal with a controlled period once a month, but bleeding without warning is very disruptive.

The good news is that after a year of continuous therapy, only 10 percent of women will continue with this breakthrough bleeding.

Comments

Once more, Wyeth-Ayerst Laboratories has taken advantage of its patents for Premarin and Cycrin and has put them together in one pill, which is packaged in a punch-out card: 0.625 milligram of Premarin and 2.5 milligrams of Cycrin. This new product is called Prempro. It's our first "one pill does it all" HRT.

Whether my patients are using Prempro or another form of continuous estrogen and progesterone, if they start to bleed intermittently throughout the month, they and I get nervous. It's difficult to be a "patient" patient for three to four months, but if the bleeding is not heavy (there is no sense getting anemic over this) and there is a general sense of well-being on this hormonal regimen, I encourage my patients to continue. If, after four months, this is not successful, I investigate the bleeding (with ultrasound and, if necessary, endometrial sampling or even hysteroscopy) and switch to cyclical hormones.

Because of the high incidence of breakthrough bleeding in early menopause, I usually begin with cyclical hormonal therapy and consider switching to continuous therapy after several years. The most compelling reason to start with continuous hormones is the statement "I won't take hormones if I have to have periods again." If we get past these critical first few months, we'll all be satisfied.

Tips

Don't freak if you bleed, but if it's very heavy with clots, notify your doctor. If bleeding continues or starts after four months of therapy, again, make that call.

Try to take your hormones at the same time every day, and if you miss a day or two, don't be surprised if you begin to bleed. Don't stop; just keep taking the hormones, and the bleeding should subside.

MONDAY-THROUGH-FRIDAY "CONTINUOUS" HORMONE THERAPY

Schedule

Estrogen and progesterone in the same dosage we use for regular continuous therapy are taken Monday through Friday with a "break" on the weekend. This type of regimen was developed in California and does not seem to be as widely prescribed in the other forty-nine states.

Medical Rationale for this Therapy

This doesn't copy anything we do naturally; it may have some religious significance—we stop for the Sabbath (for some, it's on a Saturday; for others, it's on a Sunday, so we have covered all bases).

Positive Aspects

Breakthrough bleeding is less than what we encounter with daily continuous hormones. Some of us want "unmedicated" weekends (although most of us just want some much-needed rest).

Negative Aspects

We are decreasing our estrogen intake by nearly 30 percent, which could impact our protection from coronary artery disease and osteoporosis. We've traded constant hormone levels for fluctuating ones, and this can cause the onset of symptoms such as weekend hot flashes or headaches.

Comments

I use this therapy if my patients break through on daily HRT and refuse to use cyclical hormones because they don't want periods. If we go this route, I usually test their bone density and lipoproteins to make sure there is enough estrogen on board to afford osteoporosis and cardiovascular protection.

Future HRT

COMBINED PATCHES

A progesterone patch has been developed, but it is quite large. Right now, we would have to wear two patches (one estrogen and one progesterone). This might "patch up" our hormone situation, but it's inelegant and can cause more skin irritation. A single combined patch would be very helpful.

OTHER HORMONAL ROUTES: NOT THROUGH OUR MOUTH, NOT THROUGH OUR SKIN—WHERE ELSE?

Vaginal rings that look like a diaphragm have been developed to release estrogen for up to three months. An estrogen-progesterone ring would also work, and some of us might prefer it to pills and patches. Estrogen and progesterone can also be "sniffed" (no, this isn't a joke). It can be given as nose drops or by nasal spray and is well absorbed. We just have to make sure we get the doses of our sniffs and drops right. Both hormones can also be absorbed sublingually, so we might put some combined product under our tongue. And finally, pellets containing estradiol do exist and can be implanted under our skin. These deliver a steady level of estrogen for up to six months; again, a combined estrogen-progesterone pellet would make life simpler and require just a biannual trip to our doctor or qualified nurse. Any or all of these devices could also include small amounts of male hormone if we felt the need to add this to our HRT.

The hormones absorbed through vaginal rings, nasal drops, or skin pellets all have the advantage of initially bypassing the liver. This may prove to be a great advantage. One day hormone pills may seem old-fashioned. We may depend on our skin and mucous membranes (vagina, nose, or mouth) as the route of hormone therapy.

Hormone Problem Solving

This is a quick test to help clear up the complex data I have just presented. Unless we understand *why* we are using a particular method and what to expect, we stop it, and then we really fail. So here are some theoretical problems and solutions.

1. Your period stopped three months ago. You have hot flashes, and can't sleep. You are Caucasian, are thin, tend to have high cholesterol, and have a family history of heart attack. You should consider:

   a. Beginning cyclical hormonal therapy using oral estrogen and some form of progesterone.
   b. Using continuous-dose therapy with oral pills.
   c. Beginning Monday-through-Friday therapy (pills).
   d. Using the patch with cyclical progesterone.
   e. Using the patch with continuous progesterone.

ANSWER: "a"

Reason   You've just started menopause, and if you try continuous-dose hormones, you'll probably "bleed through." You want good absorption of estrogen to make sure your levels are high. The pills give you more of an absorption guarantee. Pills will also have a faster, more dependable effect on your lipids. If your cholesterol is high, or if you had a history of severe PMS, you might want to use natural progesterone.

2. You have been menopausal for a year. In some ways, this has been a blessing. You have always had severe menstrual or premenstrual headaches, and these have stopped. You have hot flashes, but they are not too bad. You would like to consider using estrogen because you are aware of the benefits to your future health. You should consider:

    a. Using cyclical oral estrogen and progesterone.
    b. Using cyclical patch and progesterone.
    c. Using Monday-through-Friday oral estrogen and progesterone.
    d. Using continuous oral estrogen and progesterone.
    e. Using continuous estrogen patch and progesterone.

ANSWER: "e"

Reason   The ups and downs (especially the downs) of estrogen and cyclical therapy may trigger your headaches. The blood level of estrogen stays a bit more constant with the patch (the pill's estrogen peaks and falls fourteen to eighteen hours after we take it). Not cycling progesterone may also diminish headaches. If a headache does occur, switch from synthetic to natural progesterone (or just start with this).

3. You started continuous-dose HRT as soon as you were told you were menopausal. You've been on this therapy for nine months and still bleed on and off and can't go anywhere without a tampon. You should consider:

    a. Switching to cyclical hormones.
    b. Going off HRT and forgetting the whole thing.
    c. Increasing your dose of estrogen.

  d. Increasing your dose of progesterone.

  e. Getting a pelvic ultrasound and/or endometrial sampling.

ANSWER: "e"

Reason We expect bleeding for the first four months, or perhaps even the first six months. Bleeding for nine months is too long. If evaluation shows that you have no polyps, fibroids, or abnormal hyperplasia, then try switching to cyclical hormones and at least get a defined period once a month. Give this a year or more, and if you have no abnormal bleeding, you can then try continuous-dose hormones.

4. You take cyclical hormone therapy and always bleed 2 or 3 days before you finish the hormones and cycle off for five days. You should consider:

  a. Stopping your hormones, because something is wrong.

  b. Stopping the progesterone and estrogen as soon as you start to bleed.

  c. Seeing your doctor to have your uterine lining checked with ultrasound or endometrial sampling.

  d. Doubling your progesterone the day before you bleed and continuing this double dose until the end of the cycle.

  e. Ignoring it if the bleeding is slight.

ANSWER: "c" followed by "d," or "c" followed by "e"

Reason We thought we could ignore breakthrough bleeding on the progesterone part of our cycle, but some studies have shown there can be a problem. You might also have a polyp or fibroid, so a workup is warranted. If nothing is found to be wrong, you can double the progesterone; this may stop the bleeding. Or you can just ignore it but finish the cycle.

5. You are on cyclical hormonal therapy. You hate your 5 days off. You have cramps and hot flashes, can't sleep, and get depressed. Your husband tends to plan business trips between the 25th and 30th of each month. You should consider:

a. Taking continuous-dose estrogen and cyclical progesterone.
b. Insisting on traveling with your husband.
c. Eliminating your progesterone.
d. Using continuous-dose estrogen and progesterone.
e. Using Monday-through-Friday estrogen and progesterone.

ANSWER: "a" and "b," or "d" and "b"

Reason   Cycling off the estrogen is probably causing your deprivation symptoms. If you take it continuously, you'll be happier and probably have easier periods, and your husband (and everyone else) will want to be around you. If you choose "d" and take both hormones continuously, you might succeed in stopping all bleeding and cramps.

6. You use cyclical hormones, and when you begin synthetic progesterone for 10 or 12 days, you bloat, get breast tenderness and hot flashes, and generally have a return of your former PMS. You should consider:

a. Switching from cyclical to continuous-dose therapy (which means taking a lower dose of progesterone every day).
b. Stopping progesterone.
c. Switching from synthetic progesterone to natural progesterone.
d. Increasing the estrogen to "cover" for the hot flashes.
e. Taking progesterone every three months.

ANSWER: Try "c" first, then consider "e" or "a"

Reason   Natural progesterone seems to cause fewer PMS symptoms. If, however, the symptoms are still there and you promise to get good follow-up, you can decrease your progesterone term of sentence and take it every three months. A trial of the mini-pill (continuously) and estrogen might also succeed.

7. You're 60, have never been on hormones, and feel you are "over" the menopause. You recently had a bone-density, scan, which demonstrated that you've lost a considerable amount of the bone mass in your hip. You've had a hysterectomy. You should consider:

   a. Increasing your calcium to at least 1,500 milligrams a day, taking vitamin D, and doing weight-bearing and weight-resistance exercise.
   b. Beginning estrogen replacement with the pill or patch.
   c. Taking estrogen and progesterone continuously.
   d. Taking cyclical estrogen and progesterone.
   e. Being careful not to fall.

   ANSWER: "a," "b," and "e"

   Reason   You always need your calcium, vitamin D, and weight-bearing exercise. But to build up bone density and achieve a better-than-50-percent decrease in your future potential for a fracture, you should consider estrogen. Since your uterus is out, you don't need progesterone.

8. You take your hormone pills (estrogen and progesterone) religiously every morning. You're still having hot flashes, but only at night. You should consider:

   a. Taking a higher dose of progesterone.
   b. Taking a higher dose of estrogen.
   c. Taking your hormone pills at night.
   d. Switching to the patch.
   e. Switching from synthetic to natural progesterone.

   ANSWER: "c," and if that doesn't work, try "b" or "d"

   Reason   The pill gives you peak blood levels two to three hours after you take it; these levels decrease after fourteen to sixteen hours. If you take a tablet at night, the level will be good while you sleep. If, however, you then get daytime symptoms, you can try dividing the dose or increasing the total amount and then take one pill in the morning and one at night. If you don't want to increase the dose, you can try using the patch, which gives a more even release of estrogen.

9. You've been menopausal for nearly a year. You've tried all the estrogens—Premarin, Ogen, Estrace, and the patch. You've used high doses. You still have hot flashes, sleep poorly, and haven't gotten back your premenopausal "zest." You should consider:

   a. Switching from synthetic progesterone to natural progesterone.
   b. Psychotherapy.
   c. Using higher-than-normal estrogen doses.
   d. Having your thyroid function tested.
   e. Adding testosterone to your HRT regimen.

   ANSWER: "d" and "e"

   Reason   Hypothyroidism can overcome "usual hormone" relief and should be checked if your response is not what you expect. Adding male hormone as a pill or shot may diminish recalcitrant symptoms and enhance your sense of well-being.

10. You're going to begin HRT. You have a uterus. Your cholesterol is high, your LDL high, and your HDL low, but your triglyceride level is normal. Your choice of hormones should be:

    a. Oral estrogen pills and synthetic progesterone.
    b. Oral estrogen pills and natural progesterone.
    c. The patch and a synthetic progesterone.
    d. The patch and natural progesterone.
    e. Oral estrogen only.

    ANSWER: "b"

    Reason   Oral estrogen has a more immediate and pronounced effect on your lipid profile and, according to the PEPI study, natural progesterone does less to oppose this effect than synthetic progesterone.

11. You're menopausal and have very high triglycerides. The rest of your lipid profile is only slightly "off." You've had a hysterectomy. Your choice of hormones should be:

    a. Oral estrogen and synthetic progesterone.
    b. The patch and synthetic progesterone.

c. Oral estrogen alone.
d. The patch alone.

ANSWER: "d"

Reason   Oral estrogen may increase triglycerides; the patch does not. You don't need progesterone because you've had a hysterectomy.

12. You've had breast cancer, which was treated with surgery followed by chemotherapy. You are currently on tamoxifen. You can deal with the hot flashes, but sex has become so uncomfortable (even with lubricants) that you avoid it. You should consider:

   a. Finding other forms of intimacy.
   b. Going off the tamoxifen.
   c. Using male hormones.
   d. Using systemic estrogen therapy (pills or patch).
   e. Using estrogen vaginal cream.

ANSWER: "e" if you don't want to resort to "a"

Reason   Local estrogen cream will help prevent vaginal atrophy. Small amounts of relatively weak cream such as Estrace might suffice, resulting in very little absorption and probably no effect on the recurrence rate of breast cancer. (*Note:* We're not even sure that normal systemic doses of ERT have an effect on the recurrence rate of cancer.) You will, however, have some absorption, and you should discuss this with your cancer specialist.

13. You had breast cancer over four years ago, and you've been miserable ever since. You still have hot flashes and can't sleep, and to add future worry to current symptoms, there is a strong family history of osteoporosis and heart attack. Your blood pressure is up, and your cholesterol is high. Tamoxifen makes your symptoms worse. You should consider:

   a. Continuing to suffer, because hot flashes won't kill you.

b. Taking calcium, vitamins, anti-osteoporosis medications, and therapy to lower your blood pressure and cholesterol.
c. Taking high-dose progesterone (Megace) to stop the hot flashes and help prevent osteoporosis.
d. Taking male hormone.
e. Using estrogen replacement therapy with or without tamoxifen.

ANSWER: This isn't an easy one, and if you're stumped, don't worry—so are the doctors. Option "b" is definitely acceptable; "c" is partially okay; "e" will definitely help, but you and your doctor have to be willing to check it out.

Reason The combination listed in "b" will decrease your risk of future disease but won't make you feel better. Tamoxifen may help prevent heart attack and osteoporosis, but you can only take it for five years. Megace helps with hot flashes and osteoporosis, but it may have a negative effect on your lipids Estrogen will make you feel better and decrease your risk of bone fracture and heart attack. The big question is, What will it do to your risk of breast cancer? Despite all of our studies, no one knows for sure. But we do know that saving you from breast cancer so that ten years down the line you can die of a heart attack does not constitute a "cure."

14. You've had a heart attack and are now recovering. You should consider:
a. Beginning a cardiac rehabilitation exercise program.
b. Eating a low-fat diet.
c. Stopping smoking.
d. Taking low doses of aspirin daily.
e. Beginning estrogen replacement therapy.

ANSWER: All of the above

Reason "A" through "d" are obvious; "e" will help reduce your future cardiac risk.

15. You're menopausal, feel great, and have no risk factors (everyone in your family has lived into their eighties and nineties). You should consider:

a. Doing nothing and counting on your genes.
b. Using HRT to play it safe.
c. Following your bone-density and cardiac health with appropriate tests. If they show deterioration, consider HRT.
d. Exercising, taking calcium and vitamins, and feeling blessed.
e. Telling your friends to stop complaining—menopause is a breeze.

ANSWER: "c" and "d"; "b" can also be considered.

Reason You can't always count on your genes. Your ancestors may have eaten better, exercised more, and been heartier than you. So follow your heart (in this instance, not romantically) and your bones to make sure they work well for you into *your* eighties and nineties.

8

ALTERNATIVES TO HORMONES

Most of us just don't, or won't, take hormones. Depending where we live and the prevailing hormonal climate, only 15 percent (the South and Midwest) to 32 percent (California) of menopausal women are using hormone replacement therapy. The nonusers make up a very large and ignored silent majority. Funding, research, and scientific trials have not focused on alternative or complementary therapies that would offer women beneficial ways to relieve their symptoms and manage their health.

Medications that can help alleviate hot flashes have been developed for other reasons (mostly high blood pressure) and have only incidentally been found to keep us cool and dry. They may also dry us up and keep us sedated. There are therapies other than hormones that help prevent or reverse osteoporosis and coronary heart disease. Some, like aspirin, have been proven effective in extensive trials, but only in men. Others are not routinely prescribed until we are really sick.

Because pharmaceutical companies can't patent a natural herb unless they add something to it or resynthesize it, they have little financial incentive to carry out herbal research. (Let's not kid ourselves; there's an economic side to scientific studies.) Vitamins and minerals can be repackaged and sold for specific purposes (vitamins for women over 50, women with silver hair, women who are active or want to be more

active), but these are not under the jurisdiction of the FDA and, consequently, there is no need to provide controlled studies to back up "success" stories.

"Orthodox" is a term I've always associated with religious beliefs,
but it certainly describes the fanaticism with which "orthodox" medicine
demands scientific proof of a therapy. This has led to a dismissal of hundreds, or even thousands, of years of experience with the use of natural
or alternative therapies by cultures and civilizations who, believe it or
not, may have the same symptoms and medical diseases we believe to be
our own.

I've been trained in "orthodox" medicine and expect to have proof
that a therapy works. That proof is usually a double-blind crossover
study. To perform this, a tested substance and placebo are given to two
similar groups. Both the subjects and the researchers are "blind"; no one
knows what the subjects are taking. Halfway through the test period, the
therapy and placebo are switched; the responses are evaluated, and only
then are the researchers unblinded to the results. Yet, lack of double-
blind studies should not blind us to the possibility that something may
work. We want to know about all options, so I've attempted to list what
is known by the "orthodox" and the "nonbelievers." Knowing does not
equate with proof. The danger in being so committed to that which each
of us "knows" is that we ignore the proof offered by the other side. I
would hope that as we individually make health-care decisions, we rely
on the knowledge and advice of appropriate caregivers in every disci-
pline rather than on superstition, unfounded pragmatism, or ignorance.

Treatment of Hot Flashes: Cooling Down Without Hormones

MEDICAL THERAPIES

Hot flashes seem to be instigated by an increased sensitivity of the temperature control center in our brain when it is deprived of estrogen. The
hyperactivity of this center is mediated from a neuronal point of view by
noradrenergic substances. If we can lower the center's activation thresh-
old with anti-noradrenergic medications, we should decrease hot flashes.
The following medications have been used for this purpose:

Clonidine This is an adrenergic agonist that was developed to treat high blood pressure. The term "agonist" means it's similar to the "real thing" and sits on the receptors, preventing the "real thing" from doing its thing—in this case, transmitting information between nerves. Clonidine reduces the reactivity of our blood vessels and lowers the noradrenergic activity of our central nervous system. It also decreases the brain's production of norepinephrine, which is probably one of the principal substances that transmit and activate the hot flash signals. It can be taken orally or applied through the skin with a patch. In a recent double-blind study (the magic word for medical purists) of 116 women, Clonidine reduced hot flash frequency by 45 percent. But this was only 20 percent better than the improvement they felt with a placebo. The placebo effect is very important and points out the problem of touting the initial success of any therapy. Twenty-five percent of women said their hot flashes diminished with the patch that had no medication! Other studies have shown that placebos can work in the short run for 40 percent of us because we know something is being done, and consequently allow ourselves to relax and feel comforted. This increases our internal production of natural opiates, which calm down our central nervous system. (We're not fooled into feeling better—we're relaxed into it.)

The study also showed a significant rate of side effects for the medicated patch that included dry mouth, constipation, drowsiness, and dizziness. Women with normal blood pressure tend to have a greater adverse reaction to this medication than hypertensive women. They can develop a drop in blood pressure when standing and even faint. A 20 percent gain in hot flash control might not be worth these side effects. If, however, we are hypertensive and have hot flashes, this drug can manage both problems.

Aldomet (Methyldopa) This, too, is an adrenergic agonist and is used to control high blood pressure. Large doses cause about a 40 percent reduction in hot flashes, but 60 percent of women experience dizziness, nausea, and fatigue.

Bellergal This has been the physician "standard" of nonhormonal medical therapy for those of us who suffer from hot flashes, night sweats, insomnia, and restlessness. The only drug that is currently FDA-approved for these menopausal symptoms, it is composed of three med-ications. One is an ergot compound that causes muscles and blood ves-sels to contract (preventing the dilation of our skin vessels that causes the flush). Because of this action, it should not be used by women with high blood pressure or coronary heart disease. A second component, phenobarbital, relaxes us and, indeed, causes sleepiness. In this way, it may diminish the hyperactivity of the brain in general and its thermostat in particular. This component can make Bellergal addictive. The third medication is belladonna, which inhibits a part of the nervous system and can cause decreased salivation and dilated pupils. Based on these ac-tions, the side effects of Bellergal—dry mouth, dizziness, and sleepi-ness—are not surprising. These vary from woman to woman but might be tolerable if the medication works. In a study of 66 women with signif-icant hot flashes and insomnia, more than 50 percent reported that their symptoms improved after four weeks of Bellergal therapy, but 21 percent felt the same degree of improvement with placebo. By eight to twelve weeks, the relief quotient was similar for both groups! Should we pre-scribe the drug or the placebo?

VITAMINS

Vitamin E   Studies in the 1940s (yes, they were double-blind, but they included only 66 patients) indicated that vitamin E helped relieve hot flashes and vaginal dryness. Another study in 1953 (this time on 83 women) showed that E was no more effective than placebo. Both of these trials used fairly low doses of vitamin E, just 50 to 100 interna-tional units daily. We have made very little E progress (with respect to hot flashes) over the last forty years. However, without the double-blind component, we do have surveys of hundreds of menopausal women who indicate that they have experienced hot flash relief after 800 units of vit-amin E daily and that they were hot flash–free when they added 2 to 3 grams of vitamin C and one gram of calcium in divided doses. Once their hot flashes subsided, they found they could reduce the dose of vita-min E to 400 units. I suggest vitamin E supplementation to my patients, since there may be an added benefit of antioxidant activity, which could reduce their chances of developing heart disease and cancer. (I take 400 units daily.)

Hesperidin and Vitamin C   Hesperidin is a bioflavonoid found in citrus fruit. Its chemical structure actually resembles that of estradiol. A study from the 1960s found that when 900 milligrams of hesperidin and 300 milligrams of hesperidin methylcalsone (another citrus flavonoid) were taken daily in combination with 1,200 milligrams of vitamin C, 53 percent of women stopped having hot flashes and 34 percent had less frequent and less severe flashes after one month. They also had fewer leg cramps, nosebleeds, and less bruising. Their only complaints were a new, unpleasant body odor and discoloration of clothing from perspiration. If we try these vitamins, we should stock up on antiperspirant and perfume.

CHINESE AND WESTERN HERBS

I didn't study herbs in medical school, and during my residency, the closest I ever came to herbs was in the hospital cafeteria (if we count parsley). But experience in life (and medicine) prompts us to take note of the experience of others, and Chinese herbal medicine has been "experienced" for five thousand years.

We've all heard about the Chinese concept of yin and yang, the two opposite yet complementary energies that are present throughout the universe. Yin is feminine and felt to be dark, cold, heavy, and still (I'm not sure I would consider these feminine attributes). Yang is masculine and considered to be lightweight and mobile ("flighty" might be a good term). A fever or hot flash would be yang; a chill, yin. Chinese medicine also divides the human body into five elements, or energies. Each is associated with one of five main organs: the lungs, kidneys, liver, heart, and spleen. Our other organs are categorized under one of these five. Our reproductive organs and adrenals are included under the function of the kidney.

Qi is the vital energy in the body; it circulates between the different organs and also at the surface of the body in the acupuncture channels. As Qi flows from one organ to another, it supplies energy. It goes from the lung to the kidney to the liver to the heart to the spleen, and then back to the lung. So if one organ is off, the energy to other organs is affected, and they may malfunction. According to this theory, menopause is a kidney-yin deficiency. (Kidney controls or encompasses the ovaries and uterus; we're missing yin, which is feminine.) Since the kidney is low on yin and it supplies the liver, this organ likewise becomes yin-deficient. Yin and yang oppose and balance. We can now develop an excess of yang energy. This energy is hot and mobile, so how does it manifest itself? You guessed it—as hot flashes. A deficiency of yin is also felt to cause insomnia and dream-disturbed sleep (and thousands of years ago, the Chinese had no way of measuring REM sleep!). As our liver yang rises, so do our emotions (the Chinese associate anger with the liver), and we may become irritable. This increase in anger can cause the liver Qi to stagnate, causing distention, bloating, and emotional outbursts—sound familiar?

Chinese herbs are used as tonics for a particular deficiency. The herb *Rehmannia glutinosa* (called shu di huang) is the main yin tonic. It is usually given in combination with other herbs to increase its potency and decrease side effects. Yin tonic herbs of Rehmannia with six other herbs (I'll spare us the list) is called Rehmannia-6 Formula. It's supposed to decrease nervous system excitation and regulate hormonal function. If two sedative herbs are added, it's called 8-Flavor Tea. When night sweats are a major problem, a yin tonic of Rehmannia and three other herbs called da bu yin wan is suggested. Severe hot flashes, headaches, and irritability are believed to arise from increased liver yang, and the Chinese prescribe herbs of chrysanthemum and lycie (Qi jeu di huang wan). If menopausal symptoms are mainly anger (I question this symptom), irritability, and sore breasts, this is considered liver Qi stagnation, and the herb chai hu (hare's ear) is prescribed. Lack of libido is a lack of energy, or coldness, and is considered to be a kidney yang deficiency. Rehmannia is combined with dodder to increase yang energy (you gui wan). If the heart and kidney don't communicate their energy, it's believed that we can develop insomnia, nervousness, and palpitations. Emperor Tea, which is again made from Rehmannia, is supposed to correct this energy imbalance.

Finally, I'll mention the two Chinese herbs that many of us have heard about, ginseng and dong quai (Chinese angelica). When combined in a tonic called gui pi tang, they are supposed to soothe the nerves, nourish the heart, and increase energy in the spleen. Ginseng has some estrogenic properties; when used in excessive amounts or by "susceptible" women, it may cause abnormal bleeding or even ovarian cysts. It is used by the Chinese to treat everything from menstrual disorders to depression, insomnia, anemia, asthma, nervous disorders, sexual dysfunction, and general old age. Dong quai is also called "woman's ginseng" and is used to treat menstrual cramps, menstrual irregularities, and hot flashes. It is a phyto-estrogen, which means it comes from a plant with estrogenic activity. Phyto-estrogens have less than 2 percent of the estrogen potency of synthetic or natural estrogens in birth control pills or hormone replacement therapy. It is believed that if our own estrogenic activity is low, the phyto-estrogens add to what's missing. If it's high, these plant estrogens may sit on the estrogen receptors and compete with the body's estrogen. Based on this theory, phyto-estrogens can decrease (or balance) any excess hormonal effects. So the same plant may be recommended for estrogen excess and estrogen deficiency. There are a number of phyto-estrogen herbs commonly used to treat hot flashes. They have been used for hundreds and even thousands of years by both Western and Chinese cultures with reported (but not double-blind) success. I will pass on these reports but, once more, I don't have scientific data to satisfy the "orthodox."

Western Herbs

Licorice Root   This has been used by Western and Eastern cultures for thousands of years. It is used in the treatment of PMS and is supposed to affect the ratio of estrogen to progesterone. It is also said to alleviate menopausal symptoms through its estrogenlike activity.

Chasteberry   This is found in Mediterranean regions and, as the descriptive name would suggest, has been used to suppress libido. Chasteberry has been shown to affect pituitary function and may help relieve hot flashes by diminishing LH and FSH secretion.

Black Cohosh or Squaw Root   This was used by Native Americans to relieve menstrual cramps and menstrual symptoms. It has relaxant properties and may affect uterine contractions so that heavy bleeding is decreased. This herb is also believed to contain substances that act as pain relievers and sedatives. It has been shown to have an estrogenic effect and can cause a decrease in FSH levels; this may help diminish hot flashes and even improve vaginal atrophy.

Red Sage   This is a phytoestrogen that has been used to diminish menopausal symptoms.

False Unicorn Root (Helonias) This was used by Native Americans as a female tonic. When ingested, it is metabolized into weak estrogen compounds.

I am not an herb expert; I have obtained this information from several books and articles written by nutritionists, natural medicine doctors, and herbologists. Herbs can have serious side effects, which may even include miscarriage or death. The "safest" and most effective way to go the herbal route is to refer to books written by recognized authorities and/or consult with an expert in herbal or Chinese medicine. If the herbs work, there may be a placebo component, but this also occurs with our Western, nonhormonal medications (and these are regularly prescribed and considered medically kosher). Who's to say we shouldn't give herbs a similar chance?

HOMEOPATHY

This alternative medicine is based on the principle that like is cured by like. If we have symptoms similar to those caused by toxicity from a substance, we can use an extreme dilution of that substance to treat the problem. The degree of dilution (called *potentization*) is believed to increase the potency of the substance. Remedies used for menopausal symptoms depend on an overview of our body type and symptoms. Here are some of the more commonly used homeopathic remedies.

Sepia This is made from the ink of a cuttlefish. Friedrich Hahnemann, the father of homeopathic medicine, noted that one of his patients became ill, lost weight, and had no energy after licking his paintbrush to get a better point. The paintbrush had been dipped in sepia. When the artist was treated with extremely diluted sepia (the potentized form), he recovered. So if we manifest "sepia" qualities—that is, we are thin and irritable and feel worn out—the homeopathic therapy of choice would be sepia.

Pulsatilla This is prepared from the windflower and is used in Western herbalism as a sedative. It is prescribed for menopausal women who are the "pulsatilla" type—fair, blue-eyed, emotionally labile, weepy, and who tend to feel chilled.

Agnus Castus (Chasteberry) This is used in undiluted concentration in Western herbalism. In homeopathy, it is prescribed for loss of memory, anxiety, headaches, and flabby muscles.

Sage (Salvia) This is used for hot flashes.

Lachesis This is the poisonous venom of the bushmaster snake, but once diluted for homeopathic use, it has no toxic effects. It is prescribed for hot flashes, palpitations, and headaches.

Glyceryl Trinitrate and Amyl Nitrate These are "conventional" drugs that, when diluted, are used homeopathically to treat hot flashes, headaches, and palpitations.

Sulfur This is said to help hot flashes in women who tend to be messy and heavy, and consume a sweet or fatty diet.

Potassium Carbonate This is used for early-morning hot flashes and the affliction of not remembering or mixing up words (we do this all, no?).

Metallic Gold This is given for hot flashes, especially if they occur in depressed women with suicidal thoughts.

Belladonna This is a component of Bellergal and, in extreme dilutions, is used to combat redness, congestion, and sweating with facial hot flashes.

Bryonia This is prescribed to help treat vaginal dryness and atrophy.

Calcium Carbonate Made from crushed oyster shells, this is also used to treat hot flashes and water retention in overweight women.

There are many other remedies that are prescribed according to a woman's overall characteristics. Reticent, nervous women who crave salt may respond to **sodium chloride.** Anxious, irritable women who don't sleep well and overeat or drink are treated with **nux vomica.** The list goes on and, again, should only be suggested and prescribed by a trained homeopathic practitioner.

BEHAVIORAL TREATMENT OF HOT FLASHES

Who says we have to *take* something (even if it's "alternative") to treat our hot flashes? Maybe we should consider *doing* something. If our temperature control system is overactive, perhaps certain relaxation techniques can deactivate it—a sort of calmness of mind prevailing over body flushing and sweating. Slow, deep breathing may be one of these controlled actions.

In one study, 14 women were taught, over a twelve-week period, techniques of paced respiration, (taking 6 to 8 breaths a minute using their abdominal muscles) or were trained in relaxation techniques, using biofeedback from their recorded brain activity. Those who learned to pace their breathing reported that their hot flashes decreased by 50 percent. Those using biofeedback noted little change. These women were also hooked up to monitors that measured their skin temperatures for twenty-four hours before and after their training (an objective way to document hot flashes). Those who learned paced respiration demonstrated significantly fewer temperature spurts than the biofeedback group. A second study, of 24 postmenopausal women, gave similar results. This type of slow deep breathing is a component of yoga and meditation. Once more, we as Westerners with our fancy temperature monitors are verifying the effectiveness of Eastern practices.

Exercise

Can we exercise our hot flashes away? According to a Scandinavian study, we can. Over 1,300 women between the ages of 50 and 58 who lived in the same community were questioned. Those who belonged to a local gymnastics club with fitness classes (142) and exercised an average of three hours a week had significantly fewer hot flashes than those who were physically inactive. Only one active woman (6 percent) regarded her symptoms as severe, whereas 25 percent of the "couch potatoes" regarded their symptoms as severe, and 75 percent as moderate. We know that exercise increases the natural opioids (also known as *endorphins*) in our brain. Decrease of our central opioid activity may provoke hot flashes. The more we raise our opioids with exercise, the less we flush.

We are also increasing our general well-being and reducing muscle tension, anxiety, and insomnia, and I haven't even mentioned what exercise does for our hearts, muscles, bones, and, of course, weight!

Acupuncture

This technique is based on the Chinese concept of Qi energy, which flows in surface channels or meridians from one organ to another. If this energy becomes imbalanced, we develop symptoms. Fine needles inserted into specific points in these channels are supposed to restore the energy flow and balance and thus relieve these symptoms. In more scientific terms, it would appear that acupuncture points have different electrical resistance from other areas of our skin and that acupuncture therapy has an electrical basis. It's been shown to raise our nervous system's endorphins both centrally (in the brain) and peripherally (in the nerves in the rest of our body). These endorphins diminish pain, cause sedation, and increase our sense of well-being. With these effects, it's not surprising that some studies have shown that acupuncture can decrease the frequency of hot flashes (although I would imagine that controlling for a placebo effect is very difficult).

Diet

We know how to eliminate the negative—the foods we should not consume in order to diminish hot flashes. These include caffeine, alcohol, spicy foods, hot drinks, and possibly sugar. But how do we accentuate the positive? Can we eat our way out of menopausal symptoms?

To answer this question, we have to look at the diets of women who presumably have fewer symptoms. Once more we're given the example of Japanese women, who, according to a 1988 study of 1,141 women between the ages of 45 and 55, have far fewer hot flashes than Western women. Japanese physicians and women call menopause *konenki* and menopausal symptoms are *konenki shogai*, which they (especially the doctors) feel is a luxury disease of post–World War II urban housewives who have too much leisure time. Symptoms of *konenki shogai* are given a negative moral connotation. Clearly, anthropologic problems are a factor in symptom comparisons, but in this study, if symptoms did occur, they took the form of stiff shoulders, headache, backache, chills, irritability, and insomnia. Only 1 percent of women complained of having "rush of blood to the head." A group of Helsinki scientists looked at the phyto-estrogen consumption of Japanese women and men who consumed a traditional low-fat diet. They found that they excreted 1,000-fold more phyto-estrogens in their urine than those seen in the urine of "normal" omnivorous women consuming a Western diet. They concluded that this urinary excretion of phyto-estrogens was associated with their intake of soy products such as tofu, miso, soybeans, and boiled beans. These high levels of phyto-estrogens may partially explain why hot flashes and other menopausal symptoms are infrequent in Japanese women.

So "oy," can we "soy" our way out of hot flashes? (Sorry, I just had to do that!) Although the soybean plant is native to China, the United States is now its major grower, accounting for 50 percent of the world's production. Unfortunately, we don't eat our own soy, our animals do (it's a major protein added to their feed). We also export it in large quantities to other "phyto-estrogen-smarter" populations. Soy products contain the phyto-estrogen genistein, which has been shown to lower total cholesterol, raise HDLs, and lower LDLs in female monkeys and, more recently (thank goodness, we're included), in women. So in addition to feeling better, we may live longer as a result of diminished coronary artery disease. This same substance may also have a beneficial effect on our risk of breast cancer.

So how much soy do we need to add to our Western diet? And is adding sufficient, or do we need to concomitantly subtract animal protein and fat? A recent study on genistein's effect on lipid factors tested 80 grams of powdered genistein mixed in fluid twice daily. Higher doses caused bloating and abdominal discomfort. If we use Asian eating habits as our guide, it seems that only 20 grams of traditional soy foods a day will give us a phyto-estrogen edge on menopausal symptoms. "Doses" of 25 to 50 grams of soy protein (used instead of animal protein) have been found in over thirty studies on women and men to lower cholesterol and LDL cholesterol significantly. We can use soy flour instead of wheat flour for baking (breads, bagels, pancakes, etc.). Soy milk made from whole soybeans can be used in desserts and flavored drinks (chocolate soy milk tastes pretty good!). Tofu is made by adding calcium or magnesium salts to soy milk and can be substituted for cheese (and will help lower our cholesterol consumption). It can be added to sauces, casseroles, and soups, or used in vegetable stir-fries. We can also purchase frozen soybeans, boil them for five minutes, salt them, and pop them open like peas—they make a tasty snack. Dried soybeans and soy nuts are also available.

At least three hundred plants contain phyto-estrogens. They may not give as potent an estrogen punch as soy, but they help (it's not easy for most of us to switch to a traditional Japanese diet). These include fruits such as apples, cherries, and pomegranates; grains such as alfalfa, barley, hops, oats, rice, and wheat; and vegetables such as Mexican yams, peas, potatoes, green beans, red beans, and sprouts. Fennel, garlic, parsley, and sesame seeds are included in this plant estrogen list. The message is to get fruits and vegetables in and sugar, fat, and probably meat out. This not only may have an effect on our menopausal symptoms, but will help us combat cancer, heart disease, and obesity.

ANOTHER ALTERNATIVE: NONPRESCRIPTION PROGESTERONE CREAMS

Pro-Gest is a progesterone cream made from the Mexican wild yam; it requires no prescription and is classified as cosmetic or herbal (and not under FDA jurisdiction). It is purported to help PMS and menopausal symptoms. Pro-Gest is manufactured by Professional and Technical Services in Portland, Oregon. A physician in Sebastopol, California, claims he had 100 of his patients between the ages of 38 and 83 apply it daily for more than three years. After three months, they reported an improved sense of well-being and over three years, their "weight was stabilized, aches and pains diminished, mobility and energy levels rose, and normal libido (sex drive) returned and no side effects emerged." He also reported that their bone density increased by 15 percent after three years. This is not a double-blind study, the numbers are small, and the results have not been published in an "established" or peer-reviewed journal, so it doesn't qualify for our medical "social register." Documented testing could open a lot of doors, not to mention medicine cabinets.

IT'S OUR CHOICE

We don't have to deal with early or late menopausal symptoms by default. It's our fault if we decide on a course of nonaction once we've decided we don't want the "action" of hormone replacement therapy. The options are out there. Some have benefits that have withstood the test of "orthodox" medical analysis. Others have been used for generations—

even millennia—and have withstood the test of time. Newer approaches are not always off the wall, and many merit serious consideration. But they also deserve appropriate testing; if they work, we all want to know.

Over the years, we've had ample opportunities to assume that sit-com role of the silent suffering woman—for the good of our children, our families, and even mankind (especially if that meant men who were kind). We do not have to assume this role when dealing with menopausal symptoms. Let's seek out the alternatives!

III

....

Health Concerns
After 40
We Are More Than
Our Reproductive Organs

Medically speaking, are we defined as the sum total of our reproductive organs? Once their functions diminish and our bodies no longer prepare for ovulation, childbearing, and lactation, how are we perceived by gynecologists or our primary health-care providers? Unfortunately, there are many physicians whose lack of interest in women over 40 mirrors the neglect and even blatant bias that has long colored medical research, drug trials, development of high-tech surgical procedures, and project funding.

A sad example: the Physicians' Health Study, supported by grants from the National Institutes of Health, which took place from 1983 to 1988, and included 22,000 men aged 40 to 84. Before the study was scheduled to conclude, researchers determined that those who regularly took aspirin had a 44 percent reduction in their rate of heart attack. At that point the researchers stopped the study and recommended that men in this age group use prophylactic (preventive therapy) aspirin under their physicians' guidance. This was an important, historic study with findings that would save thousands of lives each year. Yet not one woman was included in this study! A shocking fact, especially when you realize that heart attack is our number-one killer.

Regrettably, we cannot simply take this or any data derived by studying men and apply it to women. There is a very real gender difference in the way our bodies react to drugs. Our stomachs empty more slowly and have less acid to break down certain substances, so absorption varies. Fluid passes through our kidneys more slowly, so that drugs excreted in our urine will accumulate at higher levels. We also have lower levels of certain liver enzymes that break down or detoxify medications. Finally, we have a greater brain blood flow than men. Now, this last fact doesn't surprise me, but before we get a brain perfusion superiority complex, we have to acknowledge that even this difference is worrisome, since it means that we are more sensitive to medications. Indeed, women have a 25 percent higher rate of adverse drug reactions than men.

The medical and research establishments have overlooked us for too long. Finally, we have started to raise our collective, majority voice and demand change. Congress, the Federal Drug Administration, the National Institutes of Health, and yes, even our own doctors, have begun to listen. The NIH Reauthorization Bill of 1993 mandates that women and minorities must be included in federally funded research projects. But exceptions are the rule and many studies have requested that women or minorities be excluded, because they present too many variables, risks (especially pregnancy), and irrelevant factors!

Perhaps we can look forward to getting some of the answers we so desperately need, in studies specifically geared to women. The Women's Health Initiative, created in 1992, will follow 163,000 women for nine to fourteen years and help determine how hormones, calcium, vitamin D, low-fat diets, or just "benign neglect" (the control group) impact on our incidence of heart attack, stroke, cancer of the breast, colon, and uterus, osteoporosis, and longevity. It will be funded with $600 million of our tax money. It's about time!

Granted, we have much less information about the effects of major diseases on women than men, but that doesn't mean we should simply sit around and passively wait decades for data that specifically apply to us. We should at least learn what we can and make educated guesses about the lifestyle changes that can help protect our health. We also need to champion the allocation of funds for research that will begin to give us female medical parity.

In Part III, I survey the most important health threats to women, so that we can familiarize ourselves with our personal risks, prevention options, and possible treatments.

9

HEART ATTACK
Not Just a Male Disease

Our Number-One Killer

In our forties, we watch our male counterparts worry about and, indeed, suffer and die from heart attacks. While arming ourselves with low-cholesterol cookbooks, exercise machines, and CPR courses—for the men in our lives—we take our own cardiac health for granted. That's a mistake. Our lifetime probability of dying of a heart attack is 31 percent. This means that we are ten times more likely to die of a heart attack than from breast cancer or from the sum total of all of the other cancers of our reproductive organs (uterus, cervix, and ovaries)—grim proof that neither our lives nor our deaths should be defined by our reproductive parts.

In the United States, 2.5 million women are hospitalized each year for heart disease. Five hundred thousand die. Heart attack accounts for 60 percent of sudden deaths in women, most occurring without prior warning. Once we suffer a heart attack we are twice as likely to die as men. To further invalidate our conception that this is a "male" disease, consider that, as of 1990, more women in this country died from heart attacks than men.

MY HEART DOES NOT BELONG TO DADDY

The only way we can improve these disheartening statistics is by reeducating our health-care providers and, even more importantly, ourselves and our loved ones. If your current health profile includes any of the risk factors discussed below and/or you are diabetic, postmenopausal and not on estrogen therapy (see chapter 7), have a close relative (parent or sibling) who died of heart disease before age 60, or have a personal history of chest pain, you are at risk.

Why Are We at Risk?

These are the unfortunate facts:

- Twenty-five percent of women are cigarette smokers.
- Thirty-five percent of women are overweight.
- Sixty percent of women over 50 have sedentary lifestyles (physical activity has not been part of our lives).
- Forty percent of women over 50 have high cholesterol levels.
- Seventy percent of women over the age of 65 have high blood pressure (a reading of more than 140/95 mmHg). (Actually, hypertension is more common with age in women than men.)

Every one of these scenarios represents a risk factor for coronary heart disease.

SMOKING

Twenty-five percent of women smoke, increasing their risk of heart attack by a factor of 4 when compared to nonsmokers. This risk increases in direct proportion to the number of cigarettes we smoke. If we quit smoking, our risk of heart attack remains high for two years, but after four years our risk is no higher than that of women who have never smoked (see chapter 17).

One fifth of all cardiovascular-related deaths in 1990 were due to smoking. The demon's brew of 4,000 chemicals that make up cigarette smoke interacts and affects our blood vessels and heart muscles in numerous ways. The Nurses' Study found that smoking just one to four cigarettes a day doubled the risk of coronary artery disease. By diminishing blood oxygen, damaging blood vessels, causing the blood to thicken and platelets to become "stickier," and raising clotting factors and total cholesterol while lowering "good" cholesterol, smoking creates a body scenario that beckons the dual diseases of heart attack and stroke.

OVERWEIGHT AND/OR "APPLE"-SHAPED

Obesity, even if it's only mild to moderate, appears to more than double our risk of heart attack. It's not just our total weight that counts, but where those pounds are situated on our bodies. A waist-to-hip ratio greater than 0.8 greatly increases our cardiac risk. The waist-to-hip ratio determines to what degree our bodies have adopted the potbelly, no-waistline, male-pattern "apple" profile. The problem with this body shape (as opposed to the more feminine "pear" profile) transcends the cosmetic, because it contributes to changes in our insulin and fatty acid production, which in turn predispose us to the development of coronary artery disease.

You can determine your waist-to-hip ratio by dividing your waist measurement by your hip measurement; for example, if you have a 30-inch waist and 40-inch hips, your waist-to-hip ratio is an acceptable 0.75.

SEDENTARY LIFESTYLE

About 70 percent of us are sedentary or only sporadically active, a shame considering the wealth of benefits even moderate exercise bestows on our cardiovascular system. It can lower our blood pressure, tone our heart muscle, help us control our weight by burning calories, improve our clotting factors, and lower insulin levels (which impact on our blood pressure, fluid retention, and formation of fatty acids, which in turn affect our hearts). Although only 7 of the 43 studies that assessed the relationship between exercise and cononary heart disease included women (I can't figure out if the researchers thought we didn't have heart disease, or dismissed our ability to exercise!), the ones that "made it through" showed that physically active women had a 60 to 75 percent lower risk of heart disease than those who were inactive.

You don't have to put on a skimpy leotard and work out to loud, headache-provoking music to have a healthy heart. Just walk at a rapid pace (or up hills) so that you raise your heart rate to your target zone and keep it there for at least thirty minutes (see Table 17.5 in chapter 17). Or find small ways to put more activity into your life so that you're active for a total of thirty minutes a day: park your car further away from the shopping center, take the stairs instead of the elevator, do your own yard work. We've spent years perfecting our inaction; let's regress to action.

HIGH CHOLESTEROL AND TRIGLYCERIDES

A high total cholesterol (over 240 mg/dl) and a poor lipoprotein and triglyceride profile puts us at risk for heart attack. It is true that thanks in part to the effective "villainization" of cholesterol (the evil clogger of arteries), many of us lose sight of the fact that cholesterol is essential to our health. Our bodies use cholesterol for building cells and formulating hormones, among other things. What most of us don't know is that our liver produces virtually all the cholesterol we need. Given this and the fact that the average American diet is chock full of cholesterol from meat, eggs, high-fat dairy products, and some forms of seafood, it's no wonder that 40 percent of us over the age of 50 have high cholesterol levels.

Cholesterol is bound to lipoproteins made by our liver. These proteins come in two forms: good, or high-density, lipoprotein (HDL) and bad, or low-density, lipoprotein (LDL). Cholesterol stuck to LDL tends to unstick in a very harmful way, by adhering to the artery walls, where it forms plaque and clogs the vessel. Cholesterol transported by HDL does not break off and thus won't block vessels. Indeed, it tends to coat the vessel walls and prevent LDL cholesterol from sticking. I call this the "Teflon effect."

High cholesterol alone does not "a heart attack make." The ratio between the amount that is allowed to roam free and adhere versus the amount that remains bound and "coating" is far more relevant. The higher our HDL cholesterol, the lower our risk of heart disease.

Low HDL and high LDL cholesterol are not the only lipid risk factors we need to worry about and control. Triglycerides, a form of fatty acid, appear to play a much greater role in causing coronary artery disease in women than in men. In two separate studies, high triglyceride levels were found to be a more important factor than cholesterol in predicting fatal heart attacks. Another study showed that even when LDL cholesterol levels were aggressively lowered with medication, high levels of triglycerides continued to contribute to the development of small to moderate-sized blockages of the heart vessels.

Yet another cardiac strike against us is diabetes, affecting 2 percent of women. Diabetic women have greater and more adverse changes in their lipoprotein levels than diabetic men. That means that the same degree of disease is much more likely to cause heart attack in women than in men.

Table 9.1 outlines desirable and high-risk readings for total blood cholesterol, HDLs, LDLs, and triglycerides.

TABLE 9.1   KNOW YOUR CHOLESTEROL RISK

	Desirable	Borderline	High Risk
Total cholesterol	Below 200 mg/dl	200 to 239 mg/dl	240 mg/dl or above
LDL cholesterol	Below 130 mg/dl	130 to 159 mg/dl	160 mg/dl or above
HDL cholesterol	50 mg/dl or above	35 to 50 mg/dl	Below 35 mg/dl
Triglycerides	20 to 140 mg/dl	140 to 190 mg/dl	Above 190 mg/dl

HIGH BLOOD PRESSURE

High blood pressure, or hypertension (a reading of more than 140/95 mmHg), puts you at risk for coronary heart disease. At least 20 million women in this country have high blood pressure; over a third of them don't even know it. In our forties 23 percent of white women and more than 40 percent of African-American women are already hypertensive. As we age and our vessels become less pliant and constrict, our incidence of high blood pressure increases. Seventy-two percent of white women and 84 percent of African-American women between the ages of 65 and 74 have high blood pressure.

Blood pressure readings measure the force blood exerts on our artery walls as the heart pumps it through the body. High blood pressure occurs when that force is increased. If the arteries are narrowed or partially blocked by fatty deposits or *plaque (atherosclerosis)*, or if they are generally less pliant and thickened *(arteriosclerosis)*, the heart has to pump harder to force blood through. This increased pressure not only damages and weakens vessels but "bruises" blood cells, making them more likely to clump together and form clots. If these clots form in the coronary blood vessels and prevent blood from supplying the heart muscle, a heart attack occurs.

In the vast majority of women who have high blood pressure, no discernable physical cause can be found, although we know that a tendency toward high blood pressure can run in families and be influenced by such factors as weight, salt intake, and the existence of other physical problems, such as diabetes.

The benefits of antihypertensive therapy have been studied in multiple drug "trials" involving 37,000 subjects, 47 percent of whom were women. Therapy was given for three to six years and the results were encouraging. A decrease of just 6 mmHg in the diastolic pressure (this is the lower or second number in our blood pressure reading and represents the pressure in our blood vessels when the heart is not contracting) reduced death from vascular disease by 21 percent, nonfatal heart disease by 14 percent, and stroke by 42 percent. Women over 65 are more prone than men to develop an elevation in their systolic pressure in the absence of a similar increase in their diastolic reading. (The systolic pressure is the first number, or nominator, in our blood pressure reading and represents the pressure in the vessels when the heart contracts.) This elevation indicates a loss of elasticity in the wall of the arteries. When women with this form of hypertension are treated with antihypertensive drugs, reports have shown a 25 percent decrease in their incidence of heart attack and a 35 percent decrease in stroke.

What we don't know is whether the side effects of antihypertensive drugs are the same in women and men.

WHAT PROTECTED OUR HEARTS IN OUR FORTIES?

Estrogen was and is our heart's best friend; once we go through menopause and our ovaries stop producing estrogen, we lose our female heart protection. We make more cholesterol, especially the "bad" cholesterol, LDL, and lose some of our "good" cholesterol, HDL. After menopause, elements in our blood called platelets tend to become stickier, and as they bind to one another and the walls of our vessels, they produce clots that can clog our coronary arteries. As blood courses through vessels that are partially blocked by these clots, turbulence occurs. That turbulence "bruises" blood cells, which leads to even more clot formation. If the platelets lack the ability to stick together, these clots dissolve or just don't form. In our forties, estrogen helped us to achieve a "Drāno" effect, keeping our vessels clear of debris and promoting smooth blood flow. To put it bluntly, once we lose our estrogen, we begin to "clog."

Alas, without estrogen, our once-elastic blood vessels also tend to constrict, become rigid, and resist blood flow. In other words, we are more likely to develop high blood pressure, another cause of heart disease.

KNOW THE WARNING SIGNS OF A HEART ATTACK

Chest Pain   If you write off chest pain or any discomfort above the waist as indigestion, anxiety, stress, or muscle ache, you could be making a fatal mistake. Too often, women have been seen in emergency rooms and physicians' offices and sent home with antacids, muscle relaxants, and Valium when, indeed, they were developing heart attacks.

Atypical Angina   Do you have recurrent pressure or a tingling feeling anyplace above the waist when you exert yourself or feel strong emotion? Does this symptom disappear once the exertion or emotion subsides? These symptoms may be much more than "emotional." The term "'angina" is used to describe chest pain due to temporary constriction of coronary vessels. The phrase "atypical angina" is a misnomer; it only means that these types of anginal symptoms don't occur in men. Fifty percent of women who develop coronary heart disease will, however, have these types of symptoms. For us they are not "atypical."

Shortness of Breath   Are you short of breath with minimal activity and chalk it up to being "out of shape"? What may be fatally misshapen are your coronary vessels.

If we are not receptive to our cardiac messages, then the song is right: Our hearts do belong to Daddy—and to the benign neglect with which Daddy's physicians treated us.

Diagnosing and Treating Our Heart Problems

There are several types of follow-up tests that should be performed if a man or woman has an abnormal EKG or *stress test* (an EKG performed while exercising on a treadmill). Either the heart is imaged with ultrasound during exercise, or a radioactive substance called thallium is injected and monitored during exercise to check blood flow to the cardiac muscles. If these tests are abnormal, *angiography* should be performed. For this, a small catheter is inserted through the vessels leading to the heart, and dye is injected. This allows us to visualize the coronary arteries with X ray and check for any abnormal narrowing or occlusions.

Women tend to have more abnormal stress EKGs than men. Unfortunately for us, the test is less likely to detect true coronary artery disease. That does not mean, however, that the results should be ignored. Follow-up is mandatory, yet we are only half as likely as men to have further tests.

To add insult to cardiac injury, we are also 6.5 times less likely to be referred for the high-tech procedures that have helped change the fatal outcome of heart disease in men: angioplasty and coronary bypass surgery.

Angioplasty   During angioplasty a catheter with an expandable balloon is threaded into the occluded coronary vessel. The balloon is expanded and pulled back so that the cholesterol buildup, called plaque, can be "Roto-rootered" out. Guess for whom these catheters and balloons were developed? Men have larger coronary vessels than we do, and women who undergo this procedure are twice as likely to die from complications. Our vessels are smaller and more easily torn by the "man-size" catheters and balloons.

Coronary Bypass Surgery   This operation replaces damaged, clogged cardiac vessels with veins from the legs. Although now commonplace, it is still an expensive and extremely invasive procedure. Women are twice as likely to die from this surgery as men, probably because they are referred later, after a lot of diagnostic procrastination. We are now sicker and older, and our vessels are more delicate and difficult to repair. It could be argued that men are having this procedure too often, but no one argues that women are having it too infrequently.

Caring for Our Hearts

Our choices about heart care will obviously affect the quality and span of our lives, but we also have to consider the awesome impact of our matriarchal roles. Studies have shown that if we overeat, become obese, don't exercise, and smoke, not only do we increase our risk of heart disease, but—by adopting the same abusive behavior—so do our spouses and children. Women set the cardiac pace, so the message is: If you don't want to do this for yourself, do it for those you care about.

1. Don't smoke.

2. Maintain a low-fat diet.

3. Avoid obesity.

4. Be physically active.

5. Get treatment for hypertension.

6. Consider estrogen replacement therapy, especially if you have any cardiac risk factors.

Estrogen replacement in menopausal women has been shown to decrease the incidence of heart attack by 50 percent. There is not one cardiac drug on the market that can boast such a response. Estrogen works by simply continuing or restarting the heart protection we had before menopause. It can not only prevent coronary artery disease but decrease the rate of recurrent heart attacks in women who already have this disease, even if it is severe. We are never "too sick," "too fat," or "too old" to benefit from estrogen. There are other factors to consider, but educate yourself and be wary of doctors who dismiss you as being too "high-risk" for estrogen replacement. (Please see the extensive discussion of hormone replacement therapy in chapter 7.)

Consider Nonprescription Therapies

Inexpensive over-the-counter supplements and medications have been shown to have a considerable effect on our cardiac risks.

VITAMIN E

Doses of at least 400 international units a day, and not exceeding 800 units, have been shown to decrease heart attacks in men and women by 40 percent (yes, women were included in this study!).

ASPIRIN

Low doses of aspirin (325 milligrams every other day) have been shown to decrease initial heart attack in men by 44 percent and recurrent heart attack in men and women by 25 percent. Just one baby aspirin (80 milligrams) has the anticlotting "punch" necessary to inhibit the aggregation or stickiness of platelets for eight to ten days. Less clot formation in test tubes should translate into less clots in our coronary vessels. Although no randomized trials of aspirin protection against heart attack in healthy women have been conducted, a review of the data from the Nurses' Study has shown that one to seven aspirin (325 milligrams) a week decreased their relative risk of a first heart attack by 32 percent.

Women who are at risk, or who do not take estrogen, might want to consider low-dose aspirin. This would seem to be a simple choice, but side effects such as ulcers and bleeding can occur, especially with years of use, so check with your doctor before starting this regimen. More prospective testing of healthy women will help us weigh the pros and cons.

FOLIC ACID

A review of 27 studies has shown that elevated blood levels of homocysteine (an amino acid used in building protein) is associated with damage to the lining of blood vessels and atherosclerosis. This excess of homocysteine may account for 10 percent of all heart attacks. Folic acid has been found to decrease homocysteine levels. Based on additional studies, some researchers have come up with the amazing statistic that folic acid deficiencies can contribute to 30 or 40 percent of all heart attacks and strokes. To ensure that we're not in this "deficient" group, we can either take 400 micrograms of folic acid as a supplement or substantially increase our consumption of fruit and vegetables.

Get "Heart Care" Checkups and Therapy

Make sure your doctor checks your total serum cholesterol, HDL and LDL levels, and triglycerides. This should be done every three years if your first test is normal; every one to three years if these values are abnormal and every one to two years if you're at risk for heart disease (remember, risk includes not taking ERT and/or being over the age of 65). This is a simple blood test; the sample should be drawn in the morning after you have fasted—in other words, have not had anything to eat since midnight. If the reading is abnormal (see Table 9.1 for range), or if you have other risk factors, make sure you have a stress test or exercise EKG. If this too is abnormal, you need to have an exercise heart ultrasound or an exercise thallium scan. If these are normal, aside from breathing a sigh of relief, you should be screened again in two to three years. If they are abnormal, you should have an angiogram to check your coronary vessels for possible narrowing. You have to go this last step to know where you and your heart stand (or pump).

Remember, early diagnosis will allow you and your cardiologist (by now, you have definitely seen a specialist) to decide on therapies that can work. These range from medications to high-tech procedures. Drugs can effectively lower cholesterol. A Scandinavian study has shown that treating men and women with coronary heart disease with a cholesterol-lowering agent cuts overall risk of death by 30 percent and coronary death by 42 percent. Other medications can also significantly decrease cardiac risk by relaxing or dilating coronary vessels, lowering blood pressure, or improving cardiac muscle performance. Unfortunately, there is a deplorable lack of primary prevention trials in women and we still do not have overwhelming evidence that lowering cholesterol in "healthy" women will affect their coronary heart disease mortality. So the simple question of what to do about an abnormal lipid profile when we're not "sick" has not been answered. We do know that a 1 percent reduction in the cholesterol level *in men* decreases their risk of heart attack by 2 to 3 percent. If we are sick and medication is not sufficient, angioplasty or coronary bypass surgery may be necessary.

WHO CARES ABOUT OUR HEARTS?

We must. We've long suspected that our hearts were different from men's, and now research bears this out. Unfortunately, those differences—in our physiology and current attitudes toward our cardiac care—often seem to work against us. For example, we know that if we put high-risk men on a very-low-fat diet and make them exercise and lose weight, we can improve their lipoprotein profile. Their HDLs go up, their LDLs go down, and *voilà*, their hearts fare better. Sadly, diet, exercise, and weight loss have much less positive impact on our lipoproteins. To add insult to injury, if we do manage to lose our unwanted fat, we reduce our natural postmenopausal source of estrogen. Fat cells convert substances produced by our adrenal glands into weak estrogens, which help our lipid profile. Earlier we mentioned two other predominantly feminine risk factors: high triglyceride levels and diabetes.

There's little we can do to change these physiologic facts of life. What we can challenge, however, is the pervasive cardiac denial that lulls us and our physicians into ignoring warning signs, forgoing tests that are standard for men and denying or delaying the most effective, most aggressive treatments.

10

STROKE
An Accident That's a Calamity

S troke, which claimed the lives of over 87,000 women in 1990, is the third leading cause of death for women in the United States. It is the number-one cause of disability. The death rates from this disease vary from 25 per 100,000 for white women to 46.6 per 1,000 African-American women. These numbers are hard to translate in terms of individual personal risk, but what we need to consider is that when we turn 50, we have an 8 percent lifetime risk of dying from stroke. Twenty-eight percent of stroke victims are under the age of 65. Men are slightly more likely than women to succumb to this disease by a factor of 1.2, probably because they have a higher prevalence of uncontrolled high blood pressure. It's not that women have lower rates of high blood pressure; the opposite is true. We just seem to tolerate it better (perhaps because we are more likely than men to listen to our doctors, take our medications, and smoke less, and we have our own or supplementary estrogen).

What Happens in a Stroke?

A stroke occurs when the blood supply to the brain is blocked. The medical term for stroke is *cerebrovascular accident* (CVA), but generally by the time we've had a stroke, cerebrovascular disease has already affected our blood vessels, allowing the "accident" to occur. Twenty percent of us will develop cerebrovascular disease in our lifetime.

A stroke results when one of four things goes wrong with the blood vessels supplying our brain.

1. *Abnormalities*. These can occur within the vessels themselves and include:

    Arteriosclerotic plaques. Congealed masses of lipids that obstruct the blood vessel.

    Dissection of the vessel. The lining of the blood vessel separates from the outer wall so that the blood flows through a false channel that either dead-ends or ultimately ruptures.

    Developmental malformations. A thinning of the wall of the vessel causing it to bulge like a balloon (*aneurysm*) or tangles of poorly structured blood vessels connecting an artery and vein (an A-V malformation).

    Venous thrombosis. A clot formed in a vein.

2. *Embolus*. Clots that form elsewhere in the body but travel through the bloodstream to lodge in the brain's blood vessels. These clots are most commonly formed in our heart or the vessels leading from the heart.

3. *Inadequate blood flow to the vessels of the brain*. This can occur from a drop in blood pressure or shock, or if the blood becomes viscous and flows sluggishly.

4. *Hemorrhage*. Rupture of a vessel within the brain or on its surface results in *hemorrhage* (bleeding).

Stroke is the sudden injury to brain tissue occurring as a result of one of these "accidents." Portions of the brain are either denied blood (*ischemia*), or are inundated with blood in the form of a hemorrhage. Both processes destroy the brain's tissue. About 80 percent of strokes are due to lack of blood flow and an ischemic cerebral infarction (a fancy term meaning that tissue dies from lack of oxygen), and 20 percent are due to brain hemorrhage.

An infarcted brain initially "becomes pale" from lack of blood supply, but just as blood cannot get in, that which is there cannot get out. The *neuronal tissue* (or gray matter) becomes congested and red, filled with blocked dilated vessels and small hemorrhages. If recirculation is established (the obstructing clot is reabsorbed), the brain injury may even increase. Blood flows to the small damaged vessels, which now bleed, and what started out as an ischemic infarction has become hemorrhagic. This, in turn, causes swelling in the confined, ungiving space in our skull, and the compressed brain suffers more damage. Conversely, if the original "accident" is directly from a hemorrhage, the brain tissue adjacent to the site of the bleed can be further damaged from compression of the expanding clot. So whether the initial injury involves no blood or an uncontrolled burst of blood, the end result is brain tissue destruction that often goes far beyond the initial and local tissue injury.

The brain is our most complex and awe-inspiring organ (although some brains inspire less awe than others). Researchers estimate that the brain contains up to 2 billion nerve cells. On each cell surface are more than 60,000 receptors, or points of contact. Using these, we can take in 100 million pieces of information in a second, but we're lucky if we concentrate on 40 of them. (I guess that means we're working at 0.4 millionth of our capacity!) This might make us think (using 40 pieces of information) that the brain has good reserves. But one portion of the brain cannot compensate for another, since each has its own unique responsibilities. One area controls our automatic essential functions such as heartbeat, breathing, blood pressure, and all organ functions. The motor area controls every movement we perform and a blending of these movements for every function we perform. Our sensations and recognition of our world are coordinated by a particular sensory part of the brain. We have the remarkable ability to remember, understand, communicate, think, and feel emotions. All of these functions are intertwined and each has its own "clearinghouse" in a particular area of the brain. When that area is destroyed, part of what we are capable of doing, sensing, feeling, thinking, or emoting is abolished. If we cut or damage our skin, muscle, or most of our other organs, the tissue can repair itself; the brain cannot. The site of brain damaged after infarction or hemorrhage can heal only in the form of a scar, and that scar is incapable of performing neuronal duties.

Our only hope of limiting the damage of a stroke is to minimize the spread of the initial infarction or hemorrhage, prevent a second stroke, and decrease swelling and edema. The most important therapy is to prevent the stroke in the first place!

What Are Our Risk Factors?

The five most important factors that we can either treat or avoid are the same as those that cause heart attacks: hypertension (high blood pressure), high cholesterol, smoking, diabetes, and obesity (see chapter 9). All cause fatty plaque to form in the blood vessels supplying our brain; the plaque partially obstructs the vessels and increases our risk of ischemic stroke.

HIGH BLOOD PRESSURE (HYPERTENSION)

This condition contributes to nearly 70 percent of all strokes. It promotes the formation of fatty plaque in our largest blood vessel, the aorta, which can then be "thrown out" and reach the vessels in our brain; it also induces on-site plaque deposits in our cerebral vessels, which have a local "clogging" effect. To add pressure to injury, it can also cause hemorrhagic stroke by increasing the fluid pressure in the blood vessels, weakening them and causing rupture. There is a 10-to-12-fold increase in our risk of stroke if our diastolic blood pressure is above 105 mmHg.

HIGH CHOLESTEROL

Cholesterol levels and the therapies to reduce them are not gender-biased when it comes to preventing stroke in men and women. A cholesterol level greater than 308 mg/dl nearly doubles the risk for nonhemorrhagic stroke during the subsequent six years (this was seen in a Danish study of over 20,000 men *and* women). The study also found that as triglycerides became elevated, the risk of stroke went up. As HDLs (our good cholesterol) increased, there was a decline in strokes. Three percent of our general population has cholesterol levels this high, but that's 3 percent too many who are at risk.

SMOKING

We've been able to evaluate the risk of smoking and stroke in women through the ongoing Nurses' Study of 120,000 women. Current smoking appears to increase our risk of stroke by a factor of 2.5 when compared to not smoking. This risk increases with the increasing number of cigarettes smoked per day. Smoking promotes vascular brain injury by raising clotting factors, increasing the stickiness of platelets, decreasing HDL cholesterol, increasing the concentration of red blood cells, damaging the walls of blood vessels, and increasing blood pressure. (This was a long sentence, but the sentence smoking can impose on our brains is longer.) A shorter but more encouraging sentence: When we stop smoking, the increased risk remains high for two years, but by the end of four years returns to near that of women who have never smoked.

CARDIOVASCULAR PROBLEMS

Two conditions can increase our risk of stroke from traveling clots, or *emboli*. In the first, the heart beats irregularly and abnormally, so that the heart valves tend to quiver. This can lead to formation and release of clots and pieces of clots that end up traveling to the brain. This occurs with an arrhythmia called *atrial fibrillation*. The second involves generalized arteriosclerosis, or hardening of the arteries. Not only does this condition increase our chance of heart attack, but as a heart attack occurs, clots may be projected into the bloodstream, go to the brain, and cause embolic stroke. There is also a strong association between arteriosclerotic disease of the aorta (our large blood vessel that carries blood from the heart to the rest of the body) and stroke. If thick plaques (greater than 4 millimeters) adhere to the aortic wall, they may throw off small pieces or cause clots to develop. These then travel to the brain. The presence of these fatty "pebbles" in this major pathway from the heart increases our risk of stroke by a factor of 9.1.

DIABETES

This increases our risk of atherosclerosis and may contribute to 2 to 5 percent of all strokes.

OBESITY

Our risk of stroke can double if we're obese. Abdominal obesity may be as bad as general weight gain; it causes fatty acids and triglycerides to be "poured" into major veins from the abdominal fat cells and settle as plaque in our vessels.

Symptoms of a Stroke

"MINI-STROKES" AND WHAT THEY MEAN

Temporary or transient symptoms of a stroke are called *transient ischemic attacks,* or *TIAs.* They warn us of our impending risk of the "real thing" 50 to 75 percent of the time. *Low-flow TIAs* are just that, a low flow of blood through a tight vessel that has been partially obstructed by the plaque of atherosclerosis. Symptoms are similar to those of a stroke, but are brief; they last a few minutes to a few hours, are recurrent, and always follow the same pattern (the part of the brain being denied proper blood flow from the damaged vessel remains the same). *Embolic TIAs* can also occur. A small embolus may start in an artery or get there from the heart and travel to the brain. If symptoms last less than twenty-four hours, it means the small embolism freed itself or got broken down and didn't cause permanent damage to the brain. If the symptoms continue for more than twenty-four hours, a true ischemic stroke with death of brain tissue has occurred.

Since TIAs frequently herald stroke, they should immediately be investigated. We don't give them a chance (to warn us) unless we take note and seek help for these symptoms. Here are the warning signs:

- Sudden feeling of numbness
- Temporary paralysis in any muscles, including the face
- Development of a tremor or muscle spasm
- Problems speaking
- Confusion, or disorientation, or sudden lack of memory
- Drowsiness
- Blocking of part of our vision, or double vision
- Sudden unsteadiness
- Hallucinations

The good news is that if these symptoms go away, we are probably dealing with "just" TIAs and no significant permanent damage. The bad news is that if we ignore these "off moments" and try to find frivolous excuses for the temporary misbehavior of our bodies, we may end up with an irreversible stroke.

FULL STROKES

The symptoms of a full stroke are similar to those of a TIA. They just increase in severity and duration until we may be rendered partially paralyzed, totally confused, unable to speak, and even unconscious. If our breathing center or the part of the brain that controls our heart is knocked out, this "incident" is fatal. Of the 500,000 Americans who suffer strokes every year, approximately 150,000 die.

DIAGNOSIS

Ideally, doctors want to detect narrowed vessels in "risky" brains before they cause cerebrovascular damage. One of the easiest ways to pick up a narrowing in the *carotid arteries* in the neck (which carry blood to our head and brain) is to listen to them with a stethoscope. Blood flow disturbed by a partial occlusion creates turbulence that is heard as a high-pitched "whoosh," or *carotid bruit.* So our doctors should be placing their stethoscopes not just on our chest or back, but also on our neck. If your doctor hears a bruit or you're had mild TIA symptoms, or you're at risk for a stroke, one of the following tests is warranted.

Noninvasive Ultrasound and Doppler Studies   These measure blood flow in the carotids and lower brain vessels.

Invasive Cerebral Angiography   Dye is injected into the cranial vessels from a catheter that is pushed through large veins. This invasive procedure has a 2 percent complication rate that includes damage to the vessels, bleeding, stroke, and even death.

If you have symptoms of a stroke, brain imaging is indicated. *Computed tomography* (CT) scans will show whether the brain damage is from a hemorrhage. It is not reliable in detecting infarction or lack of blood flow to certain areas of the brain during the first twenty-four to forty-eight hours. *Magnetic resonance imaging* (MRI) will image the extent and location of a stroke within one hour of its onset. It also demonstrates hemorrhage.

Therapy for Stroke: The Sooner, the Better

The best stroke therapy is to catch the process at the TIA stage before ir-reversible damage has occurred. If the carotid arteries have a greater than 70 percent stricture, the therapy of choice is now *carotid endarterec-tomy:* This is a surgery in which the occluding plaque is removed from the inner lining of the vessel. A recent study was terminated before its completion after it was found that the risk of stroke for individuals with this degree of obstruction was 26 percent lower with endarterectomy than with aspirin therapy. The study subjects who had been receiving as-pirin were advised to have the surgery.

Thirty percent of people over the age of 50 have some evidence of carotid artery disease, but do they all need to have these arteries surgi-cally "Roto-Rootered"? No. Surgery will not significantly decrease the incidence of stroke (which is less than 1 percent annually) if our occlu-sion is less than 70 percent. If we're only partially blocked, we need to lower our blood pressure, stop smoking, lower our cholesterol, and have close medical follow-up. We might consider use of aspirin to reduce platelet stickiness and clot formation, as well as other antiplatelet ther-apy. Low doses of aspirin (75 to 300 milligrams per day) have been shown to be effective in individuals (mostly men) who have had TIAs, minor strokes, angina, or previous heart attack. It can reduce their odds of additional vascular "events" (stroke, heart attack, or death from vas-cular cause) by 25 percent. Other studies, however, have shown that if there is no cardiac problem, and the TIAs or previous strokes were due to "local" problems in the brain's vessels, aspirin in either low or high doses doesn't seem to make a difference to the risk of stroke. It's not clear why clots formed in our heart are decreased by aspirin, while those pro-duced directly in our cerebral vessels are not.

A clean-out procedure or endarteretomy is now being performed in some patients in whom large plaques of arteriosclerosis are found in the aorta. There is "proclaimed" success, but we don't as yet have sufficient studies to support this as a "should-do" procedure.

If we have atrial fibrillation or an ongoing irregular heartbeat that could increase our chance of "throwing" an embolism, we should use an anticoagulant called Coumadin to prevent clot formation.

Once a stroke has occurred, it is important to prevent and reduce swelling of the bloodless brain tissue. This swelling usually begins forty-eight to seventy-two hours after the stroke and will start to resolve after two weeks. Special IV (intravenous) solutions will help "sop up" excess swelling in the brain. If the stroke is from an embolism or a traveling clot, anticoagulation is usually begun two to five days after the stroke to prevent a second embolism. New clot busters called *tissue plasminogen activator (TPA)*, which are used as therapy for heart attack, are currently being investigated as therapy for stroke. Recent studies have shown that during a stroke, there is a release of an amino acid called glutamate and that this can kill healthy cells adjacent to the damaged brain tissue. Drugs that block the flow of glutamate might limit this "seepage" damage.

If stroke is due to hemorrhage, chance of survival is determined by "where" and "how big." Surgeons may attempt to remove the clot but this, too, can lead to major neurologic damage. If the bleeding comes from a congenitally weakened vessel (an *aneurysm*, or a malformation between the arteries and veins), "closing-the-leak" procedures can be performed, either by placing X ray–directed balloons in the damaged vessel or by direct surgical approach.

Preventing Stroke

Our goal is to limit our strokes to the tennis court and golf course. We've been on the right track for the last thirty years. Our death rate from stroke has decreased by 60 percent, mostly due to prevention. The following measures will decrease our risk of becoming seriously disabled or dying from stroke.

1. Stop smoking. You will reduce your risk of stroke by 30 to 40 percent after two to five years.

2. Treat your high blood pressure. Have it checked yearly, and if it's over 140/95 mmHg, work with your doctor on making lifestyle changes and possibly taking antihypertensive medication to get it down and keep it down. If you decrease your diastolic pressure by 5 to 6 mmHg, you can reduce your risk of stroke by 42 percent.

3. Exercise. There is a 30 percent reduction in the risk of stroke for exercisers, compared to sedentary individuals. This need not be an exclusive club.

4. Lower your high cholesterol and improve your lipid profile. Again, work with your doctor to make changes in your diet, exercise, and stress-reduction efforts, and take medication if necessary.

5. Consider ERT. This will improve your lipid profile, your cardiovascular function, and in some studies has been shown to lower risk of fatal stroke by 60 percent.

6. Take anticoagulant therapy if you have cardiac conditions such as atrial fibrillation.

7. Ask your doctor if you should take low-dose aspirin if you're at cardiac risk for throwing emboli (previous heart attack or angina) or if you have general arteriosclerotic disease.

8. Get annual checkups that include evaluation of your carotid arteries and additional evaluation of your large cardiac vessels (including the aorta) if you have arteriosclerosis.

9. Seek immediate medical attention for any temporary neurologic symptoms. Never let your embarrassment at "making a fuss over nothing" stop you from getting prompt professional evaluation.

We should be actively participating in the prevention and early detection of stroke before this condition robs us of our abilities. To rephrase a misstatement made by a former vice president, "A stroke is a terrible waste of a brain. . . ."

11

OSTEOPOROSIS
Bone Care versus Bone Repair

A Crippling Killer

Osteoporosis (translated literally, it means "pores of bone") is one of our most devastating yet preventable diseases. It affects more than 20 million women in the United States, among whom over 1.5 million bone fractures occur annually. The National Institutes of Health now recognize osteoporosis as one of the four deadliest diseases among women. Our risk of hip fracture equals our combined risk of developing breast, uterine, and ovarian cancer. Once we fracture a hip, we have a 20 percent chance of dying either from the surgery (hip pinning or hip replacement) or from complications resulting from prolonged bed rest and convalescence, namely pneumonia, blood clots, skin ulcers, and, adding insult to injury, worsening osteoporosis.

Economically, socially, and personally, we can't regard osteoporosis as a problem that will be fixed with casts and slings. More than half of all women who survive hip fractures will no longer be able to walk unassisted and will require long-term nursing care, 25 percent of them for the rest of their lives!

Fifty-four percent of women will suffer an osteoporosis-related fracture in their lifetime, and 1 in every 3 women will fracture her hip by age 80; this is indeed a disease of majority but not necessarily of the elderly.

229

A British study that looked at over 7,000 "normal" women who had no idea whether or not they had osteoporosis found that 5 percent of those in their forties had lost enough bone density to place them at immediate risk for fracture. Twenty percent of women in their fifties had significant osteoporosis, 45 percent in their sixties, and 60 percent in their seventies. Not only did this study demonstrate that we cannot assume we're bone-safe simply because we're under 70; it also demonstrated how little most of us know about the real state of our invisible support system.

Osteoporosis creates other insidious and crippling problems. One half of all fractures due to osteoporosis occur in the crucial bones of our upper spine, which support our head and neck and encase and protect our spinal column. These fractures are termed compression, or crush, fractures because the porous, thin vertebral bone literally collapses under its own weight. These crushed vertebrae lose their normal, even dimensions and no longer sit squarely one on top of the other in a straight tower. This creates the curvature of the spine we call "dowager hump" and loss of inches from our height. These are not just cosmetic changes causing us to become "little old ladies." There can be nerve damage, leading to limited mobility, paralysis, and severe pain. This deformity can also cause other serious health problems. Once our ribs project down and press into our abdomen, we can develop digestive disturbances; and if our chest cavity is constricted, our heart and lungs are "entrapped" and can't function normally.

In the United States, the cost of caring for this crippling disease is currently $10 billion a year. By the year 2050, with the vast demographic shift of the baby boomers into the ranks of the elderly, the annual cost will reach at least $60 billion (in today's dollars). There is no instant cure for osteoporosis. We had better start looking at osteoporosis prevention, for both our own well-being and that of our economy.

Skeletons Are Not Dead

Our bones are living tissue. Forget the "dead" skeleton presiding over biology class, or the wind-scrubbed bones of Georgia O'Keeffe's paintings. From the moment we are conceived until the day we die, our bones are constantly being built, destroyed, and rebuilt. Bone-eating cells called *osteoclasts* are found in the soft center of our larger bones, the bone marrow. In a continuous process that takes several weeks, the osteoclasts digest the bone surface, leaving behind small erosion cavities. These are then filled with new bone by bone-building cells called *osteoblasts*. This latter process takes three to four months. We maintain healthy bones and a positive bone balance when the rate and extent of new bone formation exceed that of bone resorption. We reach our bone-density peak at around age 30. This "personal best" is not achieved without basic bone training. We need to get enough calcium and vitamin D (particularly during puberty and pregnancy and while breastfeeding), do weight-bearing exercise, have regular menstrual cycles with appropriate estrogen production, and abstain from smoking and from ingesting bone-leaching substances.

After age 30, the battle of the bone begins. As we age, our osteoblast development and function gradually decline, leaving the bone-gobbling osteoclasts (I think of them as Pac-Men, but to be politically correct, let's call them "Pac-People") to run rampant, so that their creation of new erosion cavities exceeds new bone replacement. In addition to the slow, age-related porosity, menopause and the disappearance of estrogen strike another major bone blow: Bad osteoclasts increase, good osteoblasts decrease, the drilling overcomes the filling, and we lose bone.

Preventing Osteoporosis:
Our Inner Strength Is in Our Bones

Building and maintaining healthy bones are a lifelong—and life-saving—commitment. Let's look at our two major allies in the battle for healthy bones: calcium and estrogen.

CALCIUM: THE BONE BUILDER

Calcium is the "cement" of our bones. Our bone-building cells require a constant calcium supply to do their job. Bear in mind that our bodies lose 200 to 300 milligrams of calcium a day through urine, stool, and perspiration, and that we absorb only 25 to 35 percent of the calcium we consume. The amount we need to put back in order to "keep up" can vary, depending on our age and current health status (see Table 11.1).

As we age, we need increasing amounts of calcium—as much as 1,500 milligrams a day—to help compensate for natural physical changes that undermine our bones. Our intestines get lazy and absorb less cal-

TABLE 11.1   DAILY CALCIUM NEEDS

Age Group	Minimum Daily Intake
Adolescents/young adults (11 to 25 years)	1,200 to 1,500 mg
Women (25 to 50 years)	1,000 mg
Women over 50 (postmenopausal) On estrogen Not on estrogen	1,000 mg 1,500 mg
Over 65 years	1,500 mg
Pregnant and nursing	1,200 to 1,500 mg

cium, our kidneys produce less vitamin D. We also produce more parathyroid hormone. This is a substance secreted by two small glands on the side of the thyroid (hence the term "para"). The purpose of this hormone is to regulate the level of calcium in our blood. When our bodies absorb less calcium, more parathyroid hormone is released to seek and "collect" calcium from our calcium storehouse: our bones. Between decreased calcium absorption and increased parathyroid hormone, our bones are literally "eaten up." This age-dependent process can cause us to lose 0.5 percent or more of our bone mass every year once we're in our fifties.

Although our bones become vulnerable as we get older, for most of us, bone woes begin when we're unable to supply the right building material to the job site at *any* age. Everyone knows growing infants and children need milk and dairy products for healthy bones and strong teeth, but what about us during the rest of our lives? Somewhere in our teens we began eschewing unsexy milk for the more sophisticated, and bone-leaching, beverages such as soft drinks, coffee, iced tea, and alcohol. The problem is not so much that we prefer to quench our thirst with these alternatives to milk (although they each can cause health problems) but that we often drink them instead of milk. Some of us gave up dairy products because of lactose intolerance (with its uncomfortable digestive symptoms), allergy, or adoption of a dairy-free diet; others mistakenly assume that all dairy products are fattening, which is simply not true. Not only do nonfat and low-fat dairy products contain the same amounts of calcium as their whole milk counterparts, but several nonfat and low-fat dairy products now come fortified with extra calcium.

Despite the wealth of calcium out there, 25 percent of all adult women consume 300 milligrams or less of calcium each day, and half of all menopausal women consume less than 500 milligrams a day. Unless we get a minimum of 1,000 milligrams of calcium a day (1,500 after menopause), we are demanding that our cells build us new bones out of faulty cement. If a contractor did this, his license would be revoked. We alone can enforce the "building codes" for the system that should support us for the next half century and beyond.

How to Get Over 1,000 Milligrams of Calcium in Diet and Supplements

Finding and eating sufficient quantities of calcium is not difficult if we become calcium-conscious and make the effort. First we have to figure out how much calcium we are getting in our food. Then we need to add the necessary supplements.

Dairy-free diet = 300 mg calcium/day

One serving of dairy product = 250 to 300 mg calcium

One serving of calcium-fortified foods = 160 mg calcium

To get to 1,000 or 1,500 mg, add needed calcium supplementation (as elemental calcium; see below)

CALCIUM IN FOOD

Obviously, our best sources of calcium are dairy products, but sardines and salmon (*with* those little calcium-containing bones) and certain vegetables are also high in calcium. Table 11.2 lists some calcium-rich foods.

CALCIUM SUPPLEMENTS

Those of us who are not getting enough calcium from food need to use calcium supplements. There are dozens of calcium products on the market, promising to deliver "healthy bones." Calcium supplements consist

TABLE 11.2 DIETARY SOURCES OF CALCIUM

Food Product	Serving Size	Calcium (mg/serving)
Dairy:		
Milk (nonfat)	1 cup	300
Ice cream—frozen dessert	$^1/_2$ cup	100
Powdered nonfat dry milk	1 tbsp	50
Yogurts:		
Plain	1 cup	270
Plain (low-fat)	1 cup	415
Plain (skim)	1 cup	450
Fruit (low-fat)	1 cup	314
Cheese:		
Swiss cheese	1 oz (sliced)	270
Muenster cheese	1 oz (sliced)	200
American cheese	1 oz (sliced)	180
Feta cheese	1 oz	140
Cottage cheese (2% fat)	$^1/_2$ cup	80
Parmesan cheese (grated)	1 tbsp	70
Other foods:		
Sardines (in oil with bones)	3 oz	370
Salmon (canned with bones)	3 oz	200
Black beans (dry)	1 cup	270
Collards	1 cup	270
Broccoli	1 cup	170
Soybean curd (tofu)	4 oz	150
Turnip greens (cooked)	$^1/_2$ cup	105
Kale (cooked)	$^1/_2$ cup	90
Egg	1 medium	55

of calcium plus another compound that produces a calcium salt. The type of salt mixture affects absorption and function.

Calcium Carbonate: Caltrate, generic oyster shell, Os-Cal, Tums-Ex, and Calcium Rich Rolaids

- *Absorption*. This is good as long as we produce "normal amounts" of stomach acid, which most of us do between the ages of 40 and 65. If calcium carbonate is chewed, dispersion and absorption may be better. Alternately, we can swallow a whole tablet with a full glass of water, which will dilute it for better absorption.

- *When to take*. With meals and no more than 500 milligrams at a time.

- *Advantages*. This is our most concentrated and, therefore, cheapest calcium. Each tablet contains 40 percent of elemental calcium, so we need only a few a day.

- *Disadvantages*. It can cause constipation and bloating. This can be alleviated by taking the calcium in divided doses and increasing our water intake (a healthy thing to do anyway). This form of calcium can decrease iron absorption if taken with iron at the same time.

Calcium Citrate: Citracal

- *Absorption*. This is the most easily absorbed calcium. It doesn't require high levels of gastric acid to be broken down and absorbed. As we get older, we generally lose some of our stomach acidity, and this form of calcium may be the best for women over 65. If we're younger, but need to lower our gastric acidity with antacid medications, the absorption of calcium citrate won't be blocked.

- *When to take*. It should be taken between meals. Some specialists feel we get our best calcium boost if we take it at night before sleep, because bone turnover and bone loss are greatest when we lie down.

- *Advantages*. Those of us who have had kidney stones can use it (in suggested doses) without worry. This type of calcium actually prevents stone formation. Calcium citrate also causes less gas or constipation than calcium carbonate. It too inhibits iron absorption.

- *Disadvantages*. Only 24 percent of the tablet is elemental calcium, so we have to take almost twice as many tablets as

of calcium carbonate to get our needed calcium load. This
becomes somewhat burdensome and expensive.

Calcium Phosphate: Posture. The concentration of elemental calcium is similar to that in calcium carbonate, as are its absorption and effects; it's just more expensive.

Calcium Lactate and Calcium Gluconate: Because of their low
percentage of elemental calcium and the many tablets needed per dose,
at three to ten times the price of the previously listed supplements, the
cost is unjustifiably high.

VITAMIN D: CALCIUM'S BEST FRIEND

Regardless of our age, we need to be sure that our calcium is accompanied by adequate amounts of vitamin D, a fat-soluble vitamin that helps
transport calcium from our intestines to our blood, stimulates our bone-
building cells, and improves bone mineralization. In the absence of vitamin D, a paltry 10 percent of the calcium we ingest is absorbed. If we
have limited exposure to the sun or live in a mostly sunless climate, our
internal production of vitamin D will be compromised. Normally we
need 400 units of vitamin D a day, more if we're not exposed to sunlight,
and perhaps as much as 800 units if we are elderly.

Getting sufficient amounts of calcium and vitamin D can make a
dramatic difference in the state of our bones. One study looked at a
group of women between the ages of 70 and 104 (average age 84). Half
of the women were given 1,200 milligrams of calcium and 800 units of
vitamin D. The others received no supplementation to their regular, cal-
cium-poor diet. After eighteen months, those who took calcium and vitamin D had a 43 percent decrease in hip fractures and a 32 percent
decrease in nonspinal fractures. No matter what your past or current calcium intake, it's never to late to start protecting your bones.

THE MAGNESIUM CONNECTION

Magnesium does a number of important jobs, among them helping us absorb other minerals, especially calcium. Fortunately, magnesium is found
in a lot of foods—milk, fresh green vegetables (it's an element of the

green part, the chlorophyll), soybeans, wheat germ, whole grains, seafood, figs, corn, apples, seeds, and nuts.

The suggested magnesium RDA for women is 300 milligrams, but many of us get less than 200. Our bodies probably need 250 to 300 milligrams of magnesium, and since we only absorb 50 percent of the magnesium we ingest, the suggested RDA may indeed be too low. If our diet has little fish, no milk products, and is not rich in greens and grains, we might want to add magnesium when we add our calcium. There are many calcium-magnesium combinations on the market containing 40 to 500 milligrams of magnesium; most are made with calcium carbonate. Or we can continue with our regular calcium tablets and add a separate tablet of magnesium (these come in doses of 60 to 400 milligrams). Remember, if you take a multivitamin that contains minerals, it too will provide magnesium (usual doses are 40 to 100 milligrams). In general, there should be no reason to supplement more than 500 milligrams of magnesium. Magnesium overdose could be dangerous.

HOW TO FIGURE OUT IF WE'RE ABSORBING OUR CALCIUM

We should excrete 2 to 3 milligrams of calcium per kilogram of body weight in our urine. A twenty-four-hour urine collection should contain at least 50 milligrams of calcium. This can easily be tested in most labs (the only difficult part is saving urine for twenty-four hours). If we excrete less than this, we may need higher or different calcium doses, as well as vitamin D and magnesium. Other medical factors, such as our general nutrition, kidney function, hormonal status, and bone density, should, of course, be investigated if we're excreting too little.

POTASSIUM BICARBONATE: A NEW SUPPLEMENT

Our bones not only support us, they act as a calcium reservoir that our bodies draw upon for other processes. For example, that reserve will be "dipped into" to balance and neutralize our blood pH when it becomes too acidic, often because of what we eat. A recent study showed that adding a solution of potassium bicarbonate (between 60 and 120 millimoles a day, depending on weight) to the diet of postmenopausal women between the ages of 51 and 77 improved their calcium balance, reduced bone resorption, and increased bone formation. This preliminary research suggests that we consider adding this to our calcium and vitamin D as part of an osteoporosis prevention program.

ESTROGEN: THE BONE PROTECTOR

Put simply, bone loss occurs whenever estrogen levels fall. This is because our bone-eating cells become more aggressive and create larger, more numerous cavities in the absence of estrogen. Estrogen-related bone loss can occur at a rate of 2 to 3 percent a year for the first five to ten years after menopause and then at a lower annual rate of 1 percent from our sixties. While we are experiencing this estrogen-related bone loss, we also have a relentless 0.5 percent annual loss of bone, which is simply due to aging. No matter how much calcium we consume, we can only "make up" for age-related bone loss *not for the estrogen-related bone depletion!*

Estrogen replacement restores bone resorption and formation, and returns us to our premenopausal equilibrium. This level of restoration occurs after six to twenty-four months of therapy and will continue for as long as we continue to use estrogen. (See chapter 7 for a full discussion of hormone replacement therapy.) Once we stop estrogen therapy, those aggressive osteoclasts are unleashed, and we resume losing the yearly 2 percent of bone. After five to ten years without estrogen, we've lost our edge and our bones are not any stronger than those of women who never took estrogen.

The message is clear: If we are going to take estrogen to protect our bones, we should continue taking it, if at all possible. If we take estrogen continuously through the years following our menopause, we will lose only 16 percent of our bone density between ages 50 and 80. This leaves us with a bone density that is 22 percent higher than that of women who never used estrogen, and that translates into a 73 percent decreased risk of fracture!

Even if you did not use estrogen in your fifties, you can catch up. If you begin "as late" as your sixties or seventies, you will still benefit by increasing your bone density by an initial 5 to 10 percent and then proceed to slow future bone loss from 1 to 0.5 percent a year. This means that if you start estrogen therapy at age 65, by the time you reach 85, your bone density will have been reduced by *only* 18 percent from its premenopausal level (compared to the 33 percent loss experienced by untreated women), and your fracture risk will be reduced by 57 to 69 percent. This bone protection is almost as good as if you started estrogen "the day" you became menopausal.

OTHER TREATMENTS FOR OSTEOPOROSIS: WHAT'S AVAILABLE FOR THOSE OF US WHO CAN'T OR WON'T TAKE ESTROGEN

It would be unfair to suggest that estrogen is the only approach to the treatment of osteoporosis. An estrogen "advantage" exists, but estrogen is not for every woman. There are some new and very promising drugs that can stop excessive bone resorption and also help bone regrowth.

Bisphosphonates

One such group of drugs are the bisphosphonates. Etidronate, the most common form, has been used in Europe, Japan, and Australia for the treatment of osteoporosis, but has yet to be given the "okay" for this use by the FDA. Despite that, many physicians in this country have prescribed it. The bisphosphonates are absorbed into the bone, where they prevent bone resorption. They act like our natural phosphate compounds but cannot be broken down by enzymes. Once in the bone, they are there to stay and irreversibly stop "bone eating" by the osteoclasts.

The concern among physicians and the FDA was that if etidronate was incorrectly prescribed (it should be given for only 14 days out of three months, at a dose of 400 milligrams a day), it would cause bad bone production (termed *osteomalacia*). Since bone is a living tissue and is supposed to be constantly broken down and built up, they questioned whether stopping this remodeling process will, in the long run, cause "abnormal bones." The good news is that studies showed that etidronate-treated bone is good. Bone mass, especially in the spine, increased by 5 percent after two years, and bone biopsies were normal after seven years. Most important, fracture rates, especially in women who already had osteoporosis, decreased. This drug also has few or no side effects.

A newer generation of bisphosphonate that is much more potent than etidronate in its ability to inhibit bone resorption has just received FDA approval for the treatment of osteoporosis; its generic name is alendronate and it's marketed by Merck under the brand name Fosamax. (It took me a while to figure this out, but I guess they meant to tell us this is the maximal phosphonate.) The requisite double-blind, placebo-controlled study was performed with this drug for two to three years on over 1,000 postmenopausal women with osteoporosis. They ranged in age from 44 to 84. The standard dose of Fosamax, which is 10 milligrams a day, was shown to increase their bone density by 6 to 10 percent in three years. These increases were found in their spines, hips, and total body bone, which means that the drug did not cause an increase in one type of bone at the expense of other skeletal areas. How good was this "new" bone? There was a 48 percent reduction in the rate of new verte-bral fractures in women treated with Fosamax compared with those who took the placebo. The treated women also lost less height (3 millimeters versus 4.6 millimeters) and, finally, the drug seemed to have a permanent effect on their bones: What was made, stayed. When these women dis-continued the medication, they did not experience an increased rate of bone loss. That's not to say they continued to make denser bones; they simply lost bone at the "usual" rate. This means that continuous daily treatment would be needed as long as we want to control the disease.

Fosamax sounds great (therapeutically speaking, it leaves us with-out a bone to pick). Well, not quite. This pill requires an empty playing field for its absorption. That means we need to take it first thing in the morning with 8 ounces of water and can't eat or drink anything else (not even coffee or juice) for at least one half-hour. Ideally, we should wait two hours, since half an hour gives only 40 percent of the absorption and bioavailability of a two-hour wait. Moreover, we can't set our alarm, take the pill, roll over, and go back to sleep. If we're lying down, the medica-tion won't get into our stomach and could also irritate our esophagus. We have to be up—coffee-less and hungry. There is also a list of precau-tions. We shouldn't use Fosamax if we have lowered kidney function. Doctors are advised to "use caution" when prescribing Fosamax for pa-tients with stomach problems such as ulcers or gastritis.

The final disappointment: Only a small number of women in the Fosamax osteoporosis trials were also receiving estrogen, and although the researchers found what they called "no adverse experiences" when the two therapies were combined, they did not recommend using Fos-amax if we're already on hormone replacement because of "lack of clini-cal experience." It's been shown that etidronate and estrogen have additive effects, and women who took both in early menopause had higher bone densities than those who took only one. It's possible that we'll achieve a similar synergistic effect with Fosamax. In the meantime, should we stop estrogen to take Fosamax? At this point, the answer would have to be "no." Fosamax will not protect us from cardiovascular diseases or bestow the other significant benefits we get with hormones (see chapter 7). If, however, we can't or won't take estrogen and have osteoporosis, this and other improved bisphosphonates "stand" to alter the disastrous course of this disease.

Calcitonin

Approved by the FDA for the treatment of osteoporosis, calcitonin works by stopping bone resorption; it antagonizes the bone-eating osteoclasts. Unlike estrogen, it actually stimulates the bone-forming cells to make new bone and can gradually cause a 5 to 20 percent increase in bone mass. It is also a bone anesthetic and decreases the pain associated with the compression fractures of severe osteoporosis. We produce our own calcitonin in our thyroid, but the amount is not sufficient for bone protection after menopause. Birds and fish also produce calcitonin, and scientists have copied fish (salmon) calcitonin and created a synthetic molecule that is fifteen times more potent than our own human product.

So why isn't this our first line of bone defense? First, there are some distressing side effects, including a decrease in appetite (perhaps welcomed by some of us, but clinically relevant), nausea, vomiting, diarrhea, frequent urination, and flushing. Calcitonin can't be given as an oral pill because our stomach enzymes break it down. Until recently, it could be administered only in shots, and these were very expensive. A calcitonin nasal spray has been developed and is used in other countries. It just became available in the United States under the brand name Miacalcin. We welcome this additional armament in our bone war.

Sodium Fluoride

We have all heard that fluoride helps give us good teeth and strong bones (despite the controversy of the 1960s that we were passively being drugged with this substance in our water supply). We have accepted its value, at least for our teeth. Large doses were used in the 1980s to combat osteoporosis. We knew it stimulated bone formation, but over time our initial enthusiasm waned. The fluoride-treated bone was faulty, and fracture rates rose rather than fell. Women on this therapy also developed stomach upset, ulcers, and leg pain. However, just when we expected to give up on fluoride, researchers have found a new combination of slow-release fluoride and calcium that may increase "good" spinal bone mass by more than 4 percent a year, over four years, and hip-bone density by 2.4 percent. The fluoride saga is not over, but it "walks" a fine line between toxicity and effectiveness that can be defined only after long-term clinical trials.

How Good Are Our Bones? Who Will Stand and Who Will Fall?

Since our bones are hidden under soft-tissue padding, it's not easy to determine whether they are silently becoming unstable. While there are specific medical tests to ascertain our precise bone status (see below), determining our past and current risk factors can go a long way in helping us remain erect.

GENETIC RISK FACTORS

We can't do anything about the risk factors we inherited, but it's important to recognize them so we can try to compensate.

1. *Are you Caucasian or Asian?*   Studies have shown that the lighter or more transparent your skin, the more likely you are to have poor bone mass. Skin thickness and collagen content also can be used as indicators of bone risk. For example, one study has shown that if your skin is really transparent, your risk for osteoporosis is 83 percent, as opposed to 12.5 percent if your skin is opaque. The transparency of our skin reflects the future "transparency" of our bones.

2. *Are you thin and "small-boned"?*   Being svelte may make model sense, but doesn't always make bone sense. Lack of fat cells means lack of an extra production of estrogen, which protects bone density. Lack of muscle means lack of the exercise and weight-bearing stress that also builds bone strength. If you started out with small bone structure, you have less bone to lose before you are at increased risk for fracture.

3. *Did your mother or any other close relative have osteoporosis?* They may not have announced they had osteoporosis (older

generations of women didn't even admit to menopause), but remember back. Was your grandmother or mother stooped, did she develop a dowager hump, or fracture a hip? If your mother broke her hip, your own risk of hip fracture doubles. If she broke her hip before the age of eighty, your risk is even greater. Recently, scientists have found an osteoporosis gene. There is a particular gene that codes for the production of a protein in the body that helps vitamin D transport calcium into bone cells. If you inherit a faulty version of this gene, your bone density is destined to be poor. One day, it might be possible to be screened by simply checking for this osteoporosis gene. Once your risk is unmasked, you could choose aggressive osteoporosis therapy before the disease becomes severe.

Past and Current Risk Factors

As you read the list below, you may find that some of these risk factors applied to you in your teens or twenties, while others have applied throughout your life and may even apply now.

INADEQUATE CALCIUM

Your body has required a daily minimum of 1,000 milligrams of calcium every day since adolescence, more during times when you were pregnant or nursing. Without receiving this minimum, your bones may not have reached their potential optimal mass at age 30, leaving you to begin your future years with a built-in bone deficit.

LACK OF ESTROGEN

Experiencing menopause at an early age or being post-menopausal and not on estrogen therapy will put you at risk. The younger you are when you are deprived of your estrogen—either suddenly through surgical removal of the ovaries or because of an unusually early menopause—the earlier you will begin to lose bone density and the higher your risk for osteoporosis. The risks for postmenopausal women are detailed above.

INADEQUATE SUNSHINE

You need ten to fifteen minutes of UV exposure a day to get adequate vitamin D. If you are homebound, stay out of the sun, or live in a sunless climate, you risk D deficiency and poor calcium absorption.

LACK OF WEIGHT-BEARING EXERCISE

Stress may be bad in some ways, but not for our bones. Mechanical forces, or stress, stimulate our bone-building cells. A skeleton free of mechanical stress or gravitational force loses its reason for being, and its mass quite rapidly diminishes. This phenomenon occurs with prolonged bed rest, immobilization of a limb, paralysis, and space flight (few of us can use this last excuse).

Weight-bearing exercise—walking, running, jogging, climbing stairs—is an aerobic activity that will put weight and stress on our bones. (Swimming will not, although walking in water with special resistance equipment will.) This type of exercise benefits our bones at every stage of life: It helps us reach our potential bone mass when we're young, it maintains this mass after age 30, and it reduces bone loss after menopause. In fact, menopausal women who walk, jog, or climb stairs for an hour three times a week have been found to increase their bone mass by 5.2 percent in just one year, while during this same period, their sedentary controls lost 1.2 percent.

Resistance training to build muscles will also stress our bones. If we build muscle in a particular area, the bone moved by these muscles increases in strength. In a recent study, 20 women who underwent surgical menopause were give estrogen replacement and divided into two groups. One group received resistance weight training and increased their spinal bone density by 8.3 percent, while the control group, which did not train, increased theirs by only 1.5 percent. Exercise also confers added benefits by keeping us fit and better able to maintain our balance; as "balanced" women we're much less likely to fall and sustain a fracture.

SMOKING

Women who smoke set off a domino effect: Their chemically exposed ovaries produce less estrogen, so they start off with lower bone density; they have an earlier menopause, which reduces what little estrogen protection they have; and after menopause, they lose bone mass at a faster rate. One study estimates that women who smoke one pack of cigarettes a day throughout adulthood reach menopause with a 5 to 10 percent decrease in bone loss, resulting in a 40 to 45 percent increase in their risk of hip fracture.

EXCESSIVE ALCOHOL

Alcohol can inhibit our absorption of calcium and vitamin D; it may also decrease our liver's ability to activate vitamin D. There are reports that women who have two to six drinks a week are at increased risk of suffering hip fracture. If we already have osteoporosis, any amount of alcohol can cause us to lose our balance, fall, and sustain a fracture.

EXCESSIVE CAFFEINE

Caffeine increases our urinary loss of calcium. It may also affect our bones by reducing bone remodeling and calcium turnover. The question of caffeine and calcium was addressed in the Nurses' Study. Women who were high caffeine consumers (more than four cups of coffee a day) were found to have a three-fold increase in their risk of hip fractures compared to caffeine-abstinent women. But what about those of us who are more moderate? A recent study of nearly 1,000 women between the ages of 50 and 98 (mean age 72.7) reported that those who had a lifetime coffee intake equivalent to just two cups per day had decreased bone density. However, women who drank at least one glass of milk a day had normal bone density, even though they were still having their two cups of coffee. This would seem to suggest that we can overcome (or milk away) caffeine's effect on bone loss if we just get enough calcium (or we could help "express" this by drinking café au lait). (See Table 17.9 for some surprising sources of caffeine.)

EXCESSIVE USE OF SOFT DRINKS AND OTHER PHOSPHOROUS-CONTAINING FOODS AND BEVERAGES

Soft drinks—both diet and regular—contain phosphoric acid, which leaches calcium. Effervescent mineral water and some natural juice "sodas" don't. Better yet, have a glass of milk!

EXCESSIVE WEIGHT LOSS OR EXERCISE WITH PROLONGED ABSENCE OF
MENSTRUAL PERIODS

If we quickly lose more than 10 percent of our ideal body weight or go
below a critical body fat content, our body reacts by shutting down the
brain's signals to our ovaries. This is nature's way of protecting our diminished resources from the physical stresses of pregnancy and childbirth and not wasting energy on ovulation and estrogen production. Our
periods stop or become irregular, a sure sign that our estrogen level has
dropped. Since our bones don't know how old we are, they respond to
any dramatic drop in estrogen in much the same way they would respond
to menopause. The result is a menopausal rate of bone loss years before
we actually reach menopause.

LONG-TERM OR EXCESSIVE USE OF CERTAIN MEDICATIONS

Certain drugs inhibit calcium absorption. These include therapeutic
fiber preparations such as Metamucil, antacids containing aluminum,
certain diuretics (furosemides), steroids, high doses of anticonvulsant
drugs, lithium, and excessive levels of thyroid hormone. The antibiotic
tetracycline reduces calcium absorption and, conversely, calcium reduces
uptake of tetracycline.

Most of us will find that we "qualify" for some of these osteoporosis risk
factors. Hopefully, our honest self-assessment will be our collective call
to arms (and legs and backs).

Screening for Osteoporosis: How Do We Test Our Bones?

We fail if we wait for the ultimate test of our bone strength: whether or
not we sustain a fracture with a simple fall. If you "fall" into a risk category, you can do one of two things: Immediately and aggressively embark
on a program to stop this demineralization process, or, if like many of us
you need one more incentive, get a real picture of your own bone
strength. Bone-density scans are reliable, inexpensive, and readily performed at most radiology labs.

DUAL ENERGY X-RAY ABSORPTIOMETRY (DEXA)

DEXA can measure the bone density of the spine, hip, and total body with a precision of 1 to 2 percent. The machine actually prints out a picture of our bones. Either by shades of black and white or by color, it indicates the density, and a computer gives us an appropriate reading. Radiation is very low. Just to reassure you (about the machine, not our environment), the average adult in the United States receives 3,000 uSVs (the unit of natural radiation) a year, and a spinal bone-density scan adds 1 uSV or 0.03 percent of our yearly average. You are not exposing yourself to unnecessary radiation.

The report card from this test is given in fairly complicated medical lingo. Your bone density is measured in grams of calcium per square centimeter. These values are then compared with those of an "ideal average woman" (an oxymoron) who is 30 years old and has reached her "bone best." Doctors can tell you what percentage of your bone has been lost from this ideal thirties level and whether that amount currently puts you at risk for a fracture. If at age 50 you have lost 10 percent of your bone mass, you have a lifetime fracture risk of 30 percent. If you have lost 20 percent, this risk doubles, and if it's 30 percent, it would double again, but you can't get to 120 percent, so your lifetime risk of fracture becomes 100 percent! Risk at any age is also calculated in standard deviations from the norm at age 30. A decrease of one standard deviation, which roughly corresponds to 10 percent bone loss, doubles your fracture risk. If you are 2.5 standard deviations below the mean (and it is mean to get this result), you have significant osteoporosis.

This is your bone scale. You can use it to check your baseline and make decisions about therapy. It can also be used as an ongoing check to follow your living, remodeling skeleton.

ULTRASOUND

An even simpler predictor of bone mass has recently been developed: an ultrasound of the heel bone. If the ultrasound easily passes through this bone, the bone is porous. Excellent correlations between heel-bone density and that of our hips and spines have been demonstrated in early studies. Remember in the 1950s how we stuck our feet into fluoroscopy machines to see if our new shoes fit? This was probably "radiation abuse," but with ultrasound, we are safe—there's no radiation. In the future, we may again be putting our feet into an imaging machine to see if our bones "are fit."

CHEMICAL TESTS

There also are chemical tests that can be used to assess the status of your bones, especially if you have bone loss. The amount of calcium excreted in your urine can be analyzed to see if you are absorbing calcium. Levels of certain chemical markers of bone formation and bone breakdown can also be checked in your blood and urine. These can be used to assess the immediate efficacy of any treatment.

A Message to Our Daughters

Our mothers were right but did not always prevail during our baby boomer rebellion. Maybe we can do better. Our daughters need to know that dairy products are a must. Weight-bearing exercise is invaluable. We should be sure our daughters have regular periods. If they skip periods, they need to see a doctor. It may be advisable to have them use low-dose birth control pills, not just for contraception (gulp!), but to get enough estrogen to protect their bones. If they are not eating right, we should bribe, coerce, or even try logic to get them to take calcium supplements and vitamins. If at all possible, let's not let our daughters become the newest sacrifices to cigarette ads. We, and they, can "come a long way" with straight posture by not smoking. And, anyway, who wants to be called "baby"? We also have a role in the battle of the fluids. We can serve and drink milk, juices, and water instead of coffee, tea, processed sodas, and alcohol.

Our new mother-daughter term of endearment should no longer be a simple "dear." Let's substitute "DER" (for dairy, exercise, and regular periods) and really make a difference.

12

CANCER
Our Worst Fear,
but Need It Be?

Remember when we didn't even utter the word "cancer"; we used to call it "the big C"? If we did use the full word, it was whispered, as if saying it aloud would either raise evil spirits or cause direct contamination and disease to anyone within earshot. Our past avoidance of the word, our state of denial and conspiracy of silence hurt us tremendously. Indeed, lack of prevention, screening, and treatment allowed us to succumb to our worst fear.

Science and medicine have advanced tremendously in the understanding and treatment of cancer. We have to keep up. The world is becoming computer-literate, and few want to be left out. Women have to be cancer-literate, or we will be left out with far more serious consequences.

Why Do We Get Cancer?

Each of our cells has a particular genetic structure, or architectural plan. This inner plan controls the cell's function, its ability to reproduce or multiply, and its life span. As we age, our cells are subjected to wear and tear, as well as exposure to the garbage we put into our bodies and contaminants we have placed in our environment. Genes get changed or are poorly copied or are no longer protected from the runaway effects of their mistakes by other genes (tumor-suppressor genes). This process is called *mutation*. Certain mutations result in cancer-causing genes, or *oncogenes*. The source of the mutation might be genetic (i.e., we are born with an error in place), or there might be an interplay of genetics and environment. Oncogenes may not be present at birth, but we can inherit or develop a "weakness" that permits their growth under the bombardment of bad influences (radiation, chemicals, or simply aging). Once a cell's inner plan goes awry, the usual instructions are absent, and it and its descendants change their behavior. These previously "civilized" cells undergo anarchy. They manifest uncontrolled growth and invade normal tissue and organs. Abnormal cancer cells cannot perform normal functions, and our body suffers. Without defensive treatment, we may die.

Breast Cancer: An Attack on Our Female Being

STATISTICS: THE BEST OF TIMES, THE WORST OF NUMBERS

The increased rate at which we are developing this truly female cancer (men are one fortieth less likely to develop breast cancer as women) is alarming. One in eight women is currently expected to develop breast cancer in her lifetime. This proportion has increased by 52 percent since 1950. Currently, 182,000 women develop breast cancer, and an estimated 46,000 die yearly. Is this an epidemic?

These numbers have to be put into some perspective. The actual 1 in 8 represents the likelihood of breast cancer at age 85. At 40, the figure is quite low, 1 in 223, and increases as we get older. Nearly half the increase in lifetime risk since the 1950s can be attributed to increased longevity. There is also an increase in the incidence, or rate, with which breast cancer strikes American women, but again this appears to occur when we are older. In fact, there has been no apparent change in the breast cancer rates of women under the age of 56 since 1950. If we talk to our friends or doctors, we all seem to think we are seeing more breast cancer in younger women. That's because as baby boomers enter middle age there are simply more of us, so that even with the same rate of breast cancer (200 per 100,000 women), more of us are stricken.

IS THERE A LETHAL WEAPON? WHAT CAUSES BREAST CANCER?

Do Chemicals Cause Cancer?

We blame just about every product of our modern agricultural and industrial growth for our breast cell mutations and resulting cancer. We were promised better living through chemistry; we got pesticides and harmful substances that irreversibly entered our ground, water, livestock, and food. By-products of DDT and PCBs are stored in high concentration in the fat of animals and in the fat of their milk. These resemble estrogen, and once they enter our bodies, they can easily fit into our estrogen receptors. Our breasts are loaded with these receptors. Studies have shown that women with the highest levels of pesticide residues in their breasts are four times more likely to get breast cancer than women whose breasts are "pesticide-free." There is an unreasonably high incidence of breast cancer in female farmworkers, whose exposure has been enormous. Industrial toxins pollute our atmosphere as well as our livestock. Chlorine is a component of many estrogen-binding chemicals. A study is currently being undertaken to look at its effect on our health and our estrogen-binding breasts. Congress is considering phasing out chlorine in the paper and pulp industries, but how many other chemicals bind to our breast cells, confuse our genes, and result in tumors?

Do Hormones Cause Breast Cancer?

BIRTH CONTROL PILLS AND BREAST CANCER

We have questioned the role of estrogen in various forms and its possible association with breast cancer. Most scientists feel that the widespread use of birth control pills did not cause an increase in breast cancer. According to some studies, there may be two possible exceptions: Women who used the very-high-dose pills for long periods of time, and women who develop breast cancer under the age of 45 and used the Pill for many years before delivery of their first baby. If there is a questionable risk, it might not even be due to the estrogen in the Pill, but could have been influenced by the presence of a second hormone, progesterone. Doctors are now looking at a long-acting progesterone, Depo-Provera, which is injected every three months.

HORMONE REPLACEMENT THERAPY AND BREAST CANCER

The most controversial estrogen is that which we use after menopause for hormone replacement. This differs from the estrogen in birth control pills; it is conjugated, or natural, estrogen similar to that which our ovaries produce. The amount used is only one fourth as strong as that in the lowest-dose birth control pills. It is "hormone replacement," which means it is as close as possible to the amount of estrogen our ovaries produce before menopause. There are a number of possible factors that cause us to worry about an association between estrogen replacement therapy and breast cancer.

1. Many breast cancers have estrogen receptors. Breast cancer tumors are often "differentiated"; that is, the cancer cells have not undergone complete anarchy and still "remember" their breast tissue past. They maintain their ability to connect to and be influenced by estrogen. We postulate that these estrogen-sensitive tumors may grow more quickly in an estrogen-rich environment. Estrogen replacement therapy might not cause normal cells to become cancerous, but in certain instances it could augment the growth of preexisting cancer cells. What does this mean? A tumor that might take seven to nine years to grow to a size we could detect might reach that size a few years earlier. But it was always going to be there! We can still detect and treat this cancer at an early stage. The good news (this is relative) is that these "dependent" tumors respond best to therapy, and women who develop breast cancer while taking estrogen have a much lower death rate than women who develop breast cancer while not on hormones.

2. Women take estrogen replacement therapy for many years. The effect of long-term or lifetime therapy is difficult to evaluate because we need to study a lifetime of thousands of women.

3. ERT is given at an age when we are at increasing risk for breast cancer. Our "age risk" is less likely to be blamed for breast cancer than our "hormone risk." When we're stricken, we and our physicians want to blame something. Psychologically, but not scientifically, we need to find a cancer scapegoat; often it's estrogen therapy.

4. Data from studies are confusing. There have been over fifty studies searching for a correlation between estrogen therapy and the risk of breast cancer. The results are very confusing! The data from these studies have been combined, separated, dissected, and discounted or lauded by some very fancy statistical analyses (see chapter 7).

The American College of Obstetricians and Gynecologists formed a committee (something doctors always do when we are confused) to give physicians some sort of informed opinion on the subject. Their conclusion, published in 1994, was that

> More than 50 epidemiologic studies have failed to demonstrate consistently or conclusively a detrimental impact of replacement estrogen use on the incidence of breast cancer.

These experts also made another important observation: that although current studies (up to 1994) don't show that estrogen increases rates of breast cancer, the many inadequacies of these studies and lack of long-term follow-up on a sufficiently large number of women "preclude total reassurance that ERT is safe in these women [regarding breast cancer risk]."

There is no single, definitive answer. The decision to use or not use estrogen should not be made on the breast cancer issue alone. We must weigh a questionable risk against several less questionable benefits and then come to a decision based on our own individual health needs and concerns.

Risk Factors in Breast Cancer

Can anyone predict which of us will be the "1 in 8"? Table 12.1 lists some of our relative risks, which measure the degree to which a given factor increases our chance of developing breast cancer. Each number over 1 represents the percentage of increase in risk for that factor. For example, having no first-degree relatives with breast cancer places your risk at 1, while your mother's having developed breast cancer before age 60 gives you a relative risk of 2—a 100 percent increase—in other words, your risk is doubled.

Before we can formulate an effective breast care plan, we need to acknowledge the following risk factors, some of which are avoidable.

TABLE 12.1   RISK OF BREAST CANCER (Probable)

	Risk of 1 (comparison)	Risk Factor	Relative Risk
Family history	No first-degree relatives	Mother affected before age 60	2.0
		Mother affected after age 60	1.4
Age at first period	16	Under 14	1.3
Age at birth of first child	Under 20	20 to 24	1.3
		25 to 29	1.6
		Over 30	1.9
		No children	1.9
Age at menopause	45 to 54	Over 55	1.5
		Under 45	0.7
		Ovaries removed before 35	0.4
Benign breast disease	No biopsy or aspiration	Biopsy done: benign	1.5
		Biopsy done: overgrowth of glands (proliferation)	2.0
		Atypical glands	4.0
Obesity	Thin: 10th percentile	Overweight: 90th percentile	1.2
Alcohol consumption	Nondrinker	1 drink/day	1.4
		2 drinks/day	1.7
		3 drinks/day	2.0

Note: For hormones, see chapter 7; too complicated to give numerical risk.

Adapted from Jay R. Harris, Margo E. Lippman, Umberto Veronesi, and Walter Willett.

AGE

This is the single most significant risk factor for breast cancer. The probability of breast cancer increases with age, as indicated in Table 12.2.

FAMILY HISTORY

More than 90 percent of breast cancers are "sporadic," meaning that they occur in women with no evidence of inherited susceptibility. You

TABLE 12.2   AGE-RELATED ODDS OF DEVELOPING BREAST CANCER

Age	Odds
25	1 in 19,608
35	1 in 622
45	1 in 93
55	1 in 33
65	1 in 17
75	1 in 11
85	1 in 8

should never allow yourself to feel complacent because you probably have not inherited a genetic predisposition for breast cancer. You still need to remain extremely vigilant. If you do have a family history of breast cancer on your mother's side, especially if it occurred before menopause, be aware that it places you at higher risk. If two or more relatives (mother, aunt, sisters, or grandmother) had breast cancer, you are at risk for "familial" breast cancer. Several types of breast cancer have been shown to be inherited. These appear to be due to genetic aberrations that cause the activation of tumor-promoting genes (oncogenes) and deactivation of tumor-suppressor genes. Women who develop genetic cancer are younger and more likely to have the disease in both breasts than women who develop the more common, sporadic cancer.

Recent advances in gene mapping have allowed us to begin a search for breast cancer genes. We have managed to "map" only a fraction of all human genes, so it's quite probable that there are additional, undiscovered breast cancer genes out there. Two breast cancer genes have already been identified. The first is called BRCA-1, and this gene has been fully isolated and mapped and is found on chromosome 17. Mutations of this gene predispose women to breast and ovarian cancer. If a woman with a strong family history of breast cancer has a mutated BRCA-1 gene, she has an 80 to 85 percent lifetime risk of developing breast cancer and a 50 percent risk of ovarian cancer. This mutated gene is passed down in a dominant fashion, which means that each of her children have a fifty-fifty chance of inheriting it. If they are boys, this increases their risk of prostate cancer and colon cancer. They, of course, can later pass the risk of breast cancer to their daughters.

More than one hundred mutations have been identified in the BRCA-1 gene. Some are "nonsense" changes and don't cause cancer. One serious mutation classified as 185delAG seems to have an alarmingly high incidence (1 percent) in Ashkenazi or Eastern European Jewish women. This mutation may have been passed down from a common ancestor. (Let's not point the finger at Moses—he wasn't Ashkenazi.)

It's not clear that all women (Jewish or otherwise) who have an "abnormal" BRCA-1 gene will develop breast cancer. If they have no family history, it's possible that they also possess "saving" genes that block or counteract this mutation's effects. We've recently discovered that the BRCA-1 gene instructs cells to produce (you guessed it) BRCA-1 protein. This should reside in the nucleus of the cell where it controls genetic instructions for the cell's growth and function. If the protein is abnormal or misplaced outside of the nucleus, it can't do its job, and the cell grows in a malignant fashion. The "saving" genes may in some way protect this protein.

It's possible that we can develop a mutation of BRCA-1 without a known family history. It's been found to be present in at least 10 percent of women who develop breast cancer before the age of 35. We estimate that 1 in 200 to 400 American women may be carriers of a BRCA-1 mutation. If they're Jewish, this has been calculated to confer a 20 percent risk of developing early breast cancer (under the age of 40), and if they're not Jewish, this risk is 9 percent.

A second gene, BRCA-2, has been localized on chromosome 13. Its mutations may account for one-third of our genetic breast cancers. It too confers an 80 percent lifetime risk of breast cancer, but it's less virulent to our ovaries than BRCA-1 changes. Women who harbor a defective form of this gene have "only" a 20 percent chance of developing ovarian cancer. Men, however, are not just carriers; they're afflicted with a 20 percent risk of breast cancer as well as an increase in prostate and colon cancer. If a man develops breast cancer, it may be sporadic, but it's so rare it's likely that he has a mutated BRCA-2 gene, which he can pass to his offspring. So the message is clear; breast cancer history (and ovarian cancer and probably colon and prostate cancer) have to be assessed on both sides of our families; paternal may be as important as maternal.

THE "OPEN-WINDOW" PERIODS OF OUR LIVES

There are two times in our lives when our estrogen window is open and we're exposed to estrogen without the protective effect of progesterone. In the years before puberty, our estrogen levels increase and may stay elevated for four to five years before normal and regular ovulation occurs. Once we ovulate and are exposed to progesterone or become pregnant, we close the estrogen window. When we enter a long perimenopause with irregular ovulation or a late menopause, we open the estrogen window again. Other factors that prolong duration of the open window and are associated with an increase in breast cancer are:

- Infertility due to lack of ovulation
- Obesity (being more than 20 percent above your appropriate weight); excess fat produces excess estrogen
- Delayed pregnancy (having your first child after 30)
- Early menarche (having a first period before age 12)
- Late menopause (after age 53)

Breast-feeding for at least six months helps decrease the risk of breast cancer, perhaps because it lowers estrogen production and closes the window.

SMOKING

If you smoke, you naturally have a higher risk of lung cancer, but did you know that you also increase your risk of breast cancer? A growing list of pollutants and harmful substances in this inhaled poison has been correlated with development of oncogenic mutations. We worry about external pollutants in our environment; when we smoke, we send known toxins straight to our breasts.

HIGH-FAT DIET AND OBESITY

The more overweight we are, the more prone to breast cancer we are, especially if most of our weight is in our abdomen (the "apple" shape). Overweight women may produce more insulin (making it harder to lose weight; it's a vicious cycle) and more insulinlike growth factor 1 (IGF-

1), similar to the growth factors that have been found to promote breast cancer. If you're overweight, it may be because you are eating a high-fat diet. Even if you are not obese, the hamburgers, French fries, ice cream, and other "staples" of our so-called American diet give us a concentrated dose of the pesticides stored in animal and dairy fat. Increased fat has also been found to cause molecular damage to breast cells, which can lead to cancer. Recent studies have shown a 50 percent increase in risk among women ingesting high levels of saturated fat.

We know that Japanese women who maintain a traditional diet—which has less than half the fat that we consume—have a rate of breast cancer that is one fourth of ours. When Japanese women move to Western countries and adopt our Western diet, that difference disappears within one generation. Dr. Peter Greenwald, Director of the National Cancer Institute, Division of Cancer Prevention and Control, has stated, "If the American diet were as low in fat as the Japanese was until recently (10 to 20 percent fat), then rather than the 46,000 deaths per year, we might expect our breast cancer death rate to be much lower, possibly as low as 11,000."

Ample nutrition also makes us grow taller, and we begin our periods earlier than many non-Western or Third World women. Both our height and early puberty may be risk factors for breast cancer.

LACK OF EXERCISE

Lack of exercise not only contributes to obesity but deprives us of an important opportunity to fight breast cancer. We need every form of prevention we can get! Researchers have found that even a few hours of physical activity a week can reduce our risk of developing premenopausal breast cancer by as much as 50 percent. It's been found that women with the lowest risk exercised regularly in their teens and twenties and continued to do so for four hours a week. We should be teaching our daughters to exercise to prevent cancer, and join them—a whole new purpose for "Mommy and Me" activities. Researchers are now studying the effect of continued exercise (or taking up exercise again, now that we've learned what it can do) in postmenopausal women.

ALCOHOL

In 1987 two studies published in *The New England Journal of Medicine* caused an uproar. One was the Nurses' Study, which reported a 30 to 60 percent increase in the risk of breast cancer with just 5 grams of alcohol a day (or approximately three drinks a week). The risk seemed to be even higher—250 percent—in women under 55 who had no risk factors for breast cancer and who inbibed one or more drinks a day. Another study, which looked at 7,000 women from across the country over a ten-year period, found that any amount of alcohol was associated with an increased risk of breast cancer ranging from 50 to 100 percent. The association between drinking and breast cancer was stronger in premenopausal than postmenopausal women and greater in leaner than heavier women.

A recent review of thirty-eight studies came to a less alarming conclusion: Daily consumption of one alcoholic drink was associated with an 11 percent increase in breast cancer. This rose to 24 percent with two drinks, and 38 percent with three drinks. Whether it's by 50 percent or 11 percent, however, we're not sure why alcohol increases our breast cancer risk. Several theories have been put forth based on our knowledge of how alcohol can adversely affect the liver, estrogen levels, DNA, and the immune system.

BREAST CYSTS AND PREVIOUS ABNORMAL BREAST BIOPSIES

Women who develop multiple breast cysts, especially if they are recurrent and need to be drained, do have a higher cancer risk, perhaps because the cysts tell of some abnormal breast cell activity or stress. If a biopsy shows multiplying or enlarged breast cells (*hyperplasia*) and they are irregular (*atypia*), there is also a greater chance that other areas of "irregular" breast tissue might develop into cancer.

DES (DIETHYLSTILBESTROL)

This was a type of estrogen that was given to women who threatened to miscarry during the late 1950s and 1960s. It was subsequently shown to have no effect on the miscarriage rate, and, unfortunately, may increase the rate of breast cancer in those women who took it. It appears that the risk of breast cancer becomes greater with the length of time since exposure. Current research seems to indicate that this risk may increase by 30 to 40 percent after twenty years. Daughters of women who took DES are just now entering their forties. Only time will tell if they too are at increased risk for breast cancer.

THE PROVERBIAL NEEDLE IN A HAYSTACK: SCREENING FOR EARLY BREAST CANCER

MAMMOGRAPHY: THE PICTURE THAT CAN SAVE YOUR LIFE

Until we know how to prevent breast cancer, our best weapon against it is early detection. Mammography is the mainstay of this arsenal. If we find a tumor when it's small (less than 1 centimeter) and it hasn't spread to the lymph nodes, we can survive this malignancy 95 percent of the time. The average-size lump detected through breast self-exam is greater than 1 inch in diameter; mammography can "pick up" a tumor when it is less than a quarter of this size. Despite these impressive diagnostic differences between hands and machines, less than 29 percent of American women have mammograms on schedule. What this means is that right now, 2.6 million women in the United States have breast cancer, but 1 million don't know it. Without the right picture, we lose diagnostic time and lives!

The mammogram machine squeezes our breasts from top to bottom and then from side to side, while sending X rays through them. We might assume that this machine was invented by a man. However, I have to admit that the principal researcher who stressed the importance of rigorous compression for good pictures was a woman! The X-ray films that are printed after this admittedly uncomfortable and inelegant procedure show a general picture of our breasts, their glands, fat, and blood vessels, and any changes in densities within them. Most important, they can show tumors. These may vary from small, round, even opaque areas (probably benign) to uneven, spiderlike changes that are very white against the general "blackness" of the breast fat (the older we are, the more fatty our breasts and the more easily we can see these irregular patterns). Many early breast cancers contain calcium. This is fortunate, because the smallest "dots" of calcium are starkly visualized in an X ray. An experienced radiologist can usually tell the "good" dots from the bad ones.

Our initial mammogram is termed a "screening mammogram." It both gives a baseline picture of our breasts and can pick up abnormalities. Once done, it should be saved and used to compare with future mammograms so that any change or new calcifications can be detected.

Ninety percent of screening mammograms show "no significant abnormality," and your only action will be to have continued screening. In the 10 percent of cases where an abnormality is found, doctors often do additional compression and magnification views (where our breasts are squeezed even harder!) or ultrasound. In competent imaging centers, about 2 percent of initial screens and 1 percent of repeat mammograms require some sort of biopsy to determine if the abnormal picture is breast cancer. Why is this briefly uncomfortable procedure maligned as dangerous, unnecessary, or too expensive in our cost-conscious (but not always health-conscious) society? Radiation is a scary word for all of us, and since a mammogram is an X ray, and we're supposed to do it yearly—at least after 50 (or, as many of us believe, after 40)—we worry about exposure. Let's get some perspective on our world of rays. "Natural" or background radiation from cosmic rays and our natural surroundings averages about 0.06 rads at sea level. The higher our elevation, the thinner the air, and the thinner the protective ozone layer, the greater our radiation exposure. Background radiation in Denver, Colorado, is four times that at sea level. But women who live in Denver or at other high elevations do not have an increased incidence of breast cancer. Currently, yearly mammograms cause an average dose of 0.2 rads per breast. This is less than the exposure we get by living in Denver or taking a round-trip air flight across the continent.

The usual cost of a mammogram ranges from $75 to $150. The cost of treating a woman with advanced breast cancer is $30,000 to $150,000. There is no low-cost alternative to a mammogram. Most physicians are able to pick up only 40 percent of lumps a half inch in size when placed within artificial breast models. Real breasts are much lumpier and more fibrous, and hang differently from those pert, silicone-filled teaching breasts. Mammogram alone has been credited with decreasing the death rate from breast cancer by 30 percent. We should not avoid or denigrate this picture of our breasts on the basis of cost, radiation, or discomfort.

THE AGE CONTROVERSY: ARE WE EVER TOO YOUNG OR TOO OLD FOR MAMMOGRAMS?

The younger we are, the denser and firmer are our breasts. We knew that! Remember when they used to support themselves and we burned our bras because we could?! Dense, however, is not a good term, radiographically speaking. It "clouds" the X ray's ability to focus in on abnormalities. The general consensus is that mammography in women younger than 30 is useless. Between the ages of 30 and 40, our breasts begin to accumulate more fat, which actually replaces glands, and our tissue is less solidly "packed." Mammography then begins to be able to "see" trouble spots.

In the past, many women had their first baseline mammogram between the ages of 35 and 40. The National Cancer Institute recommended that women between 40 and 49 be screened every one to two years, and after 50, yearly. We all got used to this and simply worked to achieve compliance. This screening schedule for women between 40 and 50 has been questioned after a large Canadian study and early American studies showed that mammogram screening of women in their forties did not lower their death rate from breast cancer. Another issue was the large number of false positive (indicating a possible cancer where none was present) mammograms found in younger women. Because of this increased density and "questionable findings," younger women undergo four times as many biopsies as women over 50 to detect one cancer. This also raises the financial cost of breast care. These issues caused the National Cancer Institute to state that currently it has "no opinion" and will not recommend routine mammography in women under 50.

The ensuing uproar has not been resolved. The quality of many of the Canadian mammograms and the judgment calls of the doctors reading them were criticized (especially by our now outraged American radiologists, who fought this recommendation for obvious reasons). This group also claimed that the Canadian studies used pre-1985 films that were not state-of-the-art and that recent ongoing studies with new and better equipment show a 20 percent decrease in mortality in younger women with early mammographic diagnosis of their breast cancer. A final punch to this radiographic fight: We know that breast cancers in younger women grow faster and have a shorter "preclinical" (before-we-feel-it) phase. If doctors do screen women in their forties, many experts feel it should be done annually, while mammograms every two years after the age of 50 may be sufficient to pick up the slower-growing cancers of "older" women.

So where does this controversy leave us, the X-ray consumers? There is no question that if we have risk factors, we should begin mammography in our forties on a yearly basis. If we are not "at risk" (but may be in the 80 to 90 percent of women who develop sporadic cancer— which, to most of us, is still a risk group), we should still consider early screening in our forties, but realize that we might run a greater chance of needing a biopsy to prove we don't have breast cancer. If finding breast cancer early gives us a 20 percent hedge, we should go for it. The American Cancer Society, the American Medical Association, the American College of Obstetricians and Gynecologists, and the American College of Radiology all agree.

If we establish 40 as a low-end screening age, is there an age when we can finally stop? The answer is no. The older we are, the higher our risk. Advanced age should not make us expendable to the ravages of advanced cancer. The 30 percent decrease in mortality for early pick-up is still a fact for all women. For those of us in our seventies and eighties who are generally healthy, there is no reason to skip regular mammograms. Even an 85-year-old woman can expect to live another 5.6 years.

Breast Self-Examination: Know Thyself!

Few of us over the age of 40 were encouraged to be physically self-exploratory. "Nice girls" didn't touch anything having to do with their sexual beings. We are old enough to get over this conditioned reluctance. It is time to feel, push, squeeze, and observe—our breasts. Ten percent of tumors are not "X-ray-genic"; they don't show up on mammograms. They don't contain calcium, or they grow without the usual X-ray markers, especially in younger women. Eventually, though, they can be felt, and since we are the only ones in constant "contact" with our breasts, it's worthwhile to start feeling them (see the breast self-exam shown in Figure 12.1). We will change doctors over the years, but we, our breasts, and our hands remain a constant. If you know your breasts, you can sometimes reassure a new doctor that what she or he feels has been there unchanged for many years. This will cut down (quite literally) on unnecessary biopsies.

Ideally, we're checking for a lump measuring half an inch, but most of us won't be able to feel anything smaller than one inch. The best time to check our breasts is right after a period, when the glands are less swollen and tender. Those of us who are menopausal need to set a regular date—the first of the month, a full moon, or whenever we pay our bills.

Feeling "something" is not cause to freak. See if it changes after a month or two. If a new lump appears and remains or grows, it's time to consult an "outside" expert. The current large-scale statistics don't show that breast self-examination affects cancer mortality, but it stands to reason that we would rather remove a one-inch lump than one that is three or four times larger; there is less spread, and the surgery is less disfiguring.

FIGURE 12.1

6 Simple Steps to Monthly Breast Self-Examination

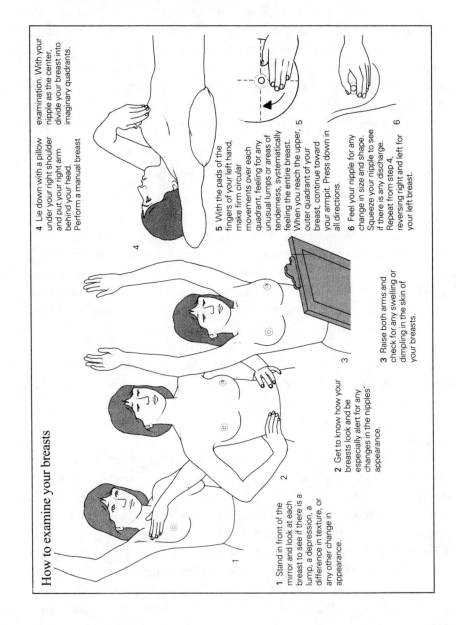

How to examine your breasts

1 Stand in front of the mirror and look at each breast to see if there is a lump, a depression, a difference in texture, or any other change in appearance.

2 Get to know how your breasts look and be especially alert for any changes in the nipples' appearance.

3 Raise both arms and check for any swelling or dimpling in the skin of your breasts.

4 Lie down with a pillow under your right shoulder and put your right arm behind your head. Perform a manual breast examination. With your nipple as the center, divide your breast into imaginary quadrants.

5 With the pads of the fingers of your left hand, make firm circular movements over each quadrant, feeling for any unusual lumps or areas of tenderness, systematically feeling the entire breast. When you reach the upper, outer quadrant of your breast, continue toward your armpit. Press down in all directions.

6 Feel your nipple for any change in size and shape. Squeeze your nipple to see if there is any discharge. Repeat from step 4, reversing right and left for your left breast.

Can Doctors Do a Better Job?
Breast Examination by the Physician

We physicians are supposedly trained to do breast examinations. Clearly, some of us are better at this than others. But give us the benefit of doubt, we do find new or undiscovered lumps, and we are objective observers. A thorough breast exam should always be part of our gynecologic checkup as well as any routine physical. If breast self-exam causes a woman continual anxiety because she always "feels things" or her breasts are difficult to examine, she shouldn't feel embarrassed to see her physician for more frequent breast checkups. I have a patient who comes in every three months for reassurance. This, combined with her yearly mammogram, has kept her anxiety level down.

Breast Ultrasound: If There Is No Radiation,
Why Can't It Be Used to Screen for Cancer?

Ultrasound is just what the word implies: high-frequency sound waves. They are projected through the breast tissue by a transducer. If the tissue is mainly composed of water (as fat is), the waves go through and we see black on the screen. If the waves hit something solid, they are bounced back and recorded as white. The process is, unfortunately, not good for screening. In a recent study, only 23 percent of early breast cancers were detected with this technique. Masses less than 1 to 2 centimeters are not "visualized," and ultrasound doesn't pick up microcalcifications, which are often the hallmark of early cancer.

What we can do is ultrasound a specific area where we either feel a lump or see an irregularity in a mammogram. If the waves bounce back from the mass and record a white area, we are dealing with a solid lump. If the waves go through, it is fluid-filled or cystic. Ultrasound can reassure us and prevent unnecessary biopsies. If a cyst is found, it can be followed or drained with a needle (*aspirated*). If an abnormal area is deemed solid and has irregular borders (also something we can delineate with ultrasound), it should be tested by needle sampling (*core biopsy*) or removal (*excisional biopsy*).

IS EXPENSIVE BETTER? NEW TECHNIQUES FOR
BREAST CANCER DETECTION

MRI (Magnetic Resonance Imaging)   This costly and confining technique (you have to lie still in a tunnel-like space for thirty to sixty minutes) is promising for several reasons: First, there is no radiation. Secondly, MRI may allow us to evaluate a "questionable lesion" found on a mammogram and determine if it is benign or malignant, theoretically sparing us an unnecessary biopsy. MRI can also help determine if a small cancer is there "by itself" or if there are other small clusters of cancer cells in the breast (a not too infrequent occurrence); this allows more appropriate choices for therapy. Finally, MRI is currently the best method to check for silicone leaks from breast implants. Doctors are concerned that these leaks can contribute to the development of autoimmune diseases in certain women. Our bodies try to figure out what to do with this leaked foreign substance, and our immune system attempts to destroy it. In the process, it may make a mistake and end up fighting our own cells and tissue. If silicone leaks are detected, doctors often consider removing the implants to prevent or diminish this complication.

A single MRI can cost up to $1,600 and obviously cannot be used to screen 50 million women annually. Also, it picks up many lesions that are not cancer, causing unnecessary biopsies. It can, however, be used in addition to mammography in very-high-risk women. The degree of risk that warrants MRI will be defined only as we test more women and analyze our "positive pick-up" in the years to come.

PET Scan (Positive Emission Tomography—Not Domestic Animals!)   This test measures the uptake of radioactive labeled sugar into cancer tissue. Cancer cells are more active and use more sugar in their cellular metabolism than normal cells. The greater the consumption of this harmless radioactive sugar (which is injected into the vein one hour prior to the test), the brighter the spot on the scan. Bright spots will pinpoint the cancer and their intensity may correlate with the degree of malignancy. This test is even more expensive than MRI and costs $2,000 to $3,000.

In the future, will we be able to get a shot, lie under a screen, and be checked for cancer "hot spots"? Sounds like science fiction now, but we may be there in the next decade.

MIBI (Scan)   Like PET, MIBI is a "glow scan." Instead of measuring sugar uptake, it looks at the uptake and use of another radioactive substance (technetium-99) by energy units in the cells. Since cancer cells are "overactive," their energy units work like crazy and concentrate the technetium. This scan could help us determine whether an irregular density seen with mammography is actually malignant. Like PET, it's expensive and may not be specific enough for small early (and perhaps less active) cancers.

The Implant Question: Can We Screen, or Are We at Higher Risk for Breast Cancer?

Amid the very public and very litigious ongoing controversy about breast implants and silicone the fact remains that over 1 million to 2 million American women have had breast augmentation. How does this impact on their breast cancer risk? Silicone itself, either as part of the gel-filled implant or when it leaks and is "free" in the breast tissue, has not been implicated in the development of breast cancer. But the mere physical presence of implants can hinder early diagnosis. Breast cancer is often found later or in more advanced stages in women who have undergone breast augmentation. Scarring around the implant and hardening of the implant can make mammography a more difficult and less perceptive screen. Some breast tissue may be hidden or compressed by the implant. Because we don't want to rupture the darn things when we press the breast, we may forfeit getting a better picture.

If you have implants, make sure you go to a radiology lab that offers special techniques for breast visualization, but under no circumstances should you avoid mammography. If you do, you have allowed your implants to have a far greater impact on your health than that decried by the press, lawyers, or our legislators.

Genetic Screening

Screening for an abnormality of the BRCA-1 gene is currently becoming available through research centers and commercial labs. It is an extremely labor-intensive test and is very expensive. It can be performed on either blood or tissue. Should this testing be "open" to anyone with a family history of breast or ovarian cancer? Some researchers argue that it should be limited to women who have already been diagnosed with these cancers in order to see if they harbor the mutation. If they do, only then should their relatives be screened for the same mutation. But remember, if we're tested and we're not found to have a BRCA-1 mutation, we still must contend with our 1 in 8 lifetime chance of developing breast cancer. This risk could be even higher if there is a mutation that the current test can't find. And if we test positive, what's the next line of action? Our options range from frequent breast exams, mammograms (and at what age should we start?—remember, these mutations can cause breast cancer before the age of 40) to MRIs or other new but as yet unproven tests and perhaps, in extreme instances, bilateral mastectomies (that means the breast tissue, skin, and nipples). Even after this radical and disfiguring surgery, some breast cells remain and can become malignant! And if we test positive, we also have a considerable risk of developing ovarian cancer. That, too, raises the need for surgery; removing both ovaries in our mid to late thirties, or after we've had our children. Once more, there are no guarantees; some women have developed ovarian cancer in the cells lining their abdominal cavity years after having prophylactic ovarian surgery.

There is one more potential problem that we'll have to face with this type of genetic fortune-telling: our health insurance coverage. Will insurers get hold of our genetic testing and, if positive, tell us we have the ultimate pre-existing condition which precludes our coverage? The geneticists, ethicists, lawyers, and lawmakers have in the past argued about our reproductive choices. They've now taken on our breast cancer options. Further studies, genetic advances, and appropriate legal protection are necessary to clarify these choices and allow us to use our personal judgment in our quest for breast health.

A BREAST CANCER DIAGNOSIS:
OUR DILEMMA, OUR CHOICES, OUR BATTLE

Each year over 180,000 of us receive this diagnosis. We suddenly become immersed in a new and frightening world filled with medical jargon—lumpectomy versus mastectomy, node resection, positive nodes, negative nodes, radiation, chemotherapy, and bone marrow transplantation. Although it is not within the scope of this book to give a full discussion of treatment choices, I want to encourage every woman to read all of the literature her doctor and local or national cancer organizations can supply (see suggested reading list). Talk to surgeons, radiotherapists, and oncologists until you feel comfortable and fully understand your options. Gone are the days when we were "put under," not knowing whether or not we would wake up without a breast. Breast conservation is possible in almost 70 percent of all breast cancers. If the breast is removed, we can have several types of reconstruction procedures. Radiation and chemotherapy have been effective in reducing recurrence and mortality. New drugs are being developed to fight breast cancer because women have become vocal and, yes, aggressive. We have made our personal fight to beat this disease a public one. The majority of us who are diagnosed with breast cancer will live out our lives without recurrence of this disease. Early diagnosis and treatment have improved, though not enough. Our personal fears should not turn us away from this disease. It should fuel our quest for knowledge and even our anger. Medicine has developed the early tools, albeit oh so slowly. We need increased funding, knowledge, and public education to enable us to become triumphant combatants in this fight that only we, as women, wage.

Lung Cancer: "You've Come a Long Way, Baby!"

Lung cancer is the number-one cause of cancer deaths for women in the United States. Those cigarette ads aimed at women really worked. As of 1987, deaths from this cancer surpassed mortality from breast cancer. In 1995, an estimated 62,000 women died of lung cancer compared to 46,000 breast cancer casualties.

ATTITUDES TOWARD LUNG CANCER

Why doesn't lung cancer strike the same chord of fear in women as breast cancer? It certainly is less curable. Early detection of lung cancer is poor because symptoms are very nonspecific (coughing, shortness of breath, fatigue, pain, and insomnia) and appear too late, when the disease has reached advanced stages. Survival rates are dreadful despite the last-ditch efforts of surgery, radiation, and chemotherapy. The five-year survival rate is only 13 percent overall for all stages of this disease. Even if we detect the disease early, the five-year survival rate is just 37 percent.

We have established screening programs for most other cancers, but there are no guidelines for lung cancer detection in women. Annual chest X rays for those of us who smoke might be helpful, but routine chest X rays in nonsmokers have generally been found to have little "positive" pick-up.

LUNG CANCER AND SMOKING

Despite the protestations of tobacco executives (who do admit that they would prefer that their own children not smoke), there is medical agreement that cigarette smoking accounts for 85 percent of all cases of lung cancer in women. In other words, at least 85 percent of our risk for lung cancer could be stopped if we didn't inhale those nicely wrapped, elegantly presented carcinogenic leaves. Once we stop smoking, we decrease our risk, though unfortunately don't eliminate it. Even if they haven't smoked for more than 15 years, long-term ex-smokers are still at a 2.2-fold increased risk of lung cancer, compared with lifetime nonsmokers. Still, this is still better than the 35-fold increased risk for current long-term smoking.

Because it takes twenty to thirty years for smoking to begin to kill us, teenage girls and young women have no fear. The immediacy of their lives and need for instant gratification overwhelms any consideration of mortality (much less what will happen five or ten years down the line). This causes us, their mothers, to wonder where we went wrong. Despite our "mature" denial, we were equally reckless at their age; we smoked, drank, rebelled, dropped out, got high, maybe even dropped acid. Some of us never quite recovered, but most of us did. We do have one excuse: We didn't have our current medical knowledge. I don't profess to know how to keep young women from succumbing to cigarette advertising campaigns. Studies show that if policies of fear don't work, cost does. High taxes on cigarettes, together with "ugly" campaigns (smoking yellows your teeth, wrinkles your skin, and makes you stink!) may be our only recourse. The young never think they'll be anything but young; smoking will put them on a fast track to old age.

WHAT ABOUT LUNG CANCER IN NONSMOKERS?

Yes, nonsmokers can get lung cancer, and over 3,800 "secondhand" smokers die of lung cancer each year. We know of some other risk factors, but none equals that of smoking or long-term secondhand smoke exposure. Environmental tobacco smoke has been classified as a known human carcinogen. The risk of lung cancer doubles for women who have forty or more years of household exposure to smoke during adulthood. Nonsmoking women married to smokers may have an increased risk for *all* cancers that is 1.5 times that of nonsmoking women married to non-smoking men. One study showed that 17 percent of lung cancer in non-smokers resulted from very early exposure to high levels of tobacco smoke during childhood and adolescence. (This gives new meaning to the term "passive smoking"; who has less control over the environment than a child?)

Chronic lung diseases such as tuberculosis, bronchitis, emphysema, and asthma may account for 16 percent of all lung cancers among non-smoking women. There may be a relationship between consumption of alcohol, particularly beer, and lung cancer. One study demonstrated that women who drank one or more beers per week had twice the risk of lung cancer. I wonder whether the beers were consumed in smoke-filled bars.

Lung cancer increases with radon exposure. Asbestos is also a known lung carcinogen. Clearly, we should ensure that our homes are free of both. Air pollution alone may not significantly increase lung cancer, but when combined with smoking, it deals us a double whammy. Translated, those of us who are "smogged-in" should not "smoke in." We have to choose what we will breathe.

WHAT PROTECTS US, ASIDE FROM GAS MASKS?

Our choice of diet may help guard us from lung cancer. The National Cancer Institute has published findings that showed that the relative risk of lung cancer in nonsmoking women increased more than 6-fold with high (as compared to very low) saturated fat consumption. A recent study from Florida indicated a strong protective effect associated with high vegetable consumption and intake of the antioxidant beta-carotene in its "natural" form in foods such as carrots, squash, pumpkin, apricots, mangoes, and peaches.

"Dying of Embarrassment": Our Delicate Denial of Colon Cancer

Many of us assume that colon cancer, like heart attack, is a male disease. We know that once the men in our lives pass 50, they have to pass some other things, including those disgusting stool and bowel tests. Women's bowel diseases may be the last holdout in our media coverage of female medical problems. Somehow, a headline SIGMOIDOSCOPY FOUND TO DE-CREASE COLON CANCER MORTALITY IN WOMEN or, to be more blunt, LOOK UP AND DISCOVER—A WAY TO LOWER OUR DEATH RATE isn't considered either news-selling or newsworthy. What we don't know or don't want to know about colon cancer can kill us.

Colon cancer is the third most common cancer diagnosed in women (after lung cancer and breast cancer). The incidence of and death rate from colon cancer is the same among women as men, or even higher—this is a gender-equal disease! We each have a 6 to 7 percent chance of developing this cancer in our lifetimes and a 3 percent chance of dying from it. In 1994, 74,000 women were diagnosed with colon cancer, and an estimated 28,000 died in 1995. More than half of us are diagnosed when it is too late, after the cancer has spread to nearby or distant organs. Caught early, colon cancer is treatable and stoppable. There is a 90 percent five-year survival if the tumor is caught when it is local, but survival falls to just 6 percent if it has sent out metastases.

Colon cancer has a unique characteristic: In most cases, it starts as a polyp and has a premalignant stage of five to ten years. If we catch it during this precancer hibernation, we can prevent subsequent cancer. *Polyps* are innocuous, soft, round projections that develop from the glands that line the colon and rectum. They may occur in one third to one half of all women over the age of 50. Thankfully, only about 5 percent of these polyps become malignant, but the more we have (and, unfortunately, if you have one, you have a 30 to 50 percent chance of having more), the higher our risk of eventually developing cancer.

Here we have a golden opportunity to find a precancer, remove it, and prevent the disease, yet few doctors and women take advantage of it. If we could do the same for breast cancer, who would refuse? I am amazed at how readily my patients accept most of the screening tests I offer—Pap smears, blood tests, mammograms, and bone-density scans. But as soon as I mention testing for colon cancer they are repulsed. They offer a large variety of reasons to indefinitely postpone stool tests ("I couldn't stay on the appropriate diet" or "The kit fell in the toilet") or sigmoidoscopy ("I couldn't possibly give myself an enema" or "You want me to have *what* put up my rectum? I'd rather die!") Let me remind all of us that if we do develop this cancer, we will end up with a lot more than a small scope invading our bowel!

SIGNS AND SYMPTOMS: AREN'T WE TOO YOUNG TO BE WORRYING ABOUT OUR BOWEL HABITS?

We joke about old people's fixation with regularity. Now we've become age-biased as well as gender-biased. Here are some signs we should not ignore.

1. Abdominal pain.

2. A change (to black) of stool color (make sure you are not taking iron or Pepto-Bismol; both of these can change the color of the stool).

3. Decreased stool caliber (thin strands).

4. Bright red blood coming from the rectum (yes, this could simply be hemorrhoids, but you can't be certain it's not from a "higher source" until you are appropriately tested).

5. Change in bowel habits.

Unfortunately, we are subjected to a lot of food contamination, whether we're eating out or cooking at home. This may result in a short-acting bacterial or viral bowel "upset" that will either pass or require antibiotics. Women also get constipated quite easily and find this to be an annoying, chronic problem. We can usually manage sluggish bowels with increased dietary fiber, eight glasses of water a day, and exercise. But if we have unexplained changes or vacillate between constipation and diarrhea, we should get checked. There is a point where our penchant for quick bowel fixes with the myriad of available over-the-counter products might delay diagnosis of a more serious problem.

RISK FACTORS

Are some of us at greater risk for colon cancer? As for so many cancers, the answer is yes. Once more, heredity is a factor, and a family history of colon cancer increases risk. It's at least 1.7 if one first-degree relative was affected and rises to 2.7 (and in some studies as high as 8) if two or more first-degree relatives had the disease. The cancer associated with this risk seems to occur at a younger age than "sporadic" colon cancer and strikes women in their thirties and forties. There is also a rare familial syndrome of multiple bowel polyps called *inherited polyposis syndrome*, which accounts for 1 percent of colon cancers. A gene that causes this problem has been identified and may help us isolate similar "faulty" genes that can mutate and place us at risk. Women with chronic inflammatory bowel disease (*Crohn's disease*, or *ulcerative colitis*) have a higher risk, probably because of the long-term effect of this illness on the lining of the bowel. Obviously, having had polyps or previous colon cancer places us at risk for recurrence. The adage "If you've had cancer, you are at risk for cancer" certainly applies, especially for women who have had breast, ovarian, or endometrial cancer in the past (or possibly have first-degree relatives with these cancers). Having one type of cancer increases our risk for another.

The most insidious risk for colon cancer is our age. The annual incidence per 100,000 women increases from 0.39 at age 50 to 4.52 at age 80. Unfortunately, we are all at risk and must overcome our "delicate" aversion to screening.

Screening for Colon Cancer: "Gentler and Kinder" Methods

Digital Rectal Examination

Every woman over 40 should have a rectal exam during her annual pelvic examination. We have already exposed our most private parts. We are lying there with our legs up and have just had a speculum inserted for our Pap smear. It is the appropriate time to get this less-than-pleasant business over with. Your gynecologist can feel polyps, tumors, or hemorrhoids along the lower three or four inches of the rectum. A pelvic exam is totally inadequate without a rectal exam, since the rectum and lower colon are part of the pelvis. I have found at least three precancerous polyps and one cancerous tumor in just the past year. These women were treated and are all doing well just because they were examined with one finger!

Occult Blood Screening

The second simple test is to check stool for occult, or hidden, blood. Polyps and tumors tend to bleed as they are buffeted by the passage of our bowel contents, but the amount of blood is miniscule and usually can't be seen. The most commonly used test for occult blood is the Hemoccult II Sensa or HemoQuant, which you perform in the privacy of your home. You avoid red meat, raw fruits and vegetables, vitamin C, and aspirin and other nonsteroidal anti-inflammatory medications (like ibuprofen) for two days, since all of these can affect the test and produce a false positive. You should also avoid the test if you're having vaginal bleeding, because that blood can contaminate stool. Use a little wooden spatula and smear a small sample of your stool on a special card. You do this with three different bowel movements (just in case that little polyp doesn't bleed each time). You then immediately mail the kit back to the lab or your doctor, and it's checked. If the test is positive your doctor may want to confirm this with a test called HemeSelect, which tests immunologically for human hemoglobin (and will rule out false positive results from red meats or other contaminants).

If you test positive, you need a more thorough examination. You might have bled from anywhere in your digestive tract, from ulcers in the stomach and upper bowel to polyps or tumors in the colon, to simple hemorrhoids. This test for occult blood has been shown to detect anywhere from 26 to 97 percent of colorectal cancers (not all bleed) and 13 percent of polyps larger than 1 centimeter. A recent study of over 21,000 participants living in Minnesota showed a decreased mortality from colon cancer of 33 percent if the test was used and if those who tested positive underwent colonoscopy and removal of polyps. Right now, the American Cancer Society suggests that this test be done annually on all people (women and men) over 50.

Flexible Sigmoidoscopy: Put a Scope Where?

There are no more secrets! A flexible scope can now be easily inserted through the rectum and up the first 60 centimeters (more than 2 feet) of the colon. This portion of the colon, with any possible polyps or tumors, is seen in living color on a video screen. Suspicious growths can be biopsied, allowing "on-the-spot" diagnosis. Women seem to develop more polyps and cancers on the right side of their colon, which, in nonmedical terms, means higher up. About 50 percent of these can be reached with the flexible sigmoidoscope.

How awful is this test? It is a lot less uncomfortable than a dilation and curettage (D&C) or probably even a cervical biopsy. Dental work can hurt more! There are no shots, no sharp instruments, and the lower bowel is a very distendable organ. You simply need to give yourself an enema (Fleet or generic) or use medication to increase evacuation and cleanse the bowel. You then lie on your side (which is certainly more elegant than our position for gynecologic exams), and you'll feel mild pressure and uncomfortable, "gassy" sensations. I have had this procedure, and my first response was "That's it?" It took five minutes and gave me years of reassurance. Screening with sigmoidoscopy every three to five years has an incredibly large protective effect. If we remove (through the scope) those dormant polyps, they can't develop into cancer. We have this wonderful opportunity to obstruct (a questionable word to use when dealing with the bowel) a malignant transformation. We can reduce our death rate from colon cancer by 60 to 70 percent if we just get that scope "put up there."

Colonoscopy: Sometimes We Have to Go Higher

Colonoscopy is a procedure that looks at the entire colon. It will pick up polyps or tumors that are high and on the right side. This is pretty major, and we need more preparation: a special diet and medication to cleanse the bowel. The procedure is performed in an outpatient facility where we are given sedation to make us more comfortable and relax the bowel. With colonoscopy, we can find 95 percent of all growths; these can be biopsied and removed during the procedure. This is our "big gun" and is saved for those of us who are at high risk or test positive on our stool tests or screening sigmoidoscopies. If we have had polyps, it should probably be repeated every three years. The American Cancer Society suggests that we do it every five years starting from 35 to 40 if we have a first-degree relative who had colon cancer before the age of 55.

Barium Enema: A Less Expensive Screening Alternative

We currently don't have enough trained colonoscopists. (I could make a joke out of this, but it would be a cheap shot!) A barium enema will visualize the walls of the rectum and entire colon. It requires no sedation and costs 50 percent less than colonoscopy. It will show 72 percent of tumors larger than 1 centimeter. If this test is positive, we go forward (or inward) to colonoscopy in order to verify the tumor by direct visualization and biopsy.

PREVENTION: A QUESTION OF KNOWLEDGE AND ATTITUDE

What we eat ends up passing through our colon and rectum. What part does food play in our risk for colon cancer? We go back to that obnoxious component of our diet—fat, especially animal fat. The more fat we eat, the greater our risk of colon and rectal cancer. One explanation is that our gallbladder has to "attack" and break down the fat. To do so, this organ produces and excretes bile acids, which then pass through the bowel. A high concentration of these acids has been shown to disturb the cells lining the bowel and may instigate cancerous changes.

The information we have about women, dietary animal fat, and colon cancer risk is pretty persuasive. A study that followed 90,000 nurses between 1980 and 1986 found that the risk of developing colon cancer was 249 percent greater for those who ate red meat than for those who ate chicken without skin or fish. Interestingly, consumption of animal fat from dairy sources was not associated with any increase in colon cancer. As a result of this study, I quit eating red meat.

Reduction of our fat intake to 20 percent of our total calories has been shown to reduce the risk of colon cancer by two thirds and rectal cancer by one third. Certain micronutrients (vitamins and minerals) may also play a protective role against this cancer. These include beta-carotene and, to a lesser extent, vitamin E and selenium. If we compare people who consume foods rich in beta-carotene to those who don't (I call this the "War of Vegetables"), the winning beta-carotene consumers have a 38 percent decrease in colon cancer risk.

High fiber intake has been shown in several studies to be associated with a more than 40 percent reduction in the risk of developing this cancer.

One less widely touted prevention is exercise. Although our information comes from studies done on men, the figures strongly suggest that regular exercise can make a difference. Men who exercised strenuously for more than four hours a week cut their colon cancer risk by approximately half. Simply walking briskly for two to three hours a week was enough to reduce the risk by 30 percent. These benefits may be derived from several exercise-induced chemical changes in our body and an increase in prostaglandins, which stimulate the movement of waste through the bowel. The less contact between the bowel wall and the carcinogenic substances we eat, the fewer opportunities for cancer to develop.

Another way of changing our colon and rectal production or types of production of prostaglandins is through aspirin. The Nurses' Study has shown that after long-term use of four to six tablets of aspirin a week (the long term here being twenty years!) the risk of colon cancer was lowered by almost 50 percent.

The question remains, "Who's in control?" We certainly want to "control" our bowel habits (we've been taught to do this from the age of 2), and we should be in control of our bowel diseases. There's simply no excuse not to. We are far more prone to colon and rectal cancer than we are to any of the cancers of our female genital tract. The available screening success becomes our diagnostic failure if we allow embarrassment, ignorance, and fear to inhibit our participation.

Uterine (Endometrial) Cancer: Our Most Common Genital Tract Malignancy and Our Most Treatable

Thirty-three thousand American women are diagnosed yearly with uterine cancer. Because this cancer has a very distinct warning sign (abnormal vaginal bleeding) and because we are able to identify those of us at risk, "only" 5,900 women die.

OUR HORMONES: RIGHT OR WRONG?;
ENDOMETRIAL CANCER

The uterus is composed of the body (or *corpus*) and the cervix, which is the opening that leads into the vagina. The uterine body has an inner cavity (or *endometrium*), which is lined with glands. During our reproductive years, these glands respond to our estrogen and, after ovulation, to our progesterone in preparation for pregnancy. If no egg is fertilized, the endometrial lining sloughs, and we get our period. To maintain its health and happiness, the endometrium needs this rhythmic feeding and deprivation of both estrogen and progesterone. If the glands are improperly stimulated and don't have a chance to shed, they "puff up" and develop little cysts; this is called *hyperplasia*. With time, excessive stimulation may cause the cells to forget how to form proper glands; the result is *atypical hyperplasia*, a precancerous condition. In the next stage, the glandular cells are so misguided by inappropriate hormonal stimulation that they become malignant, and endometrial cancer results.

RISK FACTORS

Conditions that subject these vulnerable glands to too much estrogen, or to estrogen without proper progesterone can lead to endometrial cancer. Once we understand why this cancer develops, it's quite easy to identify our risk factors.

Obesity

Obesity seems to increase our risk for most cancers, but this is especially true for endometrial cancer. Our fat cells produce a weak estrogen that does not cycle but remains constant, unaffected by the changes of ovulation or ovarian function. Years of obesity mean years of continual estrogen bombardment, which can finally result in endometrial cancer. The incidence increases as we get older and heavier.

Infertility and Irregular Periods

When we ovulate, we produce progesterone, which has a pacifying effect on our estrogen-stimulated endometrial glands. If we don't ovulate or cycle normally during the thirty-five or so years we are supposed to menstruate (other than during pregnancy), we may have undergone years of unopposed estrogen stimulation. This increases our risk for endometrial cancer.

If a woman's infertility is hormonal, and she has not had ovulations that allowed for fertilization and pregnancy, she may also have abnormally stimulated her uterine lining. A condition known as *polycystic ovarian syndrome (PCO)* is due to abnormal estrogen production, increase in male hormone, and poor or no ovulation. Women with PCO are often overweight, have excessive hair growth, and have very irregular periods. Unless their ovaries are suppressed (usually with birth control pills) or they are treated with progesterone, they are at risk for endometrial cancer.

Even fertile women don't have perfect estrogen and concomitant progesterone cycles their entire menstrual lives. We often skip periods during puberty and our teen years, and at the other end of the spectrum, we have poor ovulation and irregular cycles in our forties, just before menopause. This latter transition and relative paucity of progesterone can upset our endometrial balance and lead to precancer (*hyperplasia*) or cancer.

High Blood Pressure and Diabetes

Both of these conditions are often linked with obesity, and we might assume that any increased risk for endometrial cancer is due to "fat" estrogen stimulation. Unfortunately, those of us who are not overweight but who have become diabetic or hypertensive independently acquire this additional cancer risk and should be appropriately screened.

Abnormal Bleeding:
Don't Just Buy Pads—Have It Checked!

We have to be grateful whenever we get clear warnings of a disease. Endometrial cancer has a simple one—vaginal bleeding. If we are postmenopausal and are not taking hormones, we should never bleed. Even spotting should be taken seriously and mandates an immediate call to a doctor.

We can't assume that if we are menopausal and are on hormones, it's okay to bleed. We should have "periods" only when we cycle off of the estrogen and progesterone—not while on them. The first four to six months of therapy don't count because it takes our body and uterus time to get accustomed to these hormones. After that, however, *any* irregular bleeding needs to be checked.

Abnormal bleeding before menopause may be due to our befuddled hormones and inconsistent ovulations. Unfortunately, we can never be sure. If, in our forties, we have frequent periods or spot so much that our panties always need to be lined with minipads, we need to be checked and treated. If we dismiss all of our bleeding complaints as perimenopausal, we will miss an opportunity for early cancer detection.

Use of "Unopposed" Estrogen:
Confusing the Endometrial Glands

In the 1960s and 1970s, our mothers were told to take estrogen pills and were promised continued youth, health, and happiness. By 1975, a big "oops" (not a word we want to hear from our physicians) was proclaimed. The link between endometrial cancer and unopposed postmenopausal estrogen had been established. We are now wiser, but many of us are also without a uterus. We know that when estrogen is presented to the uterus by itself at any point in our lives, it makes endometrial glands overgrow. Indeed, just one year of unopposed estrogen replacement causes a 20 percent incidence of endometrial hyperplasia. The risk of cancer increases with the dose of estrogen used and the duration of treatment. If the hyperplasia becomes atypical, there is a 50 percent chance that it will progress to carcinoma if it is untreated. Overall, women who take even the smallest dose of unopposed estrogen for five years or longer have a 5- to 8-fold increase in their risk of developing endometrial cancer.

Scary. But let's remember the natural physiology of our uterine glands. They need the ebb and flow of estrogen *and* progesterone. It's this latter hormone that prevents berserk overgrowth. We do not have to give up on estrogen supplementation, but if we have a uterus, we should add progesterone, just the way nature did. Progesterone, in small doses, added to daily estrogen or given cyclically, ten to twelve days a month or even fourteen days every three months, will effectively prevent estrogen-related hyperplasia and cancer.

Tamoxifen: Are We Preventing Recurrent Breast Cancer While Causing Endometrial Cancer?

Tamoxifen is an interesting drug. It sits on our estrogen receptors and turns some of them on and some of them off. We use tamoxifen to prevent recurrence of breast cancer (especially if the original cancer had estrogen receptors), and it is even being studied as a way to prevent initial breast cancer in high-risk women. While it's an anti-estrogen for breast tissue, it has a positive estrogen effect on our bones and on our cholesterol and lipoproteins. This same pro-estrogen effect is a negative for the uterus, since it stimulates endometrial gland receptors, causing overgrowth of these glands, and increasing the risk of cancer. The actual degree of risk for endometrial cancer is not clear, but it may be as high as five to seven times that of a woman who is not taking this medication (and similar to the cancer risk of women on unopposed estrogen). A confounding factor is that once we have breast cancer, we have a 1.7 percent overall risk of developing endometrial cancer, as opposed to 1.0 percent for women with no cancer history.

There are several current recommendations on how to treat or follow women on tamoxifen. One is to periodically give them progesterone so that their glands are repressed. Another is to screen them aggressively with ultrasound to see if their endometrium is abnormally thick, or perform yearly scrapings of the endometrium and directly test the glands and cells to see if they are becoming malignant.

Tamoxifen has risks, but for the first 5 years of recommended use it decreases the recurrence rate of breast cancer by 25 to 35 percent. (Note that after 5 years this cancer protection appears to "wear off.") Tamoxifen also lowers the risk of heart attack and osteoporosis.

SCREENING AND TESTING: WE CAN "SEE" WHAT'S IN THERE

Ultrasound

If endometrial glands grow abnormally, they cause the uterine lining to thicken. We can see this with ultrasound. A vaginal probe, shaped like a cylinder and 2 to 3 inches thick, is placed in the vagina (using a condom—we need to practice safe ultrasound!). The probe sends out ultrasonic waves that are reflected from our pelvic organs. We see a very clear image of our uterus and ovaries on a screen. The uterine lining is denser than the walls and shows up as a white line. Thin is good, fat isn't. If the lining measures 4 millimeters or less, we don't have to worry about cancer in a menopausal woman. Thicker "lines" have to be biopsied by more invasive (surgical) methods. This simple procedure can often eliminate the need for biopsy.

Biopsy Methods

There are situations where we must get "samples" of our endometrial glands. If we have abnormal or postmenopausal bleeding and can't reassure ourselves that all is well by performing ultrasound, we have to go to the next step. The sampling can be done in several ways.

1. *Endometrial biopsy or sampling*   (See page 365.)

2. *Traditional D&C (dilatation and curettage)*   Until the late 1970s, this was the most common hospital gynecologic procedure (for a detailed description, see page 363). Today ultrasound and simple office endometrial samplings have replaced

this surgery. We also realize that this is a "blind" procedure, and that polyps, fibroids, and cancers can be missed. If any of these entities are suspected, we really should look, first by ultrasound, which would show a thickened and uneven endometrium, and then by hysteroscopy. These pictures are worth a thousand blind scrapings.

3. *Hysteroscopy* (See page 358.)

PROTECTION AND PREVENTION WITH "HORMONE CARE"

The less we are subjected to unopposed estrogen exposure from puberty to menopause, the less likely we are to develop endometrial cancer. Birth control pills are composed of small amounts of estrogen *and* progestin (synthetic progesterone). The Pill suppresses our ovaries and, in doing this, stops ovulation so that we don't get pregnant. It will also prevent our ovaries from misbehaving and creating the wrong estrogen-to-progesterone ratio. Instead, the Pill now supplies the uterine glands with balanced hormones. As a result of this action, birth control pills protect us from endometrial cancer. Studies have shown that for women on the Pill the risk of uterine cancer decreases to 0.4 (compared with 1 for women who never used the Pill) and is even lower in women who used birth control pills for ten or more years (0.2). This risk continued to be lowered (0.7) for twenty years after stopping the Pill! Progesterone-only pills or shots of Depo-Provera seem to afford similar protection. Birth control in our forties, especially for those of us with irregular cycles, may keep us healthy (from a uterine point of view) in our fifties and sixties! Those of us who are obese, hypertensive, or diabetic, or who have irregular cycles, need protection. If we can't take the Pill, we might consider "add-back" use of progesterone to protect our glands. A synthetic or natural progesterone can be taken for the last ten days before each period. This will inhibit our glands and stop aberrant growth.

TREATMENTS AND CURES

Yes, we can cure precancer and cancer of the endometrium. It takes years for simple gland mixup (hyperplasia), or precancer (atypia) to become cancer, so we have years to make a diagnosis and bring about a cure. Simple hyperplasia can be treated medically. Common sense allows us all to understand the therapy—progesterone. Prolonged or high doses of progesterone will reverse estrogen domination of the glands. They cower and shrink, and as they become submissive, they become normal. Doctors often use a drug called Megace (which is a very potent synthetic progesterone) for three months and then resample the endometrium to ensure that the glands are normal. Women who have had hyperplasia should then be closely followed and possibly treated with intermittent progesterone or, if not menopausal, birth control pills to ensure continued hormonal "evenhandedness."

If a woman has atypia, doctors can still try to reverse it with progesterone. If this fails, or the potential for cancer is great, she should consider a hysterectomy. The need for this surgery is never good news, but at least at this stage, before cancer "has set in," it can be performed vaginally. The recovery from a vaginal hysterectomy is easier and more rapid than from one done abdominally.

Once cancer is diagnosed, an abdominal hysterectomy becomes necessary. The pelvic lymph nodes are also removed, and depending on the stage of the cancer, radiation and subsequent chemotherapy or progesterone therapy is given.

Overall, the five-year survival rate for all stages of this cancer is 90 percent. It is 98 percent at stage I, when there is no spread beyond the endometrium. All we need is sense: sense to acknowledge risk, sense to follow up on bleeding, and sense to get the right tests for diagnosis. Early detection does mean cure!

Cervical Cancer

PAP SMEARS AND WHAT THEY TELL US

Just because we've reached 40 without a serious "cervical mishap" doesn't mean we should become complacent. We still need continual cervical surveillance. Every year, over 15,000 women elude our early pick-up system of Pap smears and are diagnosed with invasive cancer of the cervix; 4,800 die. The death rate from cervical cancer is more than twice as high for black women as it is for whites (6.6 versus 2.6 per 100,000 women). This may reflect a combined failure of active screening and poor follow-up for positive results in minority women. Whatever the reason, it's inexcusable! The Pap smear has been around for over fifty years. How long does it take to introduce it into routine screening programs for all women?

Most cervical cancers take many years to develop. The Pap is less than perfect; some studies have shown a 20 to 50 percent false-negative rate (precancerous changes are not detected). If it's performed regularly, however, a positive pick-up should eventually be made before we develop invasive cancer. Despite the proclaimed imperfections of the Pap smear and our inequities of screening and follow-up, we have to acknowledge substantial success. Our mortality from cervical cancer has been reduced by 70 percent since 1950.

This test is easy and affordable. "All" we have to do is get onto a gynecologic table and open our legs. (The "all" is a joke; a lot of angst goes into positioning ourselves this way!) A speculum is used to open the vagina. A small brush (similar to an eyebrow brush) is put into the cervical opening or canal, rotated 180 degrees, removed, and then used to smear adhering cells and mucus onto a glass slide. A small wooden spatula is then gently scraped on the outer portion of the cervix, and these cells are also smeared onto the slide and fixed with an alcohol spray. At a pathology laboratory the slide is immersed in a special dye and read by a cytotechnologist (a person trained to examine cells microscopically and recognize abnormalities). Since cervical cancer doesn't just suddenly develop, but usually goes through a rigorous and defined "cancer training," we are looking for these early cellular cancer recruits. On occasion, cancer cells can rapidly become malignant, but the usual course of events is that they progress from normal to mildly abnormal (mild dysplasia—*dys* means abnormal), to moderate dysplasia, severe dysplasia, and then to carcinoma in situ. ("In situ" means that the very early cancer changes are localized in the cells and have not crossed or penetrated the membrane below the cells.) The final stage is invasive cancer. This cancer can either have minimal or micro-invasion or macro-invasion. When invasive cancer occurs (this really is a war), it is classified in stages: from I to IV, IV being the worst with far-spread metastases.

Using a classification system called the Bethesda system, we classify cervical cell changes and determine our cervical "well-being." Are our cervical cells living in peace and harmony with our vaginal flora (the bacteria and viruses that normally inhabit the vagina), or is there conflict from infection, hormonal disturbance, or cancer development? The Pap report card says it all as follows.

1. Adequacy of the Specimen

If adequate cells are not present, the Pap needs to be repeated.

2. General Categorization

This either is normal (medical term—"within normal limits"; we doctors hate to use one word when three will do) or shows "benign cellular changes" (this can occur with infection or during healing processes) or "epithelial cell abnormality" (this means something is off and will be described below).

3. Descriptive Diagnoses

BENIGN CELLULAR CHANGES

This is due to either *infection* (caused by trichomonas, fungus, bacteria, or herpes) or *reactive* changes (the result of repair of previous infection or trauma, atrophy with lack of estrogen, IUD).

EPITHELIAL CELL ABNORMALITIES

These are the cells on the surface of the cervix.

Squamous Cell   These cells "coat" the cervix outside and partially inside up to the area of glands. Such changes include:

- *Atypical squamous cells of undetermined significance.* This means we are not sure what is going on, but the cells are not quite normal.
- *Low-grade squamous intraepithelial lesion (LSIL).* This basically covers mild dysplasia, also called CIN I (an acronym standing for *cervical intraepithelial neoplasia,* which means tumor changes of epithelial cells in the cervix), and is usually correlated with HPV (*human papillomavirus* infection; see below).
- *High-grade squamous intraepithelial lesion (HSIL).* This includes moderate to severe dysplasia (also called CIN II and CIN III) and carcinoma in situ.

- *Squamous cell carcinoma*. This is self-explanatory; the cells indicate cancer.

Glandular Cell Cells that come from the glands deep in the cervix or in the endometrium of the uterus are shed and can be picked up when brushing the cervix.

- *Endometrial cells*. These are usually benign, but their presence may be abnormal and even indicate endometrial pathology in menopausal women who are not taking hormones.
- *Atypical glandular cells of undetermined significance*. Another "we're not sure what this is."
- *Cervical adenocarcinoma*. This is a rare cancer of the glands of the cervix.
- *Endometrial adenocarcinoma*. Cancer cells from high in the endometrium are shed and pass out of the cervix.
- *Extrauterine adenocarcinoma*. This is extremely rare and may signify Fallopian tube cancer.

Other Malignant Neoplasms These are unidentifiable cancer cells and can even come from the ovaries.

4. Hormone Evaluation

We can do this if we scrape the vagina and add these cells to the cervical smear. The appearance of vaginal cells can tell us if the hormonal pattern is appropriate for our age, menstrual cycle, and history (hormone use). If there are a lot of bacteria in our vagina, we cannot do this evaluation.

Few of us will have to read and interpret our own Pap smear reports. What we should expect (and be told by those who read them for us) is that the Pap shows adequate cells, allowing for appropriate scanning. We then need to know if these cells appear normal or if they are abnormal, and whether they fall into a low-risk or high-risk category. We should ascertain if there are signs of viral (HPV) infection associated with these changes. If cells that shouldn't be there (endometrial or other "unknowns") are present, is there an explanation? And, finally, if a hormone evaluation has been made, does it match our hormonal status?

HOW OFTEN DO WE NEED A PAP?

The current recommendation by a lot of very knowledgeable agencies (the American Cancer Society, the National Cancer Institute, and the American College of Obstetricians and Gynecologists) is that women begin Pap smear screening at the age of 18 or earlier if they are sexually active. (We may have long since passed this criterion, but our daughters need to be educated about their cervical health.) After the initial screening, they recommend annual exams over the next three years, and if these are perfectly normal, we can "slow down" the screening process to once every three years. With this approach, we can decrease mortality from cervical cancer by 90 percent! The cutoff age for Pap smears is frequently said to be 65, but if we look at an English study showing that 40 percent of deaths from cancer of the cervix occur in women over 65, there would appear to be no reason to stop screening as we get older.

So, you may wonder, what happened to the concept of the "routine annual Pap"—a dictum spouted by so many ob/gyns? Well, the societies didn't want to cause civil war, so they stated that more frequent Paps should be left to the discretion of the doctor and patient. Clearly, an annual Pap is necessary if we are at risk because we've had multiple sexual partners in the past or present, or have been with partners who have had multiple partners, if we have previous or current herpes, or HPV infections, smoke, or had previous cervical disease. If we consider these factors, nearly all of us are high-risk, unless we and our current partner have *always* been monogamous with each other! Even if we're not at risk, we may want to "be certain," distrusting lab accuracy (the more tests, the less likely something will be overlooked), or because we're getting an annual gynecological exam for other reasons and feel it appropriate to have a Pap done while we are up "in position."

NEW TESTS THAT LET COMPUTERS DO THE WORK

"Scanning" for abnormal cells among hundreds of thousands of normal ones in a Pap smear is tough and has to be repeated for scores of slides by one human pair of eyes and accompanying brain. I give cytotechnologists a major bow of appreciation; our demands on them are overwhelming. Computers are coming to the rescue. A system called ThinPrep takes the cells we obtain by swabbing the cervix and immerses them in a fluid that is filtered and then passed through a computer that scans them. Another system called PAPNET takes the slide that was graded as normal by human eyes and then scans through hundreds of thousands of its cells. It selects over one hundred cells that appear most abnormal and these are then displayed on a high-resolution video monitor so that the cytotechnologist can reanalyze them before a final negative report is given. PAPNET has just been approved by the FDA, and some labs are offering it as an adjunct to our regular Pap smears at, of course, an extra fee. The hope is that in the future, these or other computer-assisted tests will cut down on human mistakes and incorrect readings.

CERVICAL CANCER RISK: IS THIS JUST A WORRY FOR THOSE OF US WHO "FOOLED AROUND" WHEN WE WERE YOUNG?

Cervical cancer is a threat we can use to admonish our daughters: "The younger you are when you become sexually active and the greater the number of unprotected sexual partners you have (God forbid!), the higher your chance of getting a really ugly disease." We're usually talking about sexually transmitted diseases (STDs), but in fact this is also true of cervical cancer. Herpesvirus and the new scourge, human papillomavirus (HPV), can enter the cervical cells' genetic works, alter them, and increase the risk of developing cancer. A worldwide study has found HPV in 92.9 percent of all cervical cancers! There are over seventy types of HPV viruses, and twenty-three types can dwell in the male and female genital tract. They "hop over" to us during unprotected intercourse and remain a part of our vaginal and urinary "flora." These viruses can cause genital warts or "silent" changes of the cervix. HPV infection has been shown to increase the risk for moderate to severe dysplasia by as much as 25 percent. Types 16, 18, and 31 are more notorious and can increase the chance of cervical precancer four to five times more than other HPVs. (Not only would we hope not to get HPV, but we would certainly prefer it not be one of these "bad" types.)

HPV is not a new virus. What is new is that researchers have isolated it, typed it, and established its unfortunate correlation with cervical, vaginal, and even vulvar cancers. We were probably exposed in the past and certainly will be in the present or future if we have unprotected sex with a new or nonmonogamous partner.

Cigarette smoking is as bad as viruses for our cervix (and lovemaking isn't even involved—amazing what we can do through our lungs). Smoking is associated with a nearly 2-fold increase in risk for cervical cancer even after we adjust for age and number of sexual partners. Passive exposure to cigarette smoke for more than three hours a day may also bestow this risk. Women who smoke but who have no other high-risk factors for cervical cancer should be followed as carefully (with annual Paps) as those who have had early sex, multiple partners, herpes, warts (HPV), or previous abnormal Pap smears.

DIAGNOSIS AND TREATMENT OF PRECANCER: HPV, CIN, LSIL, HSIL—TOO MANY INITIALS, TOO MANY FACTORS—HELP!!!

The procedures for cure can be as confusing as the acronyms for disease. The goal is to search and destroy.

Search

A Pap smear is a screen; it allows us to evaluate cells. For complete diagnosis, we need actual tissue, and that is obtained by biopsy. If we could see abnormal cells or tissue with our naked eye, we could simply insert a speculum, look at the cervix, and diagnose. This doesn't work; precancer is invisible to the unaided eye. If the Pap smear is abnormal, we need to augment our naked eye with a special microscope called a *colposcope*, which magnifies the cervix. Special staining solutions are swabbed onto the cervix in order to enhance the microscopic changes of abnormal tissue. We then look to see which area to biopsy. The *endocervix*, or less visible inner cervical canal, is also scraped at this time (the procedure is called *endocervical curettage*, or *ECC*), and tissues from the biopsy and scraping are sent to the lab for final diagnosis. If precancerous changes are confirmed, we go to the next stage of treatment.

Destroy

If we remove the abnormal cells and tissue, normal cells can grow back and cancer is prevented. There are two methods of getting rid of precancerous tissue: *ablative* (destructive) and *excisional* (cutting out).

ABLATIVE METHODS

Cryosurgery   We freeze the abnormal cervical tissue with a freezing probe (extreme cold destroys cells just like extreme heat) This is usually reserved for the less severe cases of dysplasia or low-grade lesions.

Rating   This can be done in the office, is easy to perform, and does not require anesthetic, and the equipment is inexpensive (which means the charges are less).

Laser   The abnormal tissue is vaporized by a special laser beam; this is usually reserved for more advanced dysplasia or high-grade lesions.

Rating   This can be performed in the office with local anesthetic, but many doctors don't own a laser and hospitalize their patients to get access to the equipment. It is high-tech and fairly expensive.

EXCISIONAL METHODS

The abnormal tissue is removed, not just destroyed. This has the advantage of allowing us to make sure we got everything (the pathologist checks the specimen and tells us if the borders are clear). On occasion, we may find that we underestimated the pathology and hidden areas of cancer are discovered. In these cases, we won't mistakenly undertreat.

LEEP (Loop Electrosurgical Excision Procedure)   A special loop "powered" by electrosurgical current so that it can cut tissue and minimize bleeding is used to remove the abnormal portion of the cervix. A portion of the endocervical canal can also be removed (*cone LEEP*).

Rating   The loop slices through the cervix "like butter." It doesn't cause pain. The equipment is not expensive, and LEEP can be performed as an office procedure with local anesthetic. Some physicians go straight to this step once the Pap smear shows dysplasia, bypassing colposcopic biopsy. This procedure is especially appropriate for women who do not want to have two procedures to follow up on abnormal Pap smears.

Surgical Conization   This procedure is performed in an operating room; a portion of the cervix and canal is removed by either knife or laser. Sutures are often required to stop bleeding. This should be done if the Pap smear shows advanced disease and there is a possibility that invasive cancer could be present. If none is there, the therapy is complete. If invasion is found, hysterectomy, plus additional therapy (radiation and lymph node resection) might be required, depending on the stage.

Rating   This is the "big gun" and should be used judiciously. Anesthesia is needed; there can be bleeding, and although high-tech equipment is not necessary, the use of an operating room and anesthesiologist, and possible hospitalization, make this the most expensive option.

Common sense, availability, and physician training guide our selection of therapies. An abnormal Pap, even if it shows severe changes, does not mean "My God, I'll need a hysterectomy!" With active screening, the silent secrets of the cervix are exposed, and we can save our organs and our lives.

Ovarian Cancer: Diagnosis, Genes, and Dumb Luck

Ovarian cancer has the dubious distinction of being our most deadly gynecologic cancer and the fourth-ranked cause of cancer deaths in women. Most of us have only a 1.4 percent lifetime chance of developing ovarian cancer, *but* once struck, less than 40 percent of us will survive five years after diagnosis. Each year over 14,000 women in this country die from this disease. These depressing statistics are mostly due to our abysmal failure to detect ovarian cancer. Early ovarian cancer has no symptoms, and we have not established an effective way to screen for it. As a result, 70 percent of women are diagnosed too late, when the tumor has spread outside the pelvis.

About 5 percent of us have genetic bad luck with regard to ovarian cancer. Comedian Gilda Radner's death and her public efforts while struggling with the disease have helped create a legacy of awareness.

Clinics and registries have been founded to track high-risk families and study the molecular genetics of this cancer. The prevailing theory is that we need two genetic mutations to cause ovarian cancer. The unlucky "genetically programmed" victims who are born with one disturbed genetic factor need just one more mutation to cause cancer. They may then develop ovarian cancer ten to fifteen years earlier than those with non-inherited mutations (Gilda Radner was found to have ovarian cancer in her early forties). For the rest of us, it will take years and the irritation of constant ovulation before we get this double change. The majority of sporadic ovarian cancers occur after menopause in our seventh decade.

We now have information to quantify our hereditary risk. If you have one relative with ovarian cancer, your lifetime probability of developing this cancer is 5 percent. If two family members are affected, this risk can increase to 7 percent. To complicate the numbers and our assessment of risk, there are several types of familial, or hereditary, ovarian cancer. One syndrome involves a high predisposition to both breast and ovarian cancer and is caused by mutations on one of several known genes. It is inherited as a dominant trait, which means that if your mother had it, you have a 50 percent chance of inheriting this gene, and if you do inherit it, a greater than 50 percent chance of eventually developing ovarian cancer. If your grandmother had it (on either your mother's or father's side), your chance of inheritance is 25 percent. The second type of hereditary cancer is called Lynch syndrome II, and this is also inherited in a dominant fashion. This mutation gives a predisposition to ovarian, endometrial, and colon cancer. Familial cancers account for less than 5 percent of all ovarian cancers. The rest of us with no family history are, to some extent, at the mercy of bad luck. However, researchers have determined that factors including certain habits, diets, childbearing patterns, and birth control history can affect this dumb-luck factor.

OTHER THAN OUR GENES, WHAT CAN WE BLAME?

ASBESTOS AND TALC

We have been programmed by Madison Avenue and our own prudish discomfort with our private parts to believe that we must smell nice, "feel fresh" (whatever that means), and be dry "down there." Powders (put on panties, on sanitary pads, or directly on the vulva) may have kept us nice and dry, but over time they were also making a quiet journey up to our ovaries. Until recently, most talcum powders contained asbestos. This is a substance we don't want in any part of our bodies. Somehow it got to our ovaries, probably by ascending through the vagina and cervix into the uterus and out the Fallopian tubes. When it reached the ovaries, it acted as a cancer promoter. Women who used talcum powder for many years to dust their bottoms, panties, or pads may have doubled or tripled their risk for ovarian cancer.

DIET

Ovarian cancer is a disease of the middle and upper class, of "well-fed" women who consume a high-fat Western diet. Japanese women (here we go again!) have the lowest rate of ovarian cancer in the world—until they move here and adopt our diet along with our ovarian cancer rate. In a recent study, researchers calculated the risk of developing ovarian cancer based on their study of the diets of women with and without the disease. They found that for every 10 grams of saturated fat consumed each day, a woman's risk of developing ovarian cancer increases 20 percent. Egg consumption increases this risk by about 42 percent for every 100 milligrams of cholesterol consumed per day. The same evaluation found that for every 10 grams of vegetable fiber we consume we get the beneficial result of lowering our risk by 37 percent. Fruit fiber seems to make no difference.

Milk fat has also been implicated. One study showed that drinking more than one glass of whole milk per day caused a risk of 3.1 (compared with 1 for women who never drank milk). This fell if the milk was 2 percent or nonfat. Galactose (a milk sugar) in milk products may also be harmful. Women whose diets contained increased quantities of cottage cheese or yogurt (these have the highest content of galactose) had a relative risk of 1.4 to 1.7. Ice cream and whole milk might be out, but considering our national female propensity for poor calcium intake, it's not clear that our total avoidance of nonfat milk or yogurt is warranted. We don't want osteoporosis, and we have to eat something!

FERTILITY, INFERTILITY, AND CONTRACEPTION

We seem to "stress" our ovaries the longer they ovulate or are pushed to function. The ultimate result of this stress is molecular mutation followed by cancer. Therefore, factors inhibiting ovarian stimulation and trauma should decrease ovarian cancer. Indeed, they do. Pregnancy and use of birth control pills can help protect our ovaries, while lack of pregnancy, infertility, and perhaps use of infertility drugs contribute to ovarian peril.

When we are pregnant, we don't ovulate, and the high level of hormones produced by the placenta shuts down our pituitary and ovaries. If we have two children, we decrease our chance of getting ovarian cancer by 40 percent. Five or more children will give us 50 percent protection (the question of whether raising three additional children is worth the extra 10 percent decrease in risk must obviously be answered individually). The older we are at the time of our first birth, the less likely we are to develop ovarian cancer. (This is exactly the opposite of the situation with breast cancer, where risk is reduced by pregnancy before the age of 25.)

Breast-feeding also causes temporary shutdown of ovarian function and, like pregnancy, has been found to be protective. We can't stay pregnant or lactating (or barefoot!) just to prevent ovarian cancer, but we can use birth control that works just as well, or better. Because it stops ovulation, the birth control pill has a wonderful protective effect against ovarian cancer (see chapter 2). We currently recommend that all women at risk stay on the Pill for as long and as late as possible, even up to menopause. This could change a high 5 percent lifetime risk to an almost "normal" risk of 2 percent. For those of us at low risk (1.4 percent), the risk can go down to less than 0.5 percent.

Another form of birth control, tubal ligation, appears to decrease the incidence of ovarian cancer by 37 percent, but the reason for this remains an enigma. Why should closing or burning a portion of the Fallopian tubes affect this cancer? Give medicine a question, and the answers will come . . . There are three theories: It stops talcum powder or other contaminants from reaching the ovaries; it may decrease ovarian function (if the blood supply is hindered); or precancerous ovaries were seen at the time of tubal ligation and removed. However, not everyone uses talc, most women seem to have normal periods and hormonal function after tubal ligation, and the protection lasts longer than ten years, so how could precancer be detected at surgery? In short, we don't have a complete answer. What makes the issue even more confusing is that hysterectomy should have the same effect on the ovaries, but in fact it gives less protection against ovarian cancer than does tubal ligation.

THE FERTILITY DRUG CONTROVERSY: DOES IT INCREASE OVARIAN CANCER RISK?

Infertility itself predisposes us to ovarian cancer. There is a 2-fold risk for women who have failed to conceive following ten or more years of unprotected intercourse. Fertility drugs consist of pituitary hormones (FSH and LH) or drugs that cause the level of these hormones to increase. Researchers have hypothesized that higher pituitary hormones or excessive ovarian stimulation can lead to ovarian trauma and cancer. To ascertain whether the use of these drugs actually does this, we had to examine women who used these medications and developed cancer and match them with controls who did not. A recent analysis of twelve published ovarian cancer studies found that only three of these studies included a history of previous use of fertility drugs. In one small sample, investigators concluded that women who had used fertility medication had almost three times the risk of developing ovarian cancer as women with no history of infertility. If the women were *nulliparous* (the treatment didn't work and they didn't get pregnant and deliver), the risk was 12 times greater. A recent Seattle study looked at nearly 4,000 infertile women and compared them to fertile women. The women who were treated with the ovulatory drug clomiphene citrate (Clomid or Serophene) for more than a year had a relative risk of 11.1 for developing ovarian cancer. Less than a year of clomiphene citrate therapy, on the other hand, seemed to be "safe."

Not surprisingly, these statistics have struck fear in the millions of us who have used fertility medications. It should be pointed out, though, that women who have never conceived despite the use of fertility drugs or have persisted in using the drugs for a long time are at highest risk. Perhaps they had a particular hormonal profile (making them resistant to treatment) that also affected their development of cancer. Scientists are still debating this issue. When six other cases of ovarian cancer related to fertility drugs were reported to the Food and Drug Administration (FDA), the agency responded by requesting that the manufacturers of these drugs include an advisory in the package labeling. The NIH also entered the fray and recommended that women receiving fertility medications be counseled on the possible increased risk of ovarian cancer, and that after treatment, they consider using oral contraceptives for protection. In the interim, women and their doctors have been alerted. We want our babies, but have to follow up on the risks we may run when we treat our infertility.

EVALUATION AND SCREENING:
A STORY OF INEFFECTIVENESS AND COST

We have failed to produce a single test or even a set of tests that gives us reliable early detection of ovarian cancer. Being a "good patient" and having annual pelvic exams is not enough. By the time your doctor feels "something," that "something" may be advanced ovarian cancer that has spread throughout the abdomen. It has been estimated that doctors need to perform ten thousand annual physical exams to detect one early ovarian cancer.

What about blood tests or tumor markers? Such tests exist and have been extensively used in men for early diagnosis of prostate cancer. Surely, there should be a test to diagnose ovarian cancer in women. We have isolated a protein called Ca-125 that is elevated in the bloodstream in 80 percent of ovarian cancers. Unfortunately, only 50 percent of patients with early-stage disease have abnormal Ca-125 levels in blood tests; the other 50 percent are tumor-marker "silent." To make matters worse, Ca-125 is elevated in a lot of conditions other than ovarian cancer, especially in women under 50. It can be high during the menstrual cycle; during pregnancy; and in the presence of fibroid tumors, endometriosis, or benign cysts; and in up to 1 percent of normal women with none of these conditions. Other malignancies from the gastrointestinal tract, lung, breast, and blood cells also raise Ca-125 levels, so it is certainly not ovarian-specific. *Cirrhosis* of the liver (degeneration of the liver due to alcoholism or chronic infection) also causes high levels of this tumor marker. Clearly, running annual Ca-125 levels on all women over 50 won't work as a screen for ovarian cancer. If we confine this test to premenopausal women with a pelvic mass, 85 percent of the blood tests will still be false-positive, but once we have documentation of an elevated tumor marker, many of these women and their doctors will feel forced to pull out all stops and resort to unnecessary, expensive, and potentially harmful surgeries ranging from laparoscopy to total hysterectomy. If, however, we confine the test to postmenopausal women with a pelvic mass, an elevated Ca-125 will indicate ovarian cancer unless proven otherwise.

But how do we find the mass? If we can't feel it at an early stage (and most women won't have pelvic examinations every few months to catch something), can we see it during its nascence? Pelvic ultrasound allows us to "view" our ovaries. New ultrasound techniques (such as color flow Doppler) also allow us to see blood flow in the pelvis. Malignant tumors develop networks of new blood vessels with rapid flow to supply their greedy appetites. If we can ultrasound the pelvis and find an ovarian cyst or mass that has abnormal vessels, we may have diagnosed a cancer we couldn't feel or detect with Ca-125. Sounds great; why don't we simply scan all women on an annual basis? Again, we are faced with a high false-positive rate. If we perform simple ultrasound on our general population of women over 40, we will pick up a lot of general pelvic changes—cysts, benign tumors, and fibroids. Once we have run the test, we're stuck. If we can't be sure our findings are benign, we have to explore further. We estimate that 67 women will have to undergo surgery in order to find one ovarian cancer.

If we combine expensive color flow Doppler studies (these machines cost hundreds of thousands of dollars) and Ca-125 levels, we can positively predict ovarian cancer in less than 40 percent of premenopausal women, but succeed in this prediction in 94 percent of menopausal women. This latter value isn't bad, but our economically minded health-care planners feel that this kind of screening is unrealistic. If we were to screen more than 43 million women in the United States with ultrasound and Ca-125 on an annual basis, the cost would be nearly $14 billion. This negative cost-benefit analysis shouldn't apply to those of us with substantial genetic risk. These women should be screened with tumor markers, ultrasound, and color Doppler ultrasound every six to twelve months. Ninety percent of women with advanced ovarian cancer will die of their disease, whereas 90 percent diagnosed early with Stage I disease will survive. In these cases, the expense is more than justified by our gain.

WHY NOT JUST REMOVE OUR OVARIES AND ELIMINATE OUR RISK?

This would seem a simple enough question, but as you can read earlier, the answer is not always clear-cut in the absence of ovarian cancer. For those of us with a genetic predisposition to ovarian cancer, however, the question takes on a special urgency.

Prophylactic oophorectomy can be done as a surgery by itself. We can remove both ovaries by laparoscopy without making a large abdominal incision; this can be done on an outpatient basis. Women who have a verifiable history of hereditary ovarian cancer should consider this procedure after age 35 or after they have finished having their babies. For women with only one family member with ovarian cancer and a 5 percent lifetime risk, the advisability of prophylactic oophorectomy is unproven. Those of us who fall into this risk category should definitely use birth control pills. If two relatives have had ovarian cancer and our risk is 7 percent or higher, removal of the ovaries becomes more reasonable, but even this does not guarantee a lifetime cure. Women from very high-risk families have on rare occasions developed peritoneal cancer (of the cells lining the abdominal cavity) years after they've undergone prophylactic oophorectomy.

TREATMENT: CAN WE WIN?

Not yet. Treatment of ovarian cancer is fraught with tremendous challenges. Once the diagnosis is made we need extensive pelvic surgery, entailing the removal of the uterus, Fallopian tubes, both ovaries, the fat "apron" which covers the intestines (omentum), and the lymph nodes in the pelvis and lower abdomen. All metastases, even if they're small, should meticulously be excised. We'll then require chemotherapy. New drugs are being tested and used, including taxol, tumor-directed antibodies, and killer cells that are activated from our own blood. They may make a difference. Once more we're at the mercy of research funds and studies to help stop this, our most insidious gynecologic cancer.

Vulvar Cancer

Cancer of the vulvar skin is uncommon and accounts for just 5 percent of all our gynecologic malignancies. This cancer can occur in our forties and fifties (especially in conjunction with HPV infections), but it's usually diagnosed in our mid-sixties. Treatment is simple with early diagnosis, but it's the early diagnosis that poses the problem. Few of us spend any time looking "down there," and our doctors often treat irritations of our outer genitals with nonchalance, expecting to cure whatever itches, burns, or hurts us with antifungal, antibacterial, or steroid creams.

Ulcerations, raised white plaques, or any abnormal discolorations that don't go away after one month warrant medical attention. Simple visual inspection isn't enough. Doctors have to biopsy the abnormal area to make an early cancer diagnosis.

If we catch the cancer while it's still "in situ" and the abnormal cells are localized, or if the tumor invades less than 1 millimeter of tissue, a local excision is all we need. If it has grown deeper, we do a more extensive excision to clear the surgical margins and dissect out the lymph nodes in the groin on the same side. If more than one node is positive, we'll usually need radiation. The treatment becomes even more disfiguring if the tumor is larger than 2 centimeters. We need a radical dissection of the lymph glands in both groins as well as radiation if the nodes are positive. If the "right" surgery is performed, our overall five-year survival rate is 70 percent. If our nodes are negative, this rises to 90 percent.

The difference between local excision and genital disfigurement and even death is determined by time and neglect. Just because we're older doesn't mean we should expect and, therefore, ignore vulvar itching and irritation. There is no such thing as a seven-year itch.

Skin Cancer

Most of us consider our skin in cosmetic terms. In our teens, we believed that if only we could have clear skin, we would be popular and live happily ever after. But clear wasn't enough, and paleness denoted nerdiness. So we smeared ourselves with baby oil (mixed with just enough iodine to give us a tint), donned our bikinis, and baked or burned ourselves into the correct shade of brown. Our next two decades were spent worrying about stretch marks, the first laugh (or frown) lines on our face, and what skin cream manufacturers referred to as the "ravages of age." Still, we wanted to look healthy and even took steps to maintain health by participating (often with our children) in outdoor activities—swimming, biking, hiking, tennis, skiing, and, of course, getting a tan. Decked out in our bathing suits (now one-piece because of our stretch marks) and soaking up the rays, we enjoyed what we felt was a much-deserved form of relaxation.

Since we entered our forties, we've become a little wiser. We even have those rapidly expanding and deepening "wise" lines to prove it. We now know the sun is not good for our skin. It promotes wrinkles and brown spots. This cosmetic concern is, however, trivial compared with what should be an overwhelming medical concern—skin cancer. We've burned ourselves to the point where skin cancer is reaching epidemic proportions.

There are two categories of skin cancer, nonmelanoma and melanoma. Nonmelanoma skin cancer is the most common cancer in the United States, affecting a total of 600,000 women and men a year. Its incidence has risen 65 percent since 1980. Although it's rarely fatal if treated early, it can cause severe disfigurement and loss of function. Malignant melanoma (MM) runs a more fatal course. It has the horrific distinction of being the fastest-growing (in incidence) of all of our cancers, increasing 300 percent in the past forty years! In 1995, 34,000 people in the United States were diagnosed with melanoma, and 7,200 died. We project that 1 in 90 Americans will develop melanoma by the year 2000.

We'd better stop obsessing over our wrinkles and start paying attention to brown, pink, and black spots, moles, sores, and funny bumps on every part of our bodies. Change is expected as we grow older, but change in any skin lesion may signify cancer. Screening for all of our other cancers requires special tests, from Pap smears to X rays to invading tubes and scopes. Skin cancer is detected with simple observation. We may not be expert dermatologists, but we can recognize what's new or different on the outside of our body. The following is a brief summary of our risks, diagnosis, treatment, and prevention of skin cancers.

MALIGNANT MELANOMA (MM): THE CANCER THAT "INKS" ITS PRESENCE ON OUR SKIN

Our *melanocytes* are the cells that lie in the bottom of the basal layer of our outer skin (*epidermis*). They produce melanin pigment, which gives us our skin color, but also protects us against ultraviolet damage. When these cells grow or differentiate abnormally, they can become malignant.

The sun shines brightly, but also bleakly, on this cancer. Radiation in the ultraviolet-B range (which has been enhanced by our depletion of the ozone layer in the atmosphere) promotes this cancer. The "sun-blame" factor is not straightforward, but appears to be intermittent. Our risk of melanoma starts when we're young, possibly before the age of 20 and perhaps even before the age of 10. It's affected by the paleness of our skin (exactly the factor we were trying to overcome by lying in the sun!). Fair, freckled, blue-eyed girls with blond or red hair who intermittently attempt to tan and end up with blistering sunburns have a very increased risk of melanoma. Those areas of skin that have a more consistent out-door exposure to the sun, such as our face, don't seem to evince the same risk as parts of our bodies that are usually covered and tend to be burned when they are uncovered. (Remember the rows of girls lying on their stomachs with the backs of their bathing suits undone?)

Ten percent of us will develop melanoma because of genetic factors. It takes only one chromosome from either of our parents with a defective melanocyte gene to cause atypical moles (called *dysplastic nevi*), and these tend to become malignant. A new test allows us to isolate this melanocyte gene from cells we obtain from the surface of our inner cheek (a *buccal smear*). Even without gene testing, we can predict that if we have these atypical moles, and two of our family members have had melanoma, we have a greater than 50 percent lifetime risk for develop-ing this skin cancer.

The other 90 percent of us can also sporadically develop atypical moles and are at risk. The incidence of these moles is 40 percent in those of us who develop melanoma, while it's only 5 percent in the general population. Congenital birthmarks (called *nevi*), especially giant ones that cover large amounts of body surface, can also progress to cancer. The smaller ones occur along lines of skin cleavage; they are raised and brown and may have hairs. One percent of us are born with them, and many dermatologists feel it's worthwhile to remove them in our early teens to avoid future malignancy. (My daughter had one on her neck that, to her dismay, we had removed; she still thinks we just wanted to torture her!)

Seventy percent of early MM lesions spread superficially or radially without penetration; that's why they develop irregular borders, change in color, and grow in width. This is also the time when simple removal will give us a cure. Thirty percent of MM tumors are nodular; they grow up and down and tend to be invasive early in their development. They appear as dark brown, black, or blue-black nodules. Because they are growing downward, they may have a very even border and appear smooth and harmless. In general, the more pigmented marks we have on our body, the higher our risk of MM. Between 18 and 85 percent of melanomas arise from lesions we call *melanocytic nevi*, which look like brown spots, patches, or moles.

The ABCDs of Melanoma Recognition

The only way to diagnose this cancer is to look at it, get worried, and "get thee to a dermatologist" to have it examined and biopsied if necessary. The ABCD rule applies to any pigmented mark or mole we have on our body.

A = Asymmetry

B = Border irregularity

C = Color variations within the "mole"

D = Dark black color and/or diameter that is greater than 0.6 centimeter (the size of a pencil eraser)

We should add "G" for growth of either a new lesion or one that has been there "forever." I'd also add a second "C" for change. If any mark or lesion changes its size, color, shape, or surface (it gets bumpy, scaly, or crusty, forms an ulcer, or bleeds), "C" mandates "CA" (cancer alarm). Have your doctor check it out!

Therapy and Prognosis

Any lesion that is suspicious should be removed in its entirety. Once the pathologist gets the tissue and confirms it is melanoma, it must be staged. Either it's a primary tumor with no spread to lymph nodes, it has spread to regional or nearby lymph nodes, or it has distant metastases. Eighty percent of melanomas are found before spreading to the lymph nodes, but this does not mean that 80 percent of us will be easily cured. The prognosis depends on the size of the lesion and the depth of its penetration into the deeper layers of our skin. If it's a very thin lesion (less than 0.75 millimeter), we have a 96 percent chance of five-year survival. If it's thick (greater than 4.00 millimeters), that chance drops to less than 50 percent. If only one regional node is involved, the chance is again 50 percent; but if the tumor has spread to four or more nodes, it drops to between 15 and 20 percent. With distant metastases, we do very poorly and have less than a 5 percent five-year survival rate.

Therapy means more than removal of the lesion for diagnosis. We need to clear the margins to make sure there are no invisible microscopic tumor cells left. Cure rates are also much better if these margins are out, so we usually have to undergo additional resection. If necessary, the closest or regional lymph nodes are also removed to see if they are involved. Once they're out (and if they test positive), we can try several forms of chemotherapy or immunotherapy. Researchers are currently working on vaccines against metastatic melanoma.

Prevention and Control: Our "PC" against "MM"

The difference between a death sentence 95 percent of the time with metastatic melanoma and near-certain cure of early thin melanoma is what I term "pay-per-view." We need to have a dermatologist (or at least a physician with "skin experience") view our skin and check our moles, especially if we have a lot of them or we're considered at risk. Optimal monitoring would include skin examinations at least once a year. This includes the area around the vagina and anus, since pigmented lesions in these areas that we don't look at can also become malignant. Sometimes doctors will photograph these moles (what a way to preserve our image) so they can recognize subtle changes. We can't expect our doctors to remember what each of our moles looked like a year ago; we certainly don't. Anything new or different should be biopsied.

This is the easy part, because we can make an appointment and have a professional do it. The hard part is our own involvement in prevention. Here is a short list of ways to protect ourselves from skin cancer.

1. Don't go for that all-in-one-weekend or summer-vacation tan if you have nontanning skin (your red, burning skin is screaming out its sensitivity and vulnerability).

2. Remember that your children are the most susceptible. If they burn, they are more likely to get metastatic melanoma in later life. Keep them, along with yourself, out of the sun or properly protected with long pants and sleeves, sun hats, and UV-blocking sunglasses.

3. Always use sunscreen of at least SPF 15 when outdoors and exposed. Read the directions on the bottle and reapply as necessary. Remember, though, that you cannot extend the time the lotion protects you from the sun's burning rays simply by applying more sunscreen.

4. Look at your skin from head to toe (and between your toes, where we can develop dysplastic nevi). If you have worrisome, growing, or changing marks, bumps, or sores, have them checked.

Melanoma is not a "hidden" cancer. It highlights itself with pigment; all we have to do is look.

NONMELANOMA CANCERS OF THE SKIN

These cancers are far more prevalent but less visible than metastatic melanoma. More than one third of all cancers in the United States are nonmelanoma skin cancers! The incidence rates have risen drastically over the last two decades, and women (who used to have fewer of these cancers than men) have been caught up in this surge of skin malignancies. Exposure to sun is the principal cause of these cancers; not intermittent exposure or burns (which increase MM), but constant or long-term exposure to ultraviolet-B radiation. The closer we are to the equator, the higher the altitude, the more the ozone layer is depleted, and the more we spend our cumulative leisure time or work time exposed to the sun, the higher our risk. Most lesions occur on skin that is frequently exposed (face, hands, and arms). The older we are (and the more years we've had to bake), the higher our incidence of these skin cancers. It rises 4- to 8-fold in our fifties to seventies as compared with our thirties and forties.

Ultraviolet-B causes damage to our skin's DNA and its repair system and alters our immune system. Longer-wavelength ultraviolet-A (a component of sunlight) is also capable of damaging DNA and is carcinogenic in animals. Both types of radiation cause mutations and affect tumor-suppressor genes.

There are other causes of these skin cancers, though they play a minor role compared with sun exposure. These include radiation therapy, chronic skin ulcers or infections, immunosuppressed states (which can result from both diseases and therapy), and certain skin diseases that cause scars. Arsenic, which used to be an ingredient in medicinal potions, is still a component of insecticides and can cause skin cancer. Cigarette smoking (my favorite thing to blame) clearly has a role in causing cancer of the lip and has been associated with an increased risk of skin cancer at other sites. Human papillomaviruses (not touching toads) cause warts and can sometimes cause premalignant or malignant skin tumors.

There are two types of nonmelanoma skin cancers: *basal cell carcinomas*, which account for 70 to 80 percent of these cancers; and *squamous cell carcinomas*, which are less frequent (20 percent) but are considered more serious because of their ability to metastasize. The latter account for about 1,500 deaths per year in the United States.

Basal Cell Carcinoma

As the name suggests, this cancer arises from the basal (bottom) cells in the epidermis or outer layer of our skin. About 80 percent of these cancers develop in the area of our head or neck where we have had long-term sun exposure. Half begin as translucent or pink, pearly raised nodules that tend to have fine blood vessels on their surface. They grow and then ulcerate, forming small sores. Other, more superficial lesions start as red, scaly patches and often occur on our arms, legs, or torso. As they grow, they become crusty and scaly. A third type of basal cell carcinoma appears as flat, off-white, or yellow patches or elevated plaques. As these lesions enlarge, they resemble scars.

The treatment for this cancer is to remove or destroy it, by electric surgical methods (cautery), excision with a knife, cryosurgery (where it's destroyed through freezing), laser surgery, topical chemotherapy, or injection of interferon (an antiviral and immunosuppressive drug) into the lesion. Recurrence rates vary between 1 and 39 percent, depending on the extent of the lesion and on treatment. If they recur, it's usually within three years. Unfortunately, the cancers on our face are the most likely to grow back, and if we need a second surgery, we get additional scarring and disfigurement. Once we've had this cancer, half of us will get a new one within five years. The insult of our past and future exposure to sun will help determine if we join this "you've got it again" group.

Squamous Cell Carcinoma

This is a cancer of superficial cells in our epidermis or outer skin layer. Eighty percent of these cancers develop on our arms, head, and neck (where the ultraviolet rays got their chance to damage these cells).

Tumors can also develop as a result of other insults or damage to our skin—chronic inflammation or scarring, radiation, or (once more) smoking. Squamous cell carcinoma commonly starts as a reddish raised nodule that has indistinct margins and may have a cavity or an ulcer in the middle. It can also look like a warty bump or a more superficial scabby plaque. This cancer usually grows locally, but it can become aggressive, invading the deeper layers of our skin, muscle, and bone. As it grows, it may extend into blood vessels and lymph channels and, in this way, metastasize.

Depending on its size and placement, squamous cell cancer should be excised, radiated, frozen, or lasered. The overall rate of metastasis ranges from 0.3 to 3.7 percent, but 11 percent of tumors that occur on the lower lip (and are often associated with smoking) metastasize. One to 20 percent of these tumors will recur because of our old and ongoing skin misbehavior (we're still in the sun!). Men have more recurrences than women (it may take them longer to learn to get into the shade).

Prevention of Nonmelanoma Skin Cancer: Pale Is Beautiful (Or at Least Cancer-Free)

"Out, out, damn spot!" means out, out of the sun. At the least, we should stay out of the sun during the middle of the day, use sunscreens, and wear protective clothing. Doctors estimate that using sunscreens that block 90 percent of UVB radiation for the first eighteen years of our (or our children's or grandchildren's) lives should reduce lifetime risk of nonmelanoma skin cancer by 78 percent. Sunscreens with SPF of 15 block approximately 93 percent of UVB radiation. Those that are double (30) block about 96 percent. It's consistent use of these lotions, gels, and creams rather than the difference between SPF 15 and SPF 46 that counts. That means frequently applying a block under our makeup, smearing it onto our exposed areas when we're outdoors, and admonishing our kids, "You can't go out like that unless you put your sun 'goop' on."

Are tanning salons any safer than the sun when it comes to skin cancer? Most places use equipment that emits UVA light. Studies with animals show that equal tanning doses of UVA are as carcinogenic as UVB. If we use these booths and lamps to get brown, we're going to increase our risk of melanoma skin cancer. One last comment—obviously,

I'm not in favor of artificial tanning—is that the type of tan we get from UVA affords less protection against subsequent sun and sunburning than a UVB tan. So the excuse that a presummer UVA tan will protect us from UVB in summer or on a tropical vacation doesn't hold a "ray" of truth. *All* tanning is dangerous!

13

"OUR" DISEASES
Why Don't We Know More About Them?

e have effortlessly surpassed men in our proprietary rights to certain diseases. These medical disorders affect women in such disproportionate numbers—from 75 percent to 90 percent of cases—that the possessive "our" applies with few qualifications. The sexist discrimination of these diseases is hard to explain. They are almost all *autoimmune* disorders (when the body turns against itself) affecting multiple organ systems—in particular our nervous system—thyroid, joints, muscles, and vital organs. Our individual susceptibility is extremely high: About 1 in 10 of us will develop an autoimmune disease in our lifetime, and this incidence appears to be on the rise. These diseases account for approximately 15 percent of our total health-care expenditures. One would hope that if these (or, more correctly, "our") diseases are so prevalent, huge efforts would be made to investigate the causes, ameliorate the symptoms, and find a cure. Once more, however, the system of allocating research funds and attention has shortchanged women. In 1993 less than 1 percent of the total budget of the National Institutes of Health went for research directly related to these disorders.

"Our" diseases seem to share a similar immunologic defect. The *T cells*, or fighter cells, of our immune systems are not given the proper "self" antigens, and so they fail to recognize our body's own tissue. These improperly programmed T cells then attack certain normal, healthy tissues as if they were foreign invading substances. Why one disease affects our thyroid and another our skin or joints is largely unknown. What we do know is that just being women places us at risk, and unless we and our physicians recognize the multitude of symptoms that accompany these disorders, we will delay proper diagnosis and therapy.

Systemic Lupus Erythematosus (SLE)

SLE is a broad autoimmune disease (the word "broad" has no politically incorrect connotations; it simply means that many tissues and organs may be affected). It hits us when we are far too young, 80 percent of the time during our childbearing years. SLE occurs in 0.1 percent of women. The disease is caused by antibodies that attack one or more components of the core of all our cells—the nucleus. These antibodies—called antinuclear antibodies, or ANA—are found in 90 percent of patients with SLE and are present in most other rheumatic or joint diseases. They are found in small amounts in about 2 percent of the normal population (so if one of your blood tests picks up a low positive reading of ANA, don't freak). Scientists think that these multiple antibodies are formed when normal body substances or antigens are minimally altered by damage from sunlight, infection, or exposure to environmental agents capable of inciting inflammation or tissue injury. This may cause them to become "supercharged" so that they excite immune reactions. There may also be changes in a specific gene or group of genes that "blind" immune recognition. If we don't "know" our own cellular components, we attack them (our bodies are not "foreign-friendly"). This self-attack is the basis of our autoimmune diseases.

The fact that lupus occurs when our hormones are at their peak (our reproductive years) would lead us to believe that SLE is hormone-dependent, or at least hormone-aided. We know that the immune response in animals is strongly influenced by sex hormones. If we take a thymus (a gland that produces immune cells) from a mouse with lupus-like disease and graft it into another mouse, mouse number two will develop lupus—but only if it is producing or given estrogen. How estrogen affects SLE in women or whether manipulation of this hormone can affect the course of the disease has not yet been established. (How much can be done with only 1 percent of research funds?!) We do know that high-estrogen birth control pills can exacerbate active disease and should be avoided.

SYMPTOMS OF SLE

The diagnosis of SLE is made if we have three or four typical manifestations of the disease. These include a characteristic rash (a butterfly-shaped redness on our cheeks or a raised red bumpy rash on our upper trunk or areas exposed to the sun), arthritis, a lowered platelet count (*thrombocytopenia*), kidney inflammation (*nephritis*), and the presence of antinuclear antibodies. These symptoms are dutifully described in the textbooks and need to be listed during medical exams, but they may not develop the way they are supposed to when we first "get sick." One joint might get sore (*arthralgia*), or we may develop a nonspecific pattern of arthritis, vague central nervous system complaints such as chronic fatigue, disturbances in our mental acuity, and mood changes including anxiety and depression (this is depressing; it describes so many other circumstances). We may have a rash and notice that our extremities tend to turn blue or white when they are cold (*Raynaud's phenomenon*).

This is all pretty nonspecific and can go on for months or years before the disease progresses to the point where it "qualifies" for diagnosis. It can then cause a variety of illnesses, depending on which tissues are attacked. If it's the joints, we may develop episodes of severe migrating joint pain. The soft-tissue supporting structures of these aching joints may become damaged, and the joint becomes deformed. If the mouth and throat are involved, we get recurrent sore throats (without infection) and oral ulcers. If the kidneys are affected, we may develop renal failure. Central nervous system "attack" can lead to migraine headaches, fever, high blood pressure, and seizures. If the large blood vessels in our brain are involved, we might experience stroke or brain hemorrhage, which can even be fatal (thankfully, this is infrequent). One third of all women with SLE may suffer inflammation of the lung, heart, or their linings. Inflammation of the blood vessels leading to the gastrointestinal tract may diminish blood flow, causing pain and loss of function. We can develop inflammation of the pancreas (*pancreatitis*) as well as disturbances of liver function. Finally, if our platelets are attacked, it can cause complications such as thrombosis or clots forming in large vessels (*thrombophlebitis*), the lung (*pulmonary embolism*), and the brain (*stroke*).

This list sounds awful, but it includes all of the worst-case scenarios. The overall ten-year survival rate for people with lupus now approaches 90 percent. The prognosis is worse the younger we are when we develop SLE and appears to improve after we've "weathered" five years of the disease, especially if our kidneys are unaffected. Since SLE strikes many of us during our reproductive years, we may have to carefully weigh the decision to get pregnant. If the disease is active, and especially if it causes kidney inflammation or high blood pressure, there is a substantial risk that pregnancy will hasten its course and, worse yet, that the disease will cause miscarriage, premature delivery, or stillbirth. Women with SLE who have a particular antibody against cardiolipids (a type of phospholipid that is prevalent in heart tissue) have a high incidence of late miscarriage (in fact, any woman with a history of repeated late miscarriages should be tested for the presence of this anticardiolipid antibody). But there is good news about pregnancy: If our disease has been in remission for at least four to six months, our pregnancy can be as normal as that of unaffected women.

On the other end of our age spectrum, if we develop SLE after the age of 60, the disease usually runs a much more benign course. Arthritis, *pleurisy* (inflammation of the lining of the lung), rash, and anemia are the major problems, but they are rarely life-threatening.

TREATMENT OF SLE

There is no one treatment for SLE (or any of the other autoimmune diseases), and there is no cure. We haven't learned how to stop our bodies from attacking themselves. We've only figured out how to curb the attack—with steroids and immunosuppressive therapy. So if we're dealing with significant episodes of "self-attack" on our kidneys, blood vessels, or other organs, we resort to these drugs, but the therapy can ultimately cause more harm than good. People with lupus have a higher rate of coronary atherosclerosis, which seems to be related to treatment with steroids rather than the disease itself. Osteoporosis is another side effect of this drug. Both immunosuppressant and steroid medications compromise our ability to deal with infections. If our main complaint is arthritis, we can often control it with aspirin or other nonsteroidal anti-inflammatory drugs. Antimalarial drugs are used for skin problems. Clotting disorders can be controlled with anticlotting drugs. If our platelet count drops or severe anemia occurs, we can use certain forms of chemotherapy or even an anti-estrogen therapy called danazol (it helps prevent platelet destruction, but this anti-estrogen does not work against other "organ attacks"). If the worst happens and kidney failure develops, we need to resort to dialysis until we can get a kidney transplant. This procedure has been remarkably successful. Ultimately, however, scientists would rather figure out how to prevent attack on our original kidneys than overcome the potential rejection of a new one.

We are just beginning to appreciate the huge variability and the many facets of this disease. SLE is a big sister to the other autoimmune diseases. They are related, but SLE has seen it all and done it all: it attacks our organs with little specificity. Until we have answers, doctors can only diagnose, treat our symptoms, and hope for remissions.

Rheumatoid Arthritis (RA)

The chief autoimmune target of rheumatoid arthritis is our joints and, more specifically, the synovial fluid and membranes that cushion the joints. These lubricating tissues are attacked, become inflamed, and are eventually destroyed along with adjacent bone and cartilage, resulting in permanent deformities. The attack tends to be symmetrical (affecting both hands or both feet) but can also occur on one side, in the wrists, elbows, knees, ankles, and neck. If these affected joints are inactive, they get stiff. A significant symptom of RA is morning stiffness that can last not for minutes—we all have that, just overcoming the inertia of our night—but for hours.

RA occurs in approximately 1 percent of the population and attacks women three times more frequently than men. Unlike SLE, it doesn't peak until our forties or fifties, when our hormones are waning. Is there a correlation? We don't know. RA tends to run in families. We are four times more likely to develop RA if we have a first-degree relative (mother or sister) with this disease. Gene changes associated with RA have been found in an area called the HLA-D complex, but only 10 percent of women with RA have a family history. So scientists postulate that environmental factors such as viruses or bacteria play a role in increasing our autoimmune susceptibility, either by irritating the synovial membranes so that they produce "annoying" antigens or through the by-products of these infecting organisms, which produce "superantigens" that combine with a susceptible gene and cause it to order an attack.

Symptoms of RA

RA can begin with fatigue, poor appetite, and weakness, and only weeks or months later do the typical joint symptoms appear. Initially, there is swelling, redness, and severe tenderness of the joints; with time, the joints can become deformed. Bumps called *rheumatoid nodules* can appear under the skin and near the joints.

Although scientists consider RA a joint disease, its autoimmune process can attack blood vessels *(vasculitis)*; this in turn affects the organs supplied by these vessels. The lungs and *pericardium* (the sac around the heart) can become inflamed. In chronic RA, red and white cells and platelets can decrease, leaving us susceptible to infections. Finally, to add bone insult (and fracture) to joint injuries, this disease also causes osteoporosis both directly by diminishing bone mass and indirectly as a result of the steroids we use to treat it.

RA is diagnosed through blood tests that detect the presence of special autoantibodies, or rheumatoid factor, in 65 percent of us with this disease. However, 5 percent of healthy women also have this factor, and this figure increases to 20 percent once we're 65 or older.

Course of RA

RA's progression, like that of the other autoimmune diseases, varies. Twenty percent of patients have little or no joint deformity after ten years, but unfortunately 80 percent do. If we have remissions the first year, our prognosis is better. If the disease is going to misbehave, this will generally happen in the first six years. RA can shorten our median life expectancy by three to seven years, because it increases our susceptibility to infection, bleeding, bone fracture, and complications from medications.

Treatment of RA

There is no cure for RA. What doctors try to do is control the pain it causes, reduce joint inflammation, preserve the joints' "jointing," and improve healing. So we rely on aspirin and other nonsteroidal anti-inflammatory medications, analgesics, and low-dose steroids as our first line of therapy. If we need to go further, we use agents called disease-modifying anti-rheumatic drugs. These include immunosuppressants and chemotherapy, which reduce the destructive capacity of RA. Finally, to improve joint function, doctors recommend special exercises and may resort to surgery or joint replacements.

Scleroderma

Scleroderma is a disease that attacks collagen, that all-important matrix of our skin and bones. We're concerned both cosmetically and health-wise when we lose our collagen as we get older and go through menopause. Plastic surgeons even inject purified collagen into our wrinkles to smooth them out. Scleroderma can be compared to a monster plastic surgeon gone crazy with huge syringes of collagen. This disease causes an accelerated, disordered laying down of collagen, which scars our skin, blood vessels, and internal organs, especially the gastrointestinal tract, lungs, heart, and kidneys.

SYMPTOMS OF SCLERODERMA

Scleroderma affects women three times as often as men. It usually begins between our thirties and our fifties. The initial symptom may be Raynaud's phenomenon, or more aptly put, the "white and blue digit phenomenon," a condition in which cold or stress causes the small arteries in our fingers and toes to constrict and their blood supply to be severely diminished. As these digits warm up or we calm down, they become red and may hurt. As the disease progresses, the connective tissue of the skin and organs is self-attacked. Fluid accumulates under the skin, which begins to thicken like a hide. Bound down to the underlying layer of fat, this thickened skin doesn't move or give. Wrinkles are replaced by stretched, immobile skin that limits facial and even body movement. When this process occurs in the gastrointestinal tract, muscle is lost and food can't be properly propelled. If the lungs are attacked, we become out of breath with exertion, develop a cough, and are at risk for pneumonia or even cancer. If the heart is targeted, its muscle becomes scarred and unable to pump or beat properly. Finally, kidney involvement can cause high blood pressure and kidney failure.

COURSE OF SCLERODERMA

Ninety-five percent of people with scleroderma have antinuclear antibodies in their blood. The disease can be either circumscribed (local) or diffuse. Ninety-five percent of people with local scleroderma will remain stable for up to twenty years. If scleroderma is diffuse and attacks internal organs, especially as we get older, our ten-year survival ranges between 30 and 70 percent.

TREATMENT OF SCLERODERMA

As with the other autoimmune diseases, we have no cure, so treatment is given to relieve symptoms and improve functioning. Doctors prescribe immunosuppressants to reduce some of the skin and organ scarring. Low-dose aspirin helps prevent the platelets from sticking to damaged blood vessel walls and causing clots. The old standby, steroids are also called into action to treat inflammation. The only good news is that for unknown reasons (though no more unknown than the cause of the disease itself), the hidelike skin changes may spontaneously disappear after a number of years. This softening is gradual and begins in reverse order of the original scarring. Skin thickness may eventually return to normal. This is the one time we celebrate loss of collagen.

Sjögren's Syndrome (SS)

The correct spelling and pronunciation of this syndrome always stump medical students. Very few of us can enunciate "sj," but the linguists have been kind; the "sj" is pronounced like "sh," so it sounds like "Shoegren's." Pronunciation is about all we have surmounted with this disease; its cause and cure remain enigmas. This autoimmune disorder attacks our normal glands through *lymphocyte* (white cell) infiltration.

SYMPTOMS OF SS

SS attacks the salivary glands, causing them to atrophy, so that saliva decreases; the mouth, tongue, and lips become horrendously dry; and we even lose our sense of taste. It also affects the tear glands in our eyes. "No more tears" may be beneficial in children's shampoo, but persistent dryness causes the surface of the eye to become red, sore, and inflamed to the point where we can lose vision. This disease has a predilection for glands and mucous membranes in our mouth, throat, nose, and airways, and one more mucous membrane distinctive to women—the vagina. (Indeed, very few individuals without vaginas are affected; SS occurs in females 90 percent of the time!) One in 1,250 women are affected, and the mean age for diagnosis of Sjögren's is 50, which, coincidentally or not, corresponds to our menopause. Severe vaginal dryness and pain during intercourse are common complaints with SS, making it not just "our" disease, but also one with gynecologic implications. In addition to our urogenital tract, lymphocytic invasion can attack practically every other organ system, including the stomach, pancreas, gallbladder, heart, brain, blood vessels, muscles, and joints.

While 75 percent of people with SS have antinuclear antibodies, and 50 percent have rheumatoid factors, there is no single blood test to identify SS.

TREATMENT OF SS

I am getting tired of admitting defeat, but all we currently have available is therapy to help alleviate our symptoms: artificial tears for our eyes, artificial saliva for the mouth, lubricants and estrogen creams for the vagina, nonsteroidal anti-inflammatories for muscles and joints, steroids, and immunosuppressive medications for serious organ complications.

Polymyositis

In polymyositis, the autoimmune attack and lymphocyte invasion are directed toward our muscles. If the condition also affects the skin, causing a rash, it is called *dermatomyositis*. Women are affected twice as frequently as men.

SYMPTOMS OF POLYMYOSITIS

Initially, polymyositis causes a weakness of a muscle or group of muscles. Later, these muscles may atrophy and contract. This can affect our ability to swallow, breathe, or walk. Involvement of the heart muscle can be fatal. If we develop this disease after the age of 50, there is an 8 percent chance it has been caused by a malignancy, and a thorough medical search should be made for cancer of the breast, colon, rectum, chest, bone, or blood. Because the muscles are inflamed (that's what the "myositis" means), many of their enzymes are released, and their presence can easily be verified by blood tests. Fifty percent of people with polymyositis also have rheumatoid factor and 75 percent have antinuclear antibodies in their blood.

TREATMENT OF POLYMYOSITIS

Treatment is the usual—steroids to diminish muscle and skin inflammation and chemotherapy for advanced disease.

Thyroid Disease

We consider the ovaries to be our uniquely female glands. All of our other glands are bisexual, existing and functioning in men and women. However, the female thyroid is more likely to malfunction than the same gland sitting in the neck of a male. Thyroid diseases are, with a 10 percent exception (including George Bush), ours.

Endocrine glands tend to be small in size, but very large in the effect their hormones have on our entire system. The thyroid's role is enormous; its hormone influences the growth and development of all our tissues, the oxygen consumption of our cells, and our total energy expenditure. Add to this its influence on the turnover of what we consume, our vitamins, and our other hormones, and we might want to look at our thyroid with new respect. I think of it as the "mistress of all glands." This mistress can become lazy and underperform (*hypothyroidism*), be frenetic and overperform (*hyperthyroidism*), or grow lumpy with benign or malignant tumors.

HYPOTHYROIDISM:
UNDERACHIEVEMENT BY GLAND AND BODY

Three percent of us will develop clinical hypothyroidism (which means we develop obvious symptoms), and an additional 10 percent of us between the ages of 40 and 60 develop what we call subclinical hypothyroidism (certain thyroid levels are off, but clinical signs have not become apparent). Our female predilection for this disorder is poorly understood, but a few factors associated with estrogen production seem to increase our thyroid risk: early menarche (first period), late menopause, a large number of pregnancies, and weight gain.

Symptoms of Hypothyroidism

Because our thyroid controls so much, its lack of proper performance causes very broad symptoms. We can develop fatigue, lethargy, depression, irritability, impaired memory, constipation, dry skin, hair loss, muscle aches, and intolerance to cold, and we can gain weight. If we're premenopausal, our cycles may become irregular. Sounds like a nightmare; it is, and interestingly, nightmares are a symptom of this disorder! The predominant cause of hypothyroidism for 90 percent of us is the same as that of our other "female" diseases: an autoimmune reaction. In this case, antithyroid antibodies go on the attack. This thyroid destruction often accompanies other autoimmune diseases such as SLE, rheumatoid arthritis, Sjögren's, and diabetes. When the gland attack involves lymphocytic infiltration and nodules or enlargement occur (*goiter*), it's called *Hashimoto's thyroiditis*. Once these antibodies ambush the thyroid, leaving it unable to produce enough of its hormone, the "supercenter" in our pituitary is put on alert. Normally, the pituitary regulates the thyroid secretion and production of hormone by TSH (*thyroid-stimulating hormone*). It now has to work harder to push the underactive thyroid. The subsequent elevated TSH makes the thyroid cells enlarge and multiply; hence the development of nodules and swelling. Initially, this may compensate for the autoimmune attack, and our thyroid levels are normal or low-normal (at this point, we have subclinical hypothyroidism). Eventually, the inflamed gland is unable to "put out," no matter how much TSH works to prod it. Our thyroid hormone levels drop, and we have clinical hypothyroidism. The laboratory diagnosis is evident; thyroid levels (measured as *thyroxine*, or T_4) are low, and TSH is high. Autoimmune thyroiditis can be confirmed by the presence of antithyroid antibodies.

Treatment of Hypothyroidism

There is no cure, but we do have effective therapy—thyroid hormone, usually given orally in the form of thyroxine or T_4 (known as Synthroid). Daily dosages vary for weight and age (the elderly need less) and commonly range between 0.15 and 0.1 milligram. Aluminum hydroxide, present in certain antacids, and iron can affect absorption. It is important to adjust the dose to our symptoms and TSH levels. If we are given too much and our TSH is repressed below normal levels, we have a greater chance of developing osteoporosis.

There is still some controversy as to whether doctors should treat the disease when it's subclinical. We know that every year, 7 percent of us with elevated TSH (over 10 milliunits/liter) who also have high levels of antithyroid antibodies will become "overt." There is also evidence that women with subclinical hypothyroidism have a higher prevalence of coronary artery disease caused by bad lipoprotein profiles. For these reasons, it might be worthwhile treating those of us who fall into this category, even though we don't have full-blown symptoms.

HYPERTHYROIDISM: TOO MUCH CAN MAKE US NERVOUS WRECKS

Overactivity of our thyroid gland affects 2 percent of us, usually in our thirties and forties. The most common form of this disorder is *Graves' disease*. It occurs when abnormal immune proteins called *thyroid-stimulating immunoglobulins (TSI)* are produced and bind to TSH receptors in the thyroid. The thyroid responds by overproducing hormones.

Symptoms of Hyperthyroidism

What makes this disease weird, both developmentally and with regard to our appearance, is an associated change that can occur in our eyes and eye sockets. The eyeballs get pushed forward and protrude because fat accumulates behind them (*exophthalmos*), while the muscles around the eyes become inflamed and then degenerate. We're not sure why these "frog eyes" develop; perhaps we develop antibodies to specific antigens in those muscles.

The classic symptoms of hypothyroidism are fatigue, nervousness, insomnia, tremors, diarrhea, heart palpitations, rapid heartbeat, shortness of breath, excessive sweating, and intolerance to heat. We may lose weight, although sometimes we may unfairly gain weight because of an increased appetite. If we're premenopausal, our periods can space out or stop. Because the heart is beating rapidly and is overworked, older women with coronary artery disease may develop chest pain or even suffer heart attacks. When examined, we often demonstrate a fine tremor or shakiness of fingers (don't test this after excessive caffeine consumption) and increased reflex response. Our skin may be warm and moist, and some telltale changes occur in our eyes; they appear to be staring, we blink infrequently, and when we look up or down, the lids lag behind the movement of the eye. Which of these signs and symptoms helped Barbara and George Bush's doctors diagnose their disease? Whatever they were, one of "our" diseases came to public notice. There was probably a peak in the documented incidence of this disorder, as Graves' disease became the Bushes' disease.

Treatment of Hyperthyroidism

The laboratory diagnosis of this disorder is confirmed if thyroid levels and TSI are elevated, while TSH is very low or undetectable. The therapy is based on a need to calm the thyroid down, either by suppression with an antithyroid medication called propylthiouracil (PTU) or total destruction using radioactive iodine. The latter will cause permanent hypothyroidism and the need to take thyroid medication for the rest of our lives.

THYROID NODULES AND CANCER

Small lumps in this normally soft and supple gland are common and can be felt in 5 percent of women but can be demonstrated by ultrasound in more than 30 percent. Eighty percent are benign, but we need to make sure. A fine-needle, or aspiration, biopsy is easy to perform—at least for the doctor; having a needle stuck into our neck might not be so easy for us! Examination of the cells will usually determine if there is need for further biopsy.

If the nodule is associated with hypothyroidism or hyperthyroidism, appropriate therapy should cause it to shrink. Even if the nodule is a simple one, causing no hormonal abnormalities, it should shrink if we inhibit TSH secretion by giving thyroid hormone (this puts the thyroid to rest).

There is an increased risk that we'll develop thyroid cancer if, in the past, we received radiation to our neck or face. Unfortunately, this was not an uncommon therapy for acne thirty years ago. Thyroid cancer

can also have a hereditary basis and is found in families that have cancers or tumors of other glands, including the pituitary and pancreas.

Treatment   Seventy-five percent of thyroid cancers are slow-
growing and quite curable if caught while smaller than 4 centimeters.
Depending on the type and size of the tumor, a portion or all of the thyroid should be surgically removed. Sometimes radioactive iodine is also
used to destroy any residual tissue or tumor cells. It's obvious that once
this surgery is performed, lifetime thyroid therapy and monitoring are
necessary so that we can function normally, despite the absence of our
"mistress of all glands."

The prevalence of thyroid disease in women is so great that thyroid hormone therapy currently ranks fifth in the United States among all new
and refill prescriptions. Our awareness should at least be commensurate
with the profits of the drug companies!

Multiple Sclerosis (MS)

There is an ongoing medical argument as to whether multiple sclerosis is
a true autoimmune disease. It does not cross over with the other autoimmune disorders and doesn't share autoantibodies such as antinuclear,
rheumatoid, or antithyroid factors. What is clear is that MS, like the
other diseases, has a female predilection, We're at least twice as likely to
develop MS as men. It's possible that our estrogen and progesterone levels affect genetic and environmental factors that precipitate this disease,
especially when they are in flux during puberty, after pregnancy, and during menopause. Early-onset MS peaks in our teens; late-onset MS peaks
after 45. Our susceptibility to this disease is partially inherited. Increased
risk is seen in families where parents, siblings, and grandparents or even
aunts, uncles, and cousins have MS. If we have a sibling with MS, we
have a 2 to 5 percent lifetime chance of developing this disorder; if one
identical twin gets it, the second has a 30 percent chance.

We call MS a multifactorial disease, which means we are not sure
exactly what causes it, and various investigators have each found valid
evidence to support the role of their particular "favorite factor." Caucasian women living in temperate climates are more likely to be affected.
The initial insult might be a virus, but we haven't identified a specific

one. Immune factors probably come into play at some point. T cells, or immune fighter cells, attack the lining of the nerves (*myelin*), causing inflammation and subsequent degeneration of the lining (aptly termed *demyelinization*). Antibodies to the central nervous system are also present; they are either primary (that is, a misled "self" antibody that helps initiate the disease) or secondary (an antibody that "correctly" responds to chronic tissue injury and the release of new, unrecognized nervous system antigens).

SYMPTOMS OF MS

The underlying pathology of MS is demyelinization. When nerves are stripped, they can't properly conduct impulses. Areas in the brain scar and form plaques. The disease can progress in ways that vary enormously. It can start, stop, and stabilize, slowly progress, or rapidly get worse. Unfortunately, the older we are when we get MS (over 40), the more likely it will follow a more rapid, disabling course. Initial symptoms are weakness and fatigue with exertion (climbing even one flight of stairs becomes difficult), lack of dexterity, feelings of tingling or numbness in one or both legs, dizziness and blurring of vision (due to inflammation of the main optic nerve), and some visual loss. With progression of the disease, we can have memory loss and impaired judgment, trouble controlling muscle functions (including walking and swallowing), bladder and bowel problems, and even incontinence. The diagnosis of MS can be difficult, especially at the onset. (Sometimes our symptoms are so mild—a tingling here, mild dizziness there—that once they subside, we ignore them and don't seek medical attention.) There is no one clinical sign or diagnostic test that is unique to MS. Computerized axial tomography (CAT) scans and MRI of the brain and spinal cord can demonstrate plaques. A spinal tap allows the spinal fluid to be checked for special cells, antibodies, proteins, and products of myelin breakdown. It can also rule out other possible causes of symptoms, such as viral or bacterial infection, brain tumor, or stroke. No doctor can predict the course of the disease or prescribe a cure.

TREATMENT OF MS

Therapy is based on management, and MS has proved itself an especially challenging disease. What works for one patient may not work for another, and with so many episodes of spontaneous remission, it's difficult to determine the effectiveness of any treatment. The symptoms of muscle spasm and stiffness are managed with relaxants and/or physical therapy; pain with various pain medication; bowel and bladder problems with laxatives, enemas, and medication to suppress bladder contractions. Rest, stress reduction, and proper diet may also help, as can keeping cool, receiving physical or massage therapy, and maintaining good hydration.

The second part of management is to attempt to stop the disease process. For this, we use the old standbys—steroids (to reduce nerve inflammation) and immunosuppressants. More than 100 therapies have been proposed for the treatment of MS, which means that none is convincingly effective for a significant number or people. Recently, beta-interferon therapy, which has both antiviral and immunosuppressive properties, has been shown to decrease disease activity in certain patients by as much as 80 percent.

Myasthenia Gravis (MG): Another Grave Disorder

This is another autoimmune disease that affects women more frequently than men. However, the ratio of afflicted women to men is the smallest (3:2). Hence, MG appears last on the list of "our" diseases. This disorder is caused by an autoimmune attack on receptors that are present at the synapses, the junctions between our nerves and our muscles. Muscles contract only when they are "told" to do so by nerve impulses. The instruction is conveyed through a substance called *acetylcholine*, which is normally produced at the end of the nerve and stored. When the nerve is stimulated, acetylcholine is released and combines with the acetylcholine receptors. These, in turn, start an electric charge at the end of the muscle fiber that, if great enough, is repeated along the fiber, triggering muscle contraction. If receptors are destroyed and their number decreases, fewer signals can go through. The muscle may get enough impulses for a few contractions (this is not complete paralysis), but then there is a neurotransmission "silence." We "ask" the muscles to contract, but there is no initiating spark; they cannot reply.

SYMPTOMS OF MG

MG causes weakness and fatigue of our skeletal muscles. Initially, our eyelids get weak and droop, and the eye muscles function poorly, so that we see double. Facial and mouth muscles are also involved. A smile can become a snarl; chewing and swallowing may be difficult; finally, the weakness becomes generalized, so that moving our limbs demands tremendous effort. This is no ordinary fatigue. It can, in severe instances, be life-threatening, when extensive weakness of the diaphragm and respiratory muscles prevents normal breathing.

A diagnosis of MG is made by administering a rapid-acting substance that inhibits breakdown of acetylcholine. This allows the neurotransmitter to interact repeatedly with the limited receptors. If muscle action improves dramatically, we know we're on the right diagnostic track. Another test uses small electric shocks (this sounds mean, but it doesn't hurt). These are delivered to a muscle every few seconds, and in people with myasthenia, the stimulated muscle contraction quickly diminishes. The clincher for diagnosis is a test for anti-acetylcholinesterase receptor antibodies, which are found in 80 percent of people with MG.

This disease generally strikes women in their prime reproductive years (twenties and thirties). Is it hormone-susceptible? We don't know. Its course is variable. It may go into remission for a while but usually recurs, especially after infections. Since this is a true autoimmune disorder, there may be other "faulty" antibodies, such as rheumatoid factor and antinuclear factor. There is also a 3 to 8 percent incidence of hyperthyroidism with MG. The thymus, a gland located below the neck that produces fighter and immune cells, may also be enlarged in MG and may even develop tumors.

TREATMENT OF MG

Unlike our treatment of other autoimmune diseases, we have therapy for MG that, while not a cure, is good enough to allow those affected to return to full, productive lives. The chief medication is an anticholinesterase, which prevents breakdown of the neurotransmitter. An additional therapy, especially if a tumor is present, is removal of the thymus. Even if they don't have a thymus tumor, 85 percent of people with MG improve with this surgery. Finally, the usual autoimmune medications, steroids and immunosuppressants, work well, both to improve symptoms and to prevent the condition from progressing.

"Our" diseases have been shortchanged with regard to allocations for medical research. Hopefully, we won't allow the allocations of our attention and knowledge to mirror this deficiency.

14

Urinary Incontinence
The Topic That Hasn't Come Out of the (Water) Closet

We start out in diapers; we then diaper our children and may do the same for our grandchildren. Enough already! We shouldn't have to "return to the diaper" as we age. Incontinence is a taboo subject; few of us will admit to having a problem (we're still working on admitting we're menopausal). Is this reticence part of our conditioned dainty distaste of our excretory functions? Bowel changes, though, are discussed regularly in TV and magazine ads; we know what to take for gas, constipation, and diarrhea. We also see plenty of commercials touting the absorption—not to mention the "winged" aerodynamics—of sanitary pads. Why is bladder malfunction handled so much more obliquely? The ads for female "adult" protection never really refer to urine or urine loss. Instead they assure us that if we use this product, we can safely dance, hug, and lift children as we get older. If manufacturers are bold enough to graphically advertise, we're shown blue fluid being absorbed by a pad!

We may feel like laughing, but many of us have learned to contain our laughter lest we wet our panties. Meanwhile, the "adult protection" industry is making $10 billion a year selling products to help us cope with or hide incontinence. "Us" is a very inclusive term, comprising 25 million Americans. Among women aged 46 to 64, an estimated 40 percent have some degree of incontinence. Less than half of these women

seek medical help. Either they are too embarrassed to mention the problem to their doctors, or they simply take for granted that this is a "normal" symptom of aging and that they must cope and absorb. The
personal and social consequences are enormous. We start to withdraw
from life outside our homes, fearing to go anyplace where we might not
be able to find a toilet. We restrict our intimate contact and sexual activities. What could be more embarrassing than losing urine during foreplay
or intercourse? (It's not surprising that 24 to 46 percent of incontinent
women admit to sexual dysfunction.) The final humiliation—total loss
of bladder control—is one of the most frequent reasons for entering a
nursing home.

Bladder Control: What Have We Done to Lose It?

The only "plug" that our bladder has is the one-inch-long urethra, which
forms an upward angle at the lower portion, or neck, of the bladder. The
urethra is kept closed by a sphincter that should open only when
the bladder contracts and we void. The lower portion of the bladder and
the urethra are supported by surrounding pelvic tissue and muscles. Any
loss in sphincter tightness, urethral support, or angulation allows urine
to spill out "without permission." If the bladder undergoes involuntary
contractions or if it can't contract and becomes overdistended, we also
lose control. There are four major types of incontinence.

STRESS INCONTINENCE

This causes us to lose urine if there is any increase in abdominal pressure
with physical exertion: during coughing, sneezing, laughing, lifting,
pushing, jumping, or even just standing up. The fuller our bladder, the
more this additional pressure will overcome urethral resistance. Our urethral resistance can be faulty at any age. Studies have reported that up to
38 percent of young women who had not given birth had some degree of
stress incontinence. When tested, many of these women were found to
have an incompetent urethral sphincter. Three other lifetime factors affect our level of stress (from a urinary point of view): pregnancy and
vaginal delivery, estrogen deficiency in menopause, and simple aging.
Pregnancy and vaginal delivery stretch our pelvic muscles, causing us to
lose urethral and bladder support. Significant stress incontinence occurs

in 35 percent of women for six to twelve weeks after childbirth. As we and our pelvic muscles heal and tone after this extraordinarily "expanding" experience, our symptoms improve, but we may never regain perfect continence (the trade-off is that we now have our perfect children). With menopause, we lose our pelvic muscle tone, collagen, and vaginal tissue support and stress incontinence can worsen. As we age, there is loss of muscle tone and collagen. (We experience this throughout the rest of our body; why should our urologic and vaginal areas be different?) Our bladder, as well as our other pelvic organs, may prolapse down as a result of all three insults so that it balloons out and even protrudes from the vaginal opening (*cystocele*). This displaces and weakens the urethra. One final factor can affect stress incontinence: excess weight. The more we have pressing on our bladder (including the fat in and around our abdomen), the "weightier" the gravity (figuratively and literally) of our stress incontinence.

URGE INCONTINENCE

(Otherwise known as "I can't hold it.") This is clinically defined as our inability to withhold urine flow long enough to reach the bathroom (or, more precisely, the toilet; peeing on the bathroom floor does not count as a goal). Any woman who has had a bladder infection knows how awful urgency can be. This condition can occur as a result of inflammation of the bladder, bladder cancer, estrogen deficiency, neurological disorders affecting nerves that stimulate the bladder, or spinal cord injuries. Frequently, the cause is none of the above, but instead relates to our conditioning. If we've spent decades ignoring bladder fullness and waiting to void until it's convenient or the end of the day, the minute we see our home toilet, our bladder contracts as a conditioned response. The problem is that this now happens when we open our front door before we even get to the bathroom. For some of us with urge incontinence, just looking at a bathroom or hearing running water can trigger bladder spasm, and we don't make it.

MIXED INCONTINENCE

Mixed incontinence is a combination of stress and urge incontinence. It accounts for 40 percent of incontinence in women. Both our anatomy and our conditioning are conspiring to cause urinary accidents.

OVERFLOW INCONTINENCE

This is a result of a bladder that remains chronically full. It's especially common in women with cystocele, where the bladder is stretched as it balloons out of the vagina. It can't completely empty, and urine remains in the "bulge." Once we stand, bend, or do anything that exerts pressure on this out-of-shape bladder, small amounts of urine escape. Diabetes can also cause overflow problems by affecting the bladder's nerve supply and its ability to contract and empty.

Diagnosis

A plumber doesn't replace a faucet if the leak is in a lower pipe. The sad fact is that we are more likely to seek "professional" help for kitchen sink incontinence than our own urinary incontinence. To get to the underlying problem causing loss of urine, we need to examine our medical history, our voiding pattern, and obviously, our urinary tract.

The medical history portion of our workup is vital. Did we have multiple pregnancies, difficult prolonged labor and pushing, or large babies? Were we always "bladder-challenged" under certain stresses? Have we had frequent infections, neurologic problems, diabetes, or previous surgeries? Are we taking any drugs that could decrease the muscle tone of the bladder or sphincter, such as antihypertensive medications, muscle relaxants, or Valium? Diuretics can also overwhelm the bladder with fluid that is being drawn from the body.

We should keep a voiding diary for a minimum of two days. How much fluid do we consume, and when? When do we void, and how much? When do we leak? What is the amount, and what were we doing when it occurred? Did we feel an urge, or did the leak just happen?

Our physical exam needs to assess the condition of the vagina (is it atrophic because of estrogen deficiency?) and the general support of the uterus, bladder, and rectum. The urethral angle can be checked by having us push down during the pelvic exam to ascertain if urine leaks out. If this occurs, can it be stopped by mechanically supporting the urethral angle? If that corrects the problem, we have "angled" our way toward a diagnosis. The competency of the urethra and the integrity of the bladder can be checked by putting a small scope called a cystoscope through the urethra into the bladder. The bladder is examined for signs of chronic inflammation, defects, and tumors; the scope is slowly removed and the doctor can see if the urethral sphincter completely closes. Our urine should be checked for blood, white cells, bacteria, and abnormal cells (to rule out bladder malignancy). After we void, how much urine is left? (This is measured by inserting a catheter.) If more than 20 percent of what we voided is still there, we may have overflow problems. Special urodynamic tests using catheters, fluid injection, and instruments to record fluid pressure can measure contractions of the bladder during its filling, storage, and voiding. The capacity of the bladder is measured, and its ability to fill and properly contract is checked. Any involuntary or inappropriate contractions that occurred during this bladder filling and stretching are documented. Special X rays with dyes are used to demonstrate bladder defects or "lost" urethral angles. By combining history, voiding diary, and these techniques, physicians have become competent urinary detectives and, once they've diagnosed a cause, can offer us an excellent chance for cure.

Therapy: Better Dryness Without Better Absorption

Our options are numerous and range from behavior therapy to medications (including hormones), devices that support, injections that strengthen, and surgical procedures that repair and bulwark. With the right therapy, 50 percent of us can be cured, 35 percent markedly improved, and 15 percent made more comfortable. Let the pad and diaper companies beware!

Behavioral Therapy We've each grown "accustomed to our pace" and that includes when and where we void. A review of our voiding diary may show why we leak. If after waiting three hours to go, we lose control, the obvious change—voiding every two hours—should be made for at least two weeks. If this keeps us dry, we can "up it" to two and a half hours for three days, and if we have no urine loss, then go back to or surpass three hours with our new bladder training. We also have to learn to relax when we have the temporary urge to go; taking three breaths very slowly may be enough to get us through this transient bladder contraction. If our accidents occur at night in bed, we need to consume our liquids during the day and stop several hours before bedtime. If we're voiding over four quarts a day, we're drinking too much fluid (the normal amount of urine is usually between 1.5 and 2 quarts a day). We should aim for six to eight glasses of water a day. Too little fluid concentrates the urine and causes bladder irritation and urge incontinence (we can't win). Spicy foods, acidic foods (citrus fruits and tomatoes), alcohol, caffeine, Nutra-Sweet (aspartame), and chocolate can all irritate the bladder and cause frequency, urgency, and loss of control. One of my patients had been plagued by urgency and incontinence to the point where she was considering surgery. Most of her bladder symptoms subsided when she stopped drinking diet sodas and switched to water. (She brought me a bottle of Evian to celebrate her bladder freedom.)

So now we've worked on our voiding schedule and eliminated irritants. We may need to do more. If our pelvic muscles are wasted (a terrible term, but that's what childbearing, low estrogen, and years of gravity will do), we can't expect a return of urinary resiliency unless we tone those muscles. Here's where a real commitment is required. First we have to learn to twitch and contract the right muscles, and that's not so simple. You and your doctor should check with a finger or even a small plastic cone to see if you know how to squeeze the right muscles. Most of us start by contracting our buttocks or anus. We then cheat by using our abdominal muscles. A mirror might help to see what's moving; it should be only the area of the vagina. Kegel exercises help us to tone these muscles. Many physicians feel that Kegels are not enough. The muscle around the urethra has both fast-twitch and slow-twitch fibers. Rapid contractions strengthen the fast-twitch fibers, and prolonged contractions strengthen the slow-twitch fibers. So instead of the uniform Kegels, they advise women to do three sets of rapid contractions and three sets of prolonged "pulling up and in" contractions. The repetitions, or sets, should gradually increase until we do them up to 200 times a day. We will need to perform these or the regular Kegels conscientiously for at least two months before we see results, and even then we're not cured, we need to keep on doing them. As any fitness expert will tell us, muscles have a short memory. As I sit here writing, I'm trying to do my contractions. I'm bopping up and down in my chair, a sure sign that I'm doing them wrong. Who said this is easy? If you are doing Kegels right, not even your hairdresser will know for sure.

Biofeedback can also be used to help us train those muscles. A gauge that measures vaginal sphincter activity can show us if we're using the right ones, and we can use this feedback to tell us where and what to contract. There is also a more passive approach; intravaginal low-voltage electrical stimulation using a device applied by a physician will cause the pelvic floor muscles to contract and can, with time, strengthen them. We can then take over on our own.

If behavior therapy is insufficient, medical and surgical intervention may be necessary to keep us waterproof.

MEDICAL THERAPY

Estrogen in the form of replacement therapy or at least as local vaginal cream will relieve symptoms of stress incontinence in 40 to 70 percent of women who have atrophic vaginal and bladder tissue.

If our incontinence is mainly urge incontinence due to inappropriate bladder contractions, antispasmodic medications are prescribed to relax the bladder muscle. The tone of the urethral sphincter can also be improved and result in better closure with drugs called *sympathomimetics* (they stimulate certain sympathetic nerve receptors in the urethra), but these are contraindicated if we have high blood pressure or heart problems.

SURGICAL THERAPY

To fix it, it has to be anatomically broken. Thus urge incontinence cannot be corrected surgically: cutting or repositioning the bladder or urethra won't stop abnormal bladder contractions. It's imperative we know what is contributing to our incontinence before we go for (or under) the scalpel. The wrong surgery not only may be useless, it may worsen urge or overflow incontinence. There is also no reason to remove a normal, well-supported uterus during operations that are performed to correct stress incontinence. If, however, the uterus is prolapsed or is enlarged by fibroids that press on the bladder, concomitant hysterectomy is probably indicated. If you haven't undergone thorough testing and are simply told to "fix it with surgery," get a second opinion. Having said that, I don't want to diminish the 50 to 75 percent success rate of appropriate surgical procedures for non-urge incontinence.

Cystocele, which can contribute to stress and overflow incontinence, can be surgically corrected by opening the overlying vaginal tissue, folding the bulging bladder inward, and stitching it up. The excess vaginal tissue is then trimmed, and the bladder is now positioned back in the pelvis, where it belongs. If the urethra and bladder neck have been pushed down, and angulation is lost, stitches placed behind the pubic bone are brought down to the side of the bladder neck and used to anchor the neck in a higher, correct position. This can be done from an abdominal approach (an incision is made above the pubic bone) or with special vaginal techniques. If the urethral sphincter is "shot," a sling can be created from our own or artificial tissue. It's sewn below the urethra and attached above to help it to close. Artificial sphincters that are pumped open or closed using a very small cuff around the urethra have also been successfully used.

NONSURGICAL DEVICES

We don't always need surgery to push the bladder up or correct the urethral position. Pessaries made of silicone rubber or plastic can be inserted into the vagina to correct cystocele and vaginal prolapse. We can also use a bladder neck support prosthesis. It consists of a ring with two prongs that fit on both sides of the urethra. This device supports the junction between the urethra and bladder neck and, in one study, had a "dry" success rate of 83 percent.

COLLAGEN THERAPY

One thing that dwindles with age and may contribute to our dwindling bladder control is collagen. We use collagen to fill the lines in our face; why not use it to fill out an incompetent sphincter? It does work. Urethral collagen injections were approved by the FDA in 1993. When these injections are performed in women with documented sphincter deficiency, 96 percent will have their incontinence cured. The collagen material costs between $1,000 and $2,000, but if that saves us or our older relatives from having multiple unsuccessful surgeries, wearing a diaper, or having to enter a nursing home, it's well worth it!

We don't have to leak in shame and silence, nor should we need to wear an absorbent pad before we give someone a hug. These pads and diapers are not even environmentally friendly! If we are willing to analyze our bladder habits, exercise the right muscles, use appropriate medication, and avail ourselves of the devices, injections, and even surgeries that medicine has to offer, we can spend our future decades with the serenity, security, and dependability of bladder control.

···

Protecting
Our
Future Health

15

GYNECOLOGICAL SURGERIES
Which Are Really Necessary?

We've gone from the passive acceptance of "You don't need those organs anymore" to the aggressive resistance of "Don't you remove anything before I get a second or third opinion!" Our reproductive organs should never be considered "expendable." There are, of course, conditions in which they may need to be surgically repaired, altered, or removed. But can medical progress and the development of nonsurgical screening and diagnostic procedures cut down on these surgeries? When we do require these surgeries, which do we go for? The "new" procedures performed through scopes poked into our abdomens or into our vaginas, or the old route of abdominal and vaginal incisions? Each surgery has its own indications, approach, and complications. Our own approach must be one of understanding, need, and personal choice. We are the keepers and guardians of our pelvic organs and the ultimate arbiters of whether they remain, are altered, or are removed.

Hysterectomy—Our Second Most Common Surgical Procedure: Are Our Collective Uteri That "Sick"?

THE NUMBERS

Hysterectomy was once the surgical procedure most commonly performed on women, but since 1981, it has been surpassed by cesarian section, so it's now number two. Women over 40 can't win. If we do get pregnant, we "out-section" younger women and thus do our part to be included in surgical statistics.

Number two is still impressive, and it represents an extraordinary proportion of women over 40. Over 600,000 hysterectomies are performed yearly in this country (at a cost of $5 billion), and over one third of all women over the age of 60 have had a hysterectomy. The average age at hysterectomy is 42.7. We peaked (or reached an organ low, whichever way you want to look at it) in 1975, when 725,000 hysterectomies were performed. The fact that the 600,000 level has remained stable for the last few years, despite the growing population of baby-soon-to-become-menopausal-boomers seems to indicate some decline.

INDICATIONS:
DO ONE THIRD OF US REALLY NEED A HYSTERECTOMY?

There are three reasons we should consider major surgery: to save our lives, to correct a significant problem that interferes with the functioning of our bodies, and to relieve suffering. Prophylaxis, or having things removed "just in case," is no longer an acceptable reason for hysterectomy. There is no such thing as a "useless uterus syndrome." If elective hysterectomies were performed on all women over 35 to prevent endometrial and cervical cancers, we would gain very little. Lives saved would amount to 1.3 percent, and our life expectancy would increase by only 2.4 months. And these figures don't take checkups and Pap smears into account; with Pap smears and early diagnosis of abnormal bleeding, both of these cancers would be detected early and probably cured.

We grade our students, our athletes, and our politicians. We need a grading system for surgical indications. It's difficult to assign numbers or letters: are all cancers a 10, or are some a 9.4? So I've come up with the following "qualifying" levels for hysterectomy.

Irrefutable Indications

INVASIVE CERVICAL CANCER

This does not include precancers (CIN I, II, or III) or noninvasive superficial cancer (carcinoma in situ).

ENDOMETRIAL CANCER

Hysterectomy, together with removal of both tubes and ovaries, is the most important component of therapy for endometrial cancer. It can be preceded or followed by radiation therapy.

OTHER CANCERS OF THE UTERUS

These occur in the wall rather than the lining of the uterus. They are rare, *leiomyosarcoma* being the most common. They are mistakenly called malignant fibroids, but probably develop independently and not from benign fibroids.

CANCERS OF THE OVARIES OR FALLOPIAN TUBES

Since the uterus constitutes a pathway of spread, it is removed, especially in women over 40.

COINCIDENTAL HYSTERECTOMY

Hysterectomy may be necessary in order to get to or manage cancers of the colon, rectum, or bladder.

Acceptable Indications

LARGE OR RAPIDLY GROWING FIBROIDS

Certainly if these cause medical problems or severe discomfort they constitute an acceptable indication for hysterectomy. Fibroid tumors are present in 20 to 30 percent of all women over the age of 30, and these tumors are the reason (valid or not) for at least 30 percent of hysterectomies done in this country. Most fibroids are just there, causing no problems, except perhaps to the doctor, who feels a larger-than-normal, lumpy uterus. They are benign growths of smooth muscle fibers in the uterine wall. If they project outward, they are called *subserosal fibroids* (these create the most uterine disfigurement and are often responsible for large tumors). If the fibroids are within the uterine wall and don't project in or out, they are called *intramural*. If they grow into the uterine cavity, they are *submucosal fibroids*. Because the latter project into and through the endometrium, they can cause the most bleeding.

We should meet two out of three criteria to warrant hysterectomy for our fibroids: large size or rapid growth to large size; pain and/or bleeding. Gynecologists talk about uterine and tumor size in terms of pregnancy. A "12 to 14 weeks-sized" uterus is about three times its normal nonpregnant size. Our patients want more mundane comparisons, so fruit-wise, we are talking grapefruit, and sports-wise, a softball. But current size may not suffice as an indication for surgery since many fibroid tumors shrink once they are deprived of estrogen in menopause.

What constitutes rapid growth? Fibroids seem to grow in spurts, so if the uterus enlarges from "8 weeks' gestation" to "12 weeks' gestation" in a year, it means little. This does not indicate that it will continue to grow at this pace. I have many patients whose fibroids "mature" to "12 weeks" in their early forties and never grow any further. Our management is expectant watchfulness (a fancy term that means I check them every six months) and nothing more. Our worry about tumor growth has been excessive. The dreaded sentence "They're growing fast, and that might mean they're cancerous, so let's take them out now" is both unnecessarily scary and essentially erroneous. Fibroids practically never become malignant. If a cancerous tumor of the uterine wall (a leiomyosarcoma) is found during surgery for fibroids, it probably arose independently from smooth muscle tissue and not from the fibroids. Further, this coincidence occurs in fewer than 1 in 1,000 cases. The suggestion that a hysterectomy should be performed in order to prevent fibroids from becoming malignant is actually quite absurd. It makes far less sense than suggesting our breasts be removed because they can become cancerous (and our risk of that is 100 times greater!).

Size or growth is not enough, and we need another "issue" to constitute an indication for hysterectomy. Pain or significant discomfort will do. But pain is uncommon with these tumors, even when they are quite large. If the uterus can expand to house a full-term baby without causing pain (until labor), why should it hurt to have a benign tumor? The rare exception is *red degeneration,* a condition in which blood vessels of rapidly growing fibroids bleed into the tumor tissue and cause pain. The opposite *(white degeneration)* occurs when a subserosal fibroid growing on a stalk twists and cuts off its blood supply. This can result in sudden sharp abdominal pain that may mimic appendicitis.

Discomfort rather than acute pain is more often the issue. Larger fibroid tumors may press on the bladder so that we constantly feel a need to void. If the tumors press backward, we might feel rectal pressure. Rarely, the tumors can press on the ureters that conduct urine from the kidneys to the bladder. If these are partially closed, the kidneys can swell, causing pain. Ultimately, there may be kidney damage.

Excessive bleeding "propels" 30 percent of our hysterectomies. Heavy period bleeding *(menorrhagia)* is hard to quantify, but if we have to keep towels between our legs and can't get out of bed or get off the toilet, that would certainly be "heavy." Less dramatically, if we soak through large pads or tampons every hour, and we become anemic, we "qualify" in the menorrhagia category. The worst bleeding occurs with submucosal fibroids. Normally when we get our periods, the small opened blood vessels coursing through the uterus to the endometrium are at right angles to the uterine muscle. As the muscle contracts, the vessels are constricted, limiting blood loss. The regenerating endometrium also heals the damaged vessels and stops bleeding. As the lining sheds, the process of regeneration starts almost immediately. A fibroid that projects out of this lining lacks both muscle fibers, to contract and close its vessels, and endometrium, to cover it and limit bleeding.

It's important to be sure that abnormal bleeding is due *only* to our fibroids. An ultrasound should be performed to evaluate the tumors and their positions. Hysteroscopy will show us if the tumor is submucosal. If it is, it can be treated with less radical procedures such as resection. A dilatation and curettage (D&C) should be done at the time of hysteroscopy to ensure that we don't have endometrial cancer with "incidental" fibroids.

If our uterus is larger than "12 to 14 weeks' gestation" *and* we are in so much discomfort that our quality of life is diminished, *or* we bleed so heavily that we can't lead our normal lives for several days (or all month if we're fatigued from anemia), hysterectomy is reasonable but not un-equivocally the only choice. Medication to shrink the tumors, as well as procedures such as myomectomy and hysteroscopic resection and abla-tion, can allow some of us the option of keeping our uterus.

SEVERE ENDOMETRIOSIS

Severe, painful endometriosis which does not respond to medication or less invasive surgery and causes life-affecting pain can warrant hysterec-tomy. Endometriosis and a variant of this called *adenomyosis* are cited as the reason for 20 percent of all hysterectomies. This disease can cause se-vere menstrual cramps (dysmenorrhea), ovulatory pain, pain with inter-course, pain with bowel movements, chronic pelvic pain, irregular bleeding, and development of large, blood-filled ovarian cysts (*en-dometriomas*). It's a lousy disease. Our treatment depends on the severity of our symptoms. Medical therapy such as birth control pills, GnRH ago-nists (which shut down our hormone production), or anti-estrogen pills such as danazol will help by preventing spread of the disease, shrinking existing lesions, and diminishing symptoms.

If these interventions don't work, we can consider surgery, begin-ning with conservative procedures. We start with laparoscopy and re-move or laser the lesions and scar tissue. We might even remove a badly affected ovary. If we've done all of this, and scar tissue and endometriosis recur, we can remove the theoretical source of the problem, the uterus. If we leave an ovary (and we often do if we're in our early forties), there is still a chance that multipotential cells—or, more correctly, "mean" po-tential cells—will "convert" (sans uterus) and cause an endometrioma.

Adenomyosis is endometriosis within the uterus. The endometrial glands grow into the uterine muscle and cause uterine enlargement, heavy periods, and horrible menstrual cramps. This is a difficult diagno-sis to make unless we remove the uterus, section it, and look at the uter-ine wall. Sometimes ultrasound will show little cystlike structures in the otherwise dense and thickened uterine wall, and MRI may be of some help in diagnosing this disease. More than 50 percent of women in their forties have some degree of adenomyosis; so is this real pathology or an age-related evolution of gland spread? If we're bleeding heavily and have cramps, and are told we have a large boggy, or soft, uterus, we don't have to rush out and get a hysterectomy to prove the diagnosis. Medical man-agement comes first, with birth control pills and GnRH agonists. If we're still miserable and bleeding is not controlled, an attempt can be made to resect, or destroy, the uterine lining with hysteroscopic endometrial ablation.

SEVERE CHRONIC PELVIC PAIN

Ten percent of hysterectomies are performed for this indication. Not every woman with pain has endometriosis. Pain can be caused by scar tissue from previous infections (pelvic inflammatory disease), by previous surgery, and by less obvious causes such as pelvic congestion. The last refers to an increase or widening of blood vessels supplying the pelvic organs. We don't know why pelvic congestion causes pain, but in one study hysterectomy with removal of the tubes and ovaries gave relief to 35 of 36 patients with dilated vessels.

Pain in the pelvis is not always gynecologic. We've got a lot of other organs and tissues residing next to our uterus, tubes, and ovaries— the bladder, large bowel, small bowel, muscles, nerves, lower spine, and bony pelvis. Doctors and patients can make a devastating mistake if they think hysterectomy will be the cure-all for back pain, bowel cramps, radiating nerve pain, and urinary frequency, urgency, or incontinence. It's not surprising that symptoms continue postoperatively if we've operated on the wrong organ! A GI, urinary, and back workup should be performed during our pelvic pain workup.

But what happens if we can't find anything wrong? We've had ultrasounds and MRIs, swallowed barium, and had colonoscopies, cystoscopies, and other "oscopies," and we still hurt. Pain is real, even if we don't always find its organic cause. Psychosomatic factors can make us hurt. A history of childhood sexual abuse has been reported in 40 to 60 percent of women with nonorganic pelvic pain. This is not a likely reason for onset of pain in our forties, but it should not be dismissed.

If anti-inflammatory medications, birth control pills, GnRH agonists, psychotherapy, acupuncture, and stress reduction don't relieve our pain, we can resort to surgery. I prefer to first perform laparoscopy and cut or laser nerve fibers in the ligaments behind the uterus (we need to look in with the scope anyway to check for organic causes of pain). If that fails, we can reluctantly go on to hysterectomy. A recent review by the CDC of 300 women who underwent hysterectomy for pelvic pain found that 60 percent of those who had no identifiable pathology were pain-free after this surgery.

PELVIC PROLAPSE

Severe pelvic prolapse that prevents our normal activities, bladder control, or bowel control might warrant hysterectomy. This is the indication for 15 percent of all our hysterectomies. We grade prolapse by how far the uterus or vaginal mucosa with underlying bladder (*cystocele*) or rectum (*rectocele*) come down when we push. If they come down to the lower third of our vagina, we have first-degree prolapse. If the cervix, bladder, or rectum push to the opening of the vagina, it's second-degree. If a portion descends past the vagina, it's third-degree, and the worst, fourth-degree, occurs if the organs prolapse all the way out and just hang there. First-degree prolapse usually causes no symptoms. The only one aware of it is the gynecologist during our exam. We certainly don't need a hysterectomy for our doctor's symptoms (concern that our cervix is lower than "normal"—"normal" being where it was before we pushed out our progeny). Second-degree prolapse may cause some pelvic heaviness and changes in our feeling of tightness during intercourse. Bladder descent may cause some urinary symptoms such as stress incontinence. Estrogen (local cream or systemic) plus Kegel exercises will usually relieve these symptoms in three to six months. Rectocele can cause a feeling of fullness and difficulty in pushing out stool during defecation. Third- and fourth-degree prolapse are uncomfortable and even scary; we feel that our organs are protruding out of our vagina when we walk or bear down. The vaginal lining is inverted by the prolapsed organs and can get irritated, infected, and bleed. Significant pelvic prolapse can cause us to become bedridden! Vaginal hysterectomy is certainly indicated in these circumstances.

There is, however, an alternative to surgery. To put it inelegantly, we can shove the organs back and keep them there with a pessary. This is a round or oblong device placed in the vagina to support the uterus, bladder, and rectum. Estrogen cream should be used so that the vaginal tissue doesn't ulcerate with the pressure of the device. Surprisingly, some of my patients are very content with their pessary. They don't feel it and prefer to come in every three months for me to remove, clean, and replace this device rather than undergo major surgery. Those who want to be sexually active usually prefer surgical repair. They don't want to contend with a foreign body, and they prefer to have a self-supporting vagina.

Questionable Indications for Hysterectomy

SILENT FIBROIDS

If they are less than "12 or 14 weeks' gestation" in size and don't cause excessive bleeding or pain, there is no need to remove them or the uterus. We've already discounted the warning "Get them out; they may become malignant"—that rarely happens. The long-standing supposition that we should take them out now when we're relatively young and healthy, rather than wait until we're older and possibly infirm, is itself infirm and unfounded. If fibroids are silent now, why should they scream to be removed in old age? If anything, they will shrink after menopause. Some women are told they should have their fibroid-filled uterus removed so that they can safely take hormone replacement therapy. HRT does *not* appear to make fibroids grow. The tumors might make ultrasonographic visualization of the uterine cavity more difficult, but that is the only drawback—and it is certainly not enough to warrant major surgery.

Finally, we've often been told to take out our fibroid uterus vaginally before it gets too large and will necessitate abdominal surgery. It's true that vaginal surgery leaves no scar, but this is still a major procedure. We're not at all sure the fibroids will grow, and if they do, they can be shrunk by as much as 50 percent with three months of GnRH agonists. Once they are brought down to a smaller discrete size, vaginal hysterectomy is again an option.

BENIGN OVARIAN CYSTS

Twenty years ago, we would have our annual pelvic exams and, if heaven forbid, our doctor found a mass, we were rushed into the OR and "explored." During this exploration, women over 40 were encouraged to have everything out—it was safer. If their ovaries had had the temerity to form any kind of tumor or cyst, even if benign, God knows what they and the uterus would form in the next thirty years. The motto was "slash and destroy."

Ultrasound, MRI, laparoscopy, and blood-tumor markers now allow us to "explore" the dark recesses of our pelvis and diagnose many cysts and tumors without major surgery. "Simple" cysts in our forties ("simple" meaning that they are filled with fluid and have thin walls) are usually functional, especially if they are less than 5 centimeters (tangerine size). Another translation: "Functional" means that a cyst developed during an abnormal ovulation and will probably recede during the next cycle or two; so we can scan and wait. We can also make it regress by suppressing ovarian function with birth control pills or GnRH agonists.

Postmenopausal cysts are more worrisome; we have been conditioned to equate these with dreaded ovarian cancer. Actually, since we've begun to perform ultrasound on so many women for various reasons, we've found that up to 17 percent of postmenopausal women have small, "simple" cysts that we can't even feel. Doppler measurement of blood flow to the cyst (benign tumors have a less aggressive blood supply) as well as low CA-125 levels can reassure us. Exploration may be necessary, but if we have no reason to suspect cancer, this can be done laparoscopically and the ovary can be removed with the cyst. If frozen section confirms the cyst is benign, the other ovary should also be removed, since there is a 15 to 20 percent chance that it, too, might develop benign cysts in future years. The uterus is not to blame for these cysts; it can be left alone! Removal of both ovaries through a scope is an outpatient procedure. We're back to most normal activities in about a week. It is no longer excusable for a doctor to tell a woman with a nonsuspicious cyst that "If it were me, or you were my wife, I would have abdominal surgery and remove everything just to be sure!"

PRECANCEROUS CHANGES OF THE CERVIX

These do not require hysterectomy. They should be correctly diagnosed with colposcopy and biopsy and treated with freezing (cryosurgery), laser, LEEP, or cone biopsy.

PRECANCEROUS CHANGES OF THE ENDOMETRIUM

Atypical overgrowth of the glands (*atypical adenomatous hyperplasia*) can be treated medically with high doses of progestational agents such as Megace and Provera. After three months of therapy, we should repeat a D&C, and if the changes have reversed, we are spared major surgery. If the atypia remains or, for some reason, we can't take progesterone, it's reasonable to have a hysterectomy since there is a 30 percent chance that this precancer will become cancer in five years.

Avoidable Indications

DYSFUNCTIONAL UTERINE BLEEDING

I am amazed at how often I ask a new patient why she had a hysterectomy, and I am told it was performed to control heavy bleeding during her perimenopause. Twenty percent of hysterectomies are performed for dysfunctional or abnormal uterine bleeding unrelated to fibroids. Just because our ovulations are off, or our uterine response to hormonal variations is exaggerated, that doesn't mean we have to lose our uterus. It makes a lot more sense to correct the hormones or treat the source of the bleeding—the shedding endometrium. The irregular cycles of the perimenopause are easily controlled with low-dose birth control pills, medroxyprogesterone acetate, or GnRH agonists. In the few instances where controlling the cycle medically does not control bleeding, a hysteroscopy should be performed. This will allow us to go to the source of the bleeding and examine the endometrium. Chances are, we'll find a cause—polyps (benign soft tissue growths from the endometrial glands that are vascular and can bleed heavily during periods) or submucosal fibroids. These can be resected; and if we also perform ablation, our periods should be lighter or absent, but we still have our uterus.

ABNORMAL BLEEDING FROM HORMONE REPLACEMENT THERAPY

One of my patients called me frantically two months after she started continuous-dose hormone therapy (estrogen and progestin every day). She was bleeding and was sure she: (a) had cancer; and (b) would need a hysterectomy. Forty percent of women will bleed during the first four months of this therapy while their uterus "gets used to it," and generally there is nothing wrong. If bleeding continues beyond this time, or if it occurs at the wrong time on cyclical therapy, it should be investigated, but that does not necessarily mean we harbor uterine cancer. If endometrial samplings are normal, doctors should simply try to play with the hormones, switching the mode and type. If bleeding persists, we should undergo office hysteroscopy. Ninety percent of the time we'll find a reason for the endometrium's misbehavior: either a polyp or a fibroid. This can be resected with operative hysteroscopy. Even if the reason is not obvious, an endometrial ablation will scar the lining and control or stop the abnormal bleeding. Once more, the uterus can stay.

SIMPLE ENDOMETRIAL HYPERPLASIA WITH NO ATYPIA

Six percent of hysterectomies are performed unnecessarily for this benign change of the uterine lining. All that has happened is that
the glands have become swollen, most likely as a result of too much estrogen and too little progesterone (a common hormonal event in the
perimenopause). The word *hyperplasia* is scaring doctors and patients
without cause. Less than 1 percent of women with untreated simple
hyperplasia and 3 percent of those with complex hyperplasia (the glands
are swollen and more densely packed together) will ever develop cancer;
and if they are given the needed progesterone, they shouldn't develop it
at all!

STERILIZATION

Why remove the housing unit when all you have to do is shut the door?
Sterilization by laparoscopic tubal ligation is a simple, safe procedure.

TYPES OF HYSTERECTOMY: WHICH WAY OUT?

There are several routes through which we can remove the uterus: abdominal, vaginal, and a combination of both (laparoscope-assisted vaginal hysterectomy, or LAVH). When a hysterectomy is performed, it is
usually termed a *total hysterectomy*, meaning that the uterus is removed
with the cervix. It does *not* mean that either the tubes or the ovaries are
removed. I've had patients tell me that they've had a "total hysterectomy" twenty years ago, so their ovaries and tubes must be gone. They
are not, unless they also had a *bilateral salpingo-oophorectomy* (removal
of both tubes and ovaries). If, during abdominal surgery, a decision is
made to amputate the uterus above the cervix, leaving the cervix in
place, a *subtotal hysterectomy* has been performed. This is not routine. It
is usually done if the surgery is difficult or if there is significant bleeding.
Leaving the cervix shortens the time and complexity of the procedure. If
we've had a subtotal hysterectomy, we have to be screened with Pap
smears for cervical cancer. Some physicians feel that leaving the cervix
in provides better pelvic support and may affect sexual response. They
are in the minority, and there are few studies to prove or disprove this
theory.

Abdominal Hysterectomy

Seventy-five percent of hysterectomies are performed abdominally. The incision is made either transversely (usually in the bikini line) or longitudinally, in the midline (between the belly button and pubic bone). This high rate of abdominal surgery mirrors both physicians' historical attitudes and training and patients' knowledge (or lack thereof) about our surgical options. Abdominal surgery *(laparotomy)* requires opening all the layers of the abdomen. Having retractors, surgeons' hands, instruments, and sponge pads in the abdominal cavity adds insult to injury. It may take days for the bowel to function normally so that we can drink or eat, and just as long for the incisional pain to diminish so that we can walk. Postsurgical bloating and severe gas pains are common. Narcotics get us through it, but they also decrease bowel activity, so we're still not able to go to the bathroom. Most of us need three days in the hospital and four to six weeks' rest at home to recover. Hysterectomy is usually performed abdominally if:

1. We have uterine, ovarian, or tubal cancer, or the surgeon needs to remove adjacent tissue and lymph nodes.

2. We have very large fibroids that can't or won't shrink with GnRH agonists and would be technically difficult to remove vaginally.

3. We've had severe endometriosis, infections, or pelvic scarring from previous surgeries, and dissection of our organs is best done in an open, hands-on fashion.

4. Our surgeon is uncomfortable with vaginal or LAVH surgery, and we don't have the ability or opportunity (community-wise or health insurance–wise) to find someone who is.

COMPLICATIONS OF ABDOMINAL HYSTERECTOMY

The worst complication is death. Thankfully, mortality rates for abdominal hysterectomy have dropped from 80 percent (in the early 1800s) to 0.06 to 0.11 percent in the 1990s if the procedure is not performed for cancer. The rate goes up to 0.7 to 2 percent when hysterectomy is performed as part of cancer surgery, because the procedure is more radical, and patients tend to be older and sicker.

The incidence of "other" complications from abdominal surgery can run as high as 43 percent. Luckily, most are minor. These include fever, bladder infections, wound infections, and lung infections (it hurts to take deep breaths or cough after abdominal surgery, so our breathing becomes shallow, and we may collapse a portion of the unfilled lung and develop pneumonia). Major complications include hemorrhage requiring transfusion, need for a second major surgery because of bleeding or trauma to the "wrong" organ (bladder, uterus, or bowel), and life-threatening pulmonary clots or heart attack. The rate of these major complications is about 4 percent.

We also have to consider the long-term adverse effects of hysterectomy performed abdominally or otherwise. How do we feel months, or even years, after our uterus has been removed? Most of us feel better if the surgery was done for the right reason (cancer, large tumors, pain, or prolapse). The preponderance of bad press about hysterectomy has been aimed at procedures that include the removal of both ovaries (performed in 68 percent of women over the age of 45). We've been told that we'll never "be the same," we'll gain weight, become depressed, suffer terrible hormonal imbalance, lose our libido, and continue our lives as "pelvic cripples."

Let's separate the issue of hysterectomy from oophorectomy (removal of ovaries). If we're not menopausal, losing our ovaries will cause rapid withdrawal of estrogen, progesterone, and testosterone. We can preempt this by taking these hormones immediately after the surgery (I usually have the OR nurse put an estrogen patch on my patients at the time of surgery and supplement testosterone as soon as they can take the pills). Removal of the uterus alone, however, should *not* cause hormonal shock. Of course, there are always exceptions to the rule, and some premenopausal women do go through early ovarian failure if the blood vessels supplying their ovaries have been injured or scarred during their surgery.

Much has been made of our psychological response to hysterectomy. We've been told how poorly we should feel once the "core" of our femininity has been removed, that we should invariably mourn the symbolic value of our uterus. But fact does not bear that out. When women who had hysterectomies for benign conditions were followed for several years, there was no evidence that the operation led to depression or greater psychological distress. Indeed, in many of these women the prevalence of psychiatric symptoms was higher before hysterectomy than after the procedure. They were probably responding to their pain, bleeding, tumors, and anticipation of surgery. There can be a risk of poor psychiatric outcome, but it appears to be limited to women with significant preoperative psychiatric disorders. If we haven't been plagued by severe neuroses or psychoses before indicated hysterectomy (and I stress the word "indicated"), we shouldn't suffer from them as a consequence of this surgery.

What role does our uterus, or the absence of the uterus, play in our sexuality? If pelvic disease caused intercourse to be painful, removal of the source of this pain should improve sexual function. A study that followed over 400 women between the ages of 25 and 50 before, during, and one year after hysterectomy found that most felt sex improved or was the same after hysterectomy, and only 7 percent complained of a decrease in libido. Other studies have found that for the majority of women, if sex was good before hysterectomy, it remained so after. In general, less than 20 percent of women complain of posthysterectomy sexual dysfunction. For some, this is due to loss of estrogen and vaginal atrophy (when the ovaries are removed). It's possible that in other women, nerve fibers are interrupted when the cervix is removed and the vagina closed, or the vagina has been shortened, making it too small for intercourse. Although we don't all mourn the loss of our uterus, there is no question that for some of us this causes a change in our body image and our sense of sexual identity. Our fantasies feed our sexuality, and they don't always lend themselves to manipulation in order to fit the surgical changes in our pelvis.

Vaginal Hysterectomy

This is the indicated route of surgery for vaginal prolapse. An incision is made around the cervix, and the vaginal tissue is pushed away so that the pelvic cavity is entered between the rectum and the lower part of the uterus. The bladder is then separated from the front part of the uterus, and clamps are placed on ligaments and blood vessels on both sides of the uterus. These are cut and tied off with ligatures, allowing the uterus to be freed and removed. We now have a hole in the top of the vagina; this is closed, and the new vaginal roof is fixed to some of the ligaments on the side. Because prolapse frequently involves the bladder (cystocele) and the rectum (rectocele), we often combine this hysterectomy with repair of these defects. This is termed an *anterior* (the bladder) and *posterior* (the rectum) repair, or *colporrhaphy.*

The chief advantage of this surgery is obvious—"Look, Ma, no scar!" Our abdomen hasn't been opened, our intestines haven't been handled, and our fascia and muscles are intact. We can eat almost immediately, our pain is not too bad, we can walk, bend, and even laugh. Many women go home from the hospital the same or next day. We have fewer postoperative problems (24 percent for vaginal hysterectomy versus 43 percent for abdominal), and most of these are minor—fever and infections. There is a 2 to 3 percent chance of significant bleeding, and a 1 to 2 percent chance of injuring the bladder. We can get infections in the area where the vaginal cuff is sutured, but we won't get infections in skin incisions. We're less likely to have lung problems, because it doesn't hurt to take deep breaths or cough. Most women can return to normal activities in less than three weeks.

There is no question that vaginal hysterectomy is the easiest route for us. But it's not always so for the surgeon, who must work in a small area with a limited view: The vessels are difficult to see; if there is scar tissue, she can't delineate the ligaments; clamps can slip off; and there can be problems with pulling the uterus out through the vagina. Sometimes the procedure is begun vaginally, but because of technical difficulty, it has to be completed abdominally. We usually need to meet the following criteria to benefit from a vaginal procedure:

1. The uterus is less than "12 to 14 weeks" in size.

2. We have no history of infections, diseases, or surgeries that have caused significant scarring.

3. We have a surgeon who is comfortable doing vaginal surgery. If the surgeon is technically very comfortable, she or he can also remove a fibroid uterus larger than "14 weeks" by literally splitting the uterus into sections and taking the fibroids out piece by piece before attempting to pull down the now "cored" body of the uterus and remove it through the vagina.

Laparoscopic-Assisted Vaginal Hysterectomy (LAVH)

This allows us to see what's going on from above in the abdominal cavity while removing the uterus from below, vaginally. The abdomen is first inflated by inserting a needle in the area of the belly button and instilling CO_2 gas. A scope is then placed through an incision in the belly button and attached to a video camera, and our insides are now projected in living color on a video screen. Two or three additional small incisions (each smaller than an inch) are made in the lower abdomen, and long, specially designed instruments are placed through *trocars* (metal or plastic tubes put through these incisions). Using these instruments while viewing the video screen (this does require good hand-eye coordination, but then so do video games), we can place ligatures or clips on ligaments and vessels, cut, cauterize, and even stitch. Once the uterus is free, we make an incision in the top of the vagina and push it out. We get the advantage of direct viewing and dissecting without the disadvantage of opening the abdomen. We can see scar tissue and cut it, aspirate cysts, remove ovaries, and even remove fibroids before we push the uterus out of the vagina. We are able to overcome some of the guesswork and "blindness" that cause many surgeons to avoid "pure" vaginal surgery.

The advantages of this technique are obvious. We don't have large incisions, just a few small, less painful ones. We decrease the likelihood of bowel problems or lung complications. We can go home the same day or the next, and we generally recover in three weeks. But there can be intraoperative complications: perforation of organs as the trocars are pushed in; bleeding from a vessel while the surgeon is attempting to clamp or tie without directly using fingers; even an inability to complete the procedure because there is too much scar tissue. This surgery can be lengthy and, since most of the instruments are disposable, costly. We might save in days of hospitalization, but we often lose these savings with high OR costs. The real advantage is patient satisfaction.

Can most hysterectomies be done this way? It depends whom you ask. The enthusiasts say yes, though they would probably exempt most cancers. LAVH can certainly be performed for early uterine cancer. The problem is that the enthusiasts are an elite group who have spent years training as laparoscopic surgeons. Many other surgeons are still learning the technique or are uncomfortable tackling major pathology in this fashion. It might be better to consider three extra weeks of safe recovery than four or five hours of general anesthesia while your surgeon attempts uncomfortable acrobatics that could result in complications. I hope this word of caution will require revision in the future, as more of us become skilled laparoscopic surgeons.

Alternatives to Hysterectomy: The Uterus You Save May Be Your Own!

Six hundred thousand is a figure we need to reduce! New advances in medical and surgical technologies should allow us to lower this prodigious number of hysterectomies that are performed yearly on American women. The nature of the problem, or disease, will determine our available alternatives.

Alternative Treatment for Fibroids

MEDICAL THERAPY

Our fibroids can be shrunk with medications called GnRH agonists. (They have nothing to do with "agony"—I prefer to call them antagonists.) They are administered as shots (Lupron) or nasal spray (Synarel). These agonists are similar to the GnRH produced in our brain, but they are "faulty" and mislead the system, preventing the real GnRH from activating the pituitary receptors to release FSH and LH. Without FSH and LH, the ovary is not stimulated, and neither estrogen nor progesterone is produced. We've induced a temporary menopausal state. Once we're deprived of estrogen, our fibroid tumors shrink as much as 50 percent in three months.

There are three potential problems with this medication. The first is that we feel menopausal and may develop significant hot flashes. The second is that, unlike the sweater we shrank in the dryer, the diminution in size is not permanent; the fibroids grow back within three months once we stop the therapy. Third, there can be long-term adverse effects; with estrogen deprivation, we begin to lose bone mass and might eventually increase our risk of coronary artery disease. Fibroids don't kill us; osteoporosis and heart attacks do. Consequently, we limit therapy to six months (at that point, if we stop, bone mass returns and we've had no impact on our cardiac health), but now our fibroids can "pooch out" and return to their original size. So where's the gain? If we had serious bleeding problems, the GnRH agonist corrected this by stopping our periods. If we were anemic, we can build up our blood count (although taking iron will also do this), and if we require surgery, we are hematologically ready and can even donate our own blood. By shrinking the fibroids, we can avoid an abdominal procedure and use a vaginal one, or we can shrink submucosal fibroids so that they are easily resected with hysteroscopy, avoiding the need for hysterectomy.

There is one more potential use for this drug: long-term administration with add-back therapy. We've found that we can prevent osteoporosis and coronary problems of both real menopause and pseudomenopause with estrogen. If we add hormonal replacement therapy to GnRH agonists, the fibroids don't grow back (the doses are probably too low), and we don't have hot flashes. Our bones and heart are also protected. Women in their forties may be able to continue with this combined "take-away and give-back" therapy until they reach menopause, at which time they can proceed to simple "give-back" therapy (HRT) without ever having surgery on their "controlled" fibroids. Right now, the major drawback to this long-term therapy is its cost. Lupron or Synarel costs more than $250 a month. If we expect to use it for years, we should at least buy stock in the company that produces it!

Another medical therapy is RU-486. This controversial antiprogesterone, which can be used to prevent implantation of a pregnancy and cause early abortion, will also shrink fibroids. It does not put us in a pseudomenopausal state and probably has fewer side effects than GnRH agonists. However, RU-486 is currently not available for antifibroid use.

ALTERNATIVE SURGICAL THERAPY

Myomectomy This procedure entails removal of the fibroids while conserving the uterus. Most physicians recommend this only if we want to "use" our uterus; that is, get pregnant. Many women have a more expansive approach to uterine conservation that can be summed up with two phrases: "You never know" and "I just don't want it out." I think surgeons need to respect our wishes. The few women whom I've seen suffer depression after hysterectomy had been talked into the procedure by their doctors.

Most myomectomies are performed through an abdominal incision. Electrosurgery or laser is used to dissect these tumors from normal uterine tissue; then the defects are carefully closed with sutures. Operative time, hospitalization, and recovery time are similar to those for abdominal hysterectomy, so as far as we're concerned, the "only thing" we're saving is our uterus. If our tumors are on a stalk (*pedunculated*) or not very deep in the uterine wall, they can be removed with laparoscopic procedures. This may result in a deformed uterus that might not be strong enough to carry a full-term pregnancy.

Myomectomy has a high rate of success (80 percent) in reducing heavy bleeding, pelvic pain, and pressure. Fibroid tumors grow back about 20 percent of the time, especially if we are relatively young and have a lot more years of ovarian "encouragement." But we've gained years of having and possibly "using" our uterus. If the new tumors cause distressing symptoms, we're now much older and might be psychologically more willing to consider hysterectomy. By then, who knows? We could have better medical therapies.

Fibroid Coagulation   This is very new (it was developed in 1990) and should be considered experimental. The procedure is performed through a laparoscope. Each fibroid is literally drilled in multiple areas with special electrocautery needles or a laser beam. The tumor's blood supply is destroyed, and it blanches. If it loses its blood vessels, it shrinks to about 50 percent of its original size. Two-year follow-ups have shown no redevelopment of new blood vessels and no regrowth of the "drilled" fibroids. How this will affect future fertility and pregnancy has not been determined, but it is an exciting alternative to more aggressive surgeries.

Alternative Treatments for Heavy Bleeding

About 200,000 hysterectomies are performed yearly to control bleeding. Medical therapies might be enough to control this bleeding, especially in our forties. But if these don't work, we still have the opportunity to avoid major surgery with operative hysteroscopy that resects and/or *ablates* (scars) the uterine lining.

HYSTEROSCOPY RESECTION

The marvel of this outpatient procedure is that it allows us to go home the same day and return to normal activities in three to four days. It is usually performed under general or epidural anesthesia. The cervix is dilated to allow a fairly wide scope (10 millimeters, or about $^1/_2$ inch) to be put into the uterine cavity. This operating hysteroscope has multiple channels. The central one houses the optical lenses through which we view the uterine lining. (We attach a camera to the end of this instrument and actually do the viewing on a video screen.) A side channel has a light source so that we can see. The third channel allows fluid to flow into the uterus and distend it, keeping the walls apart. The fourth is used to suck the fluid out so that there is a constant fluid exchange. Operating "tools" are put through the fifth channel. When we resect, our tool is a metal loop connected to a special electric current. We can move the loop back and forth from the top of the scope and literally cut off pieces of tumor, polyp, or endometrial wall. This is termed *resection*. If bleeding is due to a submucosal fibroid or polyp, we remove or resect it. If no source of bleeding is found, a superficial layer of the endometrium can be resected so that it scars and can no longer react to our fluctuating hormones and shed abnormally. We often combine GnRH agonist therapy with this procedure. It's started in the middle of our cycle, at least one month before we're scheduled for surgery. It shrinks tumors or polyps and thins the lining, making the resection easier and more effective. There is a 90 percent success rate in reducing abnormal bleeding with this procedure, meaning it could eliminate about 180,000 hysterectomies a year! I love what operative hysteroscopy "has done for us lately." I've had patients call me the day after their surgery—in disbelief—because they feel so good. (One questioned whether she had even had surgery!) Whenever I successfully perform it on a woman who was told by another doctor that she needed a hysterectomy, I count it as a victory for both of us.

The major complication rate for operative hysteroscopy is about 3 percent and is chiefly due to uterine perforation (1 percent) or fluid overload. The latter occurs if the fluid we push into the uterus is absorbed into our body and doesn't come out the suction channel; if this happens and is not corrected, we can develop severe electrolyte imbalance, which can affect our lungs and heart. If a perforation or hole is created (and this happens if the loop is placed too deeply into the uterine wall), it might necessitate a laparoscopic procedure to assess the damage and stop the bleeding, or even a laparotomy to close the defect. Rarely, a hysterectomy has to be done. The mortality rate is calculated to be 0.024 percent, versus 0.1 percent for all types of hysterectomy.

Long-term follow-up has shown that about 20 percent of women who have this procedure will need additional treatment five to ten years after resection because the fibroids, polyps, or adenomyosis grew back. We can attempt a second hysteroscopic resection or, after this period of managed procrastination, consider hysterectomy.

ENDOMETRIAL ABLATION

We use the same operating hysteroscope, but this time our "tool" is a rollerball or roller cylinder. This is attached to a special electrosurgical current, and as we roll it back and forth, the current cauterizes the lining. The lining chars and subsequently scars so it can't shed and bleed. This is often performed after a fibroid or polyp has been resected. Some surgeons prefer to first shave off the top layers of the endometrium with a loop and then rollerball the tissue underneath. Ablation alone can take less than twenty minutes and has a 90 percent success rate in stopping or diminishing abnormal bleeding.

I am often asked by my patients if scarring the uterine lining and preventing its shedding can cause any long-term consequences. We're not completely sure. It's possible that after many years, glands buried in the uterine wall could develop cancer, and since they are covered with scar tissue, we wouldn't have the usual warning sign of bleeding. Certainly, if we take estrogen replacement therapy, we should add progesterone to prevent this from happening.

Other Gynecologic Procedures: There Is More to Remove Than Our Uterus

OVARIAN SURGERY

We can perform three surgical procedures on our ovaries: Remove them (oophorectomy), remove cysts from them (cystectomy), or destroy abnormal areas (endometriosis or scar tissue) with laser or electrosurgery. Each procedure has its own indications, route, and, yes, complications.

Oophorectomy

Both ovaries should always be removed for ovarian and tubal malignancies. They are usually removed in women over 45 when hysterectomy is performed for uterine cancer. But should they automatically come out when hysterectomy (especially abdominal) is performed for other reasons?

The decision "to leave, or not to leave" (our ovaries) should be based on three simple criteria:

1. What will they do for us in the future, and for how long?

2. What is the chance that they will require future surgery?

3. Will leaving them ultimately shorten our life?

First, our future ovarian benefits will be the production of estrogen until we're menopausal and the production of male hormone (although diminished) for years after this transition. The closer we are to menopause (average age is 51), the less time we have to reap these benefits, and after a certain point we may not get them at all. Some studies have shown that hysterectomy may diminish ovarian function or even hasten ovarian failure by as much as four years. If we're in our early forties, removal of our ovaries means we are menopausal a decade too early. If we don't use estrogen replacement therapy, we will advance our risk of coronary artery disease and osteoporosis. These diseases could hit us in our sixties rather than our seventies or eighties. We are also hit by the shock of surgical castration, with severe hot flashes, vaginal atrophy, and possible changes in mood and libido unless, once more, we immediately compensate with estrogen and even testosterone.

Second, the chance that we will need to remove our "preserved" ovaries in the future is 1 to 5 percent. Half of these surgeries are needed in the first five years after hysterectomy. Having a second procedure so soon after the first might be considered surgical abuse. It's usually performed for endometriosis (especially if that was the original reason for the hysterectomy), ovarian cysts, or a condition called *residual ovary syndrome*. The latter occurs if the ovary is buried behind the *peritoneum* (which lines the abdominal cavity) or gets covered by scar tissue during the hysterectomy. The ovary swells and causes pulling of the peritoneum, and this in turn causes chronic pelvic pain.

The third reason for going back to remove the ovaries is the possibility of ovarian cancer. After age 50, we have a 0.8 percent lifetime risk of dying of ovarian cancer (but remember that we reach this figure only in our eighties). Hysterectomy, even without removing the ovaries, probably lowers that risk. It prevents "contaminants" from reaching the ovaries (there is no access from the outside if the uterine pathway is gone) and may decrease the life span of ovarian activity.

On the basis of these three criteria, most women and their surgeons will opt to remove their ovaries if possible (it can be difficult during vaginal hysterectomy) once they are over the age of 50, and indeed 65 percent do. Women under the age of 45 are generally encouraged to leave their ovaries. Between 45 and 50, we enter a "gray area" (not our hair color) and have to individually make our own decisions. I call it the battle of the fears—the fear of early traumatic menopause and need to take hormones versus the fear of future ovarian cancer.

Route of oophorectomy   If we need surgery "just" on our ovaries, it usually can be done with laparoscopy. Even if there are large cysts (and we're fairly certain that they are benign), they can be punctured, the fluid aspirated, and the now "deflated" ovary removed using clips or sutures placed through the scope. After menopause, if we develop a cyst in one ovary, there is a 15 to 20 percent chance we'll do so in the other, so both ovaries should be removed with this outpatient procedure, ensuring future pelvic harmony (or more precisely, lack of pathology).

Ovarian Cystectomy

This is generally reserved for those of us who are premenopausal and who want our ovaries to continue to produce hormones. Once more, we have to be as certain as possible that the cyst is benign and be prepared to convert the procedure to an abdominal hysterectomy and removal of both ovaries if a frozen section shows that it's malignant. Cysts can be filled with fluid, blood (common in endometriomas), or a combination of fluid and solid material. Most fluid- and blood-filled cysts should first be watched for one to two cycles to see if they disappear or be treated medically with birth control pills or GnRH agonists to suppress ovarian activity. If they don't shrink, but grow or cause pain, they should come out. Most can be removed through a laparoscope. After the scope is placed, operating instruments are put through trocars inserted through small incisions in the lower abdomen. The cyst is aspirated, the ovary is partially opened, and the cyst capsule is teased away from normal tissue. The ovary usually folds over this defect and heals nicely.

If a cyst has solid elements, it may be a *dermoid cyst*. Dermoids are fascinating tumors. They originate in germ cells that develop during our early embryonic life. These cells create our ovaries and oocytes. On occasion, some cells wait and attempt to develop after puberty. At this point, they don't know what they're supposed to be and crazily grow tissue that may include fat, hair, glands, and even teeth. It's as if these cells were trying to form a new being without being fertilized. Dermoid tumors are the most common benign ovarian tumors in our twenties and thirties, but on occasion they aren't diagnosed or don't develop until our forties. They should be removed, and this can often be done with laparoscopy. Some surgeons prefer an open incision if the tumor is larger than 7 or 8 centimeters. Rarely will these tumors occur or first be diagnosed in menopause. Once we're over 50, tumors that have cystic and solid components are more likely to be cancerous and probably should be removed (with both ovaries) through an abdominal incision. If they are malignant, a hysterectomy will be necessary.

Ablation (Destruction) of Abnormal Tissue on the Surface of the Ovary

Endometriotic implants or scar tissue can coat the surface of the ovary, causing (together with the disease that put this tissue there) pain, infertility, and abnormal ovarian function. Surgery for this problem resembles a video game. We can buzz or vaporize the superficial "bad stuff" with electrosurgery (cautery) or laser beam. Both types of "zapping" procedures can be done through a laparoscope.

DILATATION AND CURETTAGE (D&C)

Up to ten years ago, D&C was the mainstay of hospital gynecology wards. If we bled abnormally in perimenopause (and who didn't?), if we had heavy periods, or if, more ominously, we had postmenopausal bleeding, we were hospitalized for a D&C. Once ensconced in an institution, we were taken to the OR, where we were given a general anesthetic, had our cervix dilated, had the uterine cavity scraped, and then remained hospitalized one or two nights to recover from this "onslaught" to our uterine integrity. Today, this type of D&C has, for the most part, become obsolete. It has three major flaws:

1. There is rarely a need to undergo hospitalization and general anesthesia to perform a D&C. It can usually be undertaken as an office procedure with local anesthetic (a numbing shot in the cervix called a paracervical block) and, if necessary, some intravenous "calming" medications. If a patient has a very scarred cervix that can't be dilated in the office, she'll need a general anesthetic, but even this can be administered in an outpatient facility.

2. D&C alone gives us inadequate information—it's "blind." Once the curette is in the cavity, we scrape "by feel," and studies have shown that we can miss up to one third of the endometrial wall surface. That means we could miss an area with precancer or cancer. Doctors don't feel polyps (they're soft and bend) and might not feel fibroids; these common causes of bleeding are left undetected, and we continue to bleed. A 1983 study of 500 women undergoing D&C showed that this blind procedure was unable to yield a pathology diagnosis 60 percent of the time, and only two women under the age of 40 were diagnosed with endometrial cancer.

To become "unblinded," we simply need to add a method of seeing "up there"; this is done with hysteroscopy. This small scope is placed through the cervix. We then visualize the abnormal area and only then scrape to get a sample of the tissue. To make sure "we got it," we put the scope back in and look. Most hysteroscopy D&Cs can be performed in the office using a paracervical block and mild intravenous medications. A study of 276 women with bleeding problems who underwent D&C and hysteroscopy showed that hysteroscopy gave far more information (demonstrating fibroids and polyps) than the actual D&C.

3. D&C is not a cure; it's merely a diagnostic procedure. By providing the pathologist with tissue samples from the lining, it will let us know if our bleeding is from unopposed estrogen (*cystic hyperplasia*) or if precancerous or cancerous changes are present. But all we've done is scraped off superficial glands from the endometrium. Generally, these will grow back after one cycle if we're still menstruating. The D&C may remove some polyps, but the large ones usually remain. Fibroids certainly won't get scraped off. Unless we destroy the lower layer of the endometrium and remove polyps or fibroids, chances are our abnormal bleeding will continue to be an "issue." This is especially valid if we're postmenopausal and have persistent bleeding that is not precancerous.

In this case, 90 percent of us will have either polyps or fibroids. In the past, we dealt with this "issue" by undergoing several D&Cs (if one didn't work, maybe the second would) and, finally, hysterectomy. Today we have hysteroscopic resection and ablation.

ENDOMETRIAL SAMPLING

Sampling is a much nicer word than "biopsy." It seems like a kinder, gentler thing to do than the cutting or scraping we associate with biopsies. To sample our endometrial cells, we put a small cannula through the cervix and move it around the uterine cavity as we apply suction. The yield of superficial cells and glandular tissue from all the surfaces of the endometrial wall may be as good as, and in some cases better than, that obtained with the scraping of a D&C. It's technically easier (the cannula is much smaller in diameter than the curette used for D&C) and faster, and causes less cramping. It's ideal for a quick evaluation of the endometrium if we have abnormal perimenopausal bleeding or abnormal bleeding on hormone replacement therapy, or are at high risk for endometrial hyperplasia (obesity or irregular cycles with suspected unopposed estrogen). If, however, this procedure shows no pathologic changes and our abnormal bleeding persists, hysteroscopy should be done. Conversely, if cancer or precancer is picked up, the staging and degree of the disease are better evaluated with hysteroscopy and careful unblinded scraping of all suspicious endometrial surfaces.

Informed Consent and Second Opinions: These Are for Us, Not Our Lawyers

The degree of complications varies with the invasiveness of what we're doing. (I compare it to the adage "Little children cause little problems; big children, big problems.") Unless we know what can go wrong as well as what will go right or be fixed, we haven't been informed; our decision making is faulty, and our consent has not been properly obtained. This ultimately makes lawyers very happy, but it's never good for us. We can't right a wrong medical outcome in the courtroom; we should concentrate our efforts on ensuring that we get the appropriate medical care in the first place.

We need to ask and consider the following when we contemplate any major or even minor surgery:

1. What is the risk of death?

2. What is the risk of serious complications that could affect our future health? These would include, among others: hemorrhaging and need for multiple blood transfusions, shock, possible kidney or brain damage, heart attack, stroke, lung complications, anesthetic calamities, and nerve damage. Every procedure has known possible complications. We just want to share in this "known" part; we're not asking for a lot of rare and unusual calamities that can occur and would warrant mention in some sort of "Ripley's list of surgical horrors."

3. How long can we expect to be in the OR, the outpatient facility, or the hospital?

4. How long will it be before we can return to work, resume our normal activities, exercise, and, yes, even have sex?

5. How much will all of this cost? What does the insurance company cover, and what's our personal cost? (We have to add to this our days of sick leave, lost pay, and the cost of hired help at home or in the office.)

6. Are we sure our symptoms and problems will be fixed by the surgery?

7. Are there less aggressive surgical alternatives or nonsurgical methods that can prevent, delay, or even temporarily diminish the need for surgery?

8. What, if any, are the long-term psychological changes that have been correlated with this surgery?

9. Do other doctors agree with this assessment, and will a second or third opinion confirm the need for this procedure?
    Studies have shown that there is a 7 to 40 percent decrease in surgery if we obtain a second opinion! When a second opinion is mandatory (the insurance company requires it before authorizing payment), 8 to 19 percent of surgeries are deemed unnecessary. In voluntary programs (we can choose

to get a second opinion and have it reimbursed by the insurance company), the rate of disagreement is 5 to 25 percent.

The surgeon isn't always the "bad guy" or "bad gal." Doctors are biased by their training or may get pressured into a certain course of therapy because of their patients' demands. As patients, we want certain results, and we want them now. It sometimes takes a new perspective by an uninvolved expert who has not been a part of our long-term care to come up with an alternative therapy. We might reject it, but at least we've heard the words "There is another way."

10. Do we feel that our symptom or disease is bad enough to justify items 1 through 8 in order to reach our ultimate goal—getting on with our lives with improved health, unencumbered by pain and suffering? If the answer is yes, the surgery is necessary.

16

OUR MATURING PSYCHE
Sex, Hormones, and Rock and Roll

Are you sexually active? What a simple, straightforward question, yet it has raised havoc with our past veracity (if this question was asked by our mothers), our current desire for a negative response (as we ask our teenage daughters), and our future expectations of ourselves (as we deal with our sexuality in the second half of our lives). The wonder of sex is ever present: Our children wonder how it's done, young lovers wonder if anyone other than themselves has reached such a "superior" level of intimacy, married couples with young children wonder if they will ever have the time or energy to regain their sexual ecstasy, and all of us wonder whether "older" people do it! "Older," of course, being the generation ahead of us.

Approximately 70 percent of women aged 45 to 55 (definitely an older group for our children) are sexually active. If we look at our later life stages, our activity rate is still up, paralleling the rate of "up" partners in our lives. Studies show that at least 60 percent of women aged 60 to 70 continue to be sexually active (the recent Janus Report found that this number was 74 percent). The sexual statistics for women over 70 are meager (our medical profession spends more time looking at age-related male impotence than age-independent female sexual competence). However, one study of "subjects" over 60 found that 55 percent of males had intercourse at least once a week. The average frequency of intercourse for sexually active females ages 60 to 91 was 1.4 per week. (It would seem from this that they were having more frequent sex than the men; I'm not quite sure whom they were having it with.)

In another study of healthy women over 80, 30 percent had partners who were impotent, and 20 percent had insufficient opportunities for sexual encounters. Only 23 percent complained of decreased libido, whereas 30 percent had decreased vaginal lubrication, which made intercourse painful. Thirty percent complained that they were not achieving orgasm. Looking at these statistics, we have to conclude that if these women had partners capable of an erection and if they were treated for vaginal dryness, they would have continued (or bettered) the sexual activity rate of "younger" women under 70.

Our late-life sexuality has not been portrayed in conventional rock and roll, but music has not totally forsaken us. There is a wonderful song stating that "older women do it better." We can, and many of us do . . .

Sexual Function in Our Forties

HAVE WE PEAKED?

The media are finally allowing some women in their forties to have on-screen romances and, yes, sexual encounters. Of course, they all look better than most of us did in our thirties, but Hollywood has never felt that we could be sexually represented by anyone with weight problems, gray hair, or wrinkles. The real issue is whether we have allowed the media experts to misshape our sexual self-image with the "look-and-he-will-come" expectation. If our bodies are not perfect, will the proverbial "he" or, for lesbians, "she" be turned on? Do we continue to fit into our own sexual fantasies? (I'm not even going to address the fantasies of men, or this chapter will go on forever. Suffice it to say that most men's arousal seems to become less visual and more tactile with age.) Since we usually enter our forties after our mates, we have to deal with major body changes that they may already have undergone—wrinkling, balding, graying, weight gain, potbellies, and medical problems such as high blood pressure and heart disease. They no longer fit the "stud" category (though their actor counterparts can still be cast in movies as leading men). Our sexual self-image, as well as the physical presence of our partner, shapes our desire. Without a mature understanding that sexuality is more than superficial looks, we degrade one of our major sources of expression, affection, and pleasure.

There are certainly other psychological issues (other than our physical perceptions) that may invade the sexual harmony of our forties. Couples often weather years of marriage by dealing with issues and events—buying and decorating a house, raising children, and mapping career advances. In our forties, these events may have reached some sort of culmination—the house is fine, the children are older and want less contact with us, and our careers are set. Unless we really like each other, communicate, and enjoy being together, we begin to feel stuck and bored. Keeping the sexual part of our relationship going becomes a tiresome task. Some women respond to the tedium of their marriage by denying their sexuality and claiming that it's unimportant. They blame PMS, perimenopause, and their hormones for what they perceive as diminished libido. Others look for new relationships or use methods of self-stimulation. This course may be complicated by both trepidation and guilt. But for many women, midlife represents a time where they and their partners can experience a new level of intimacy as they look at their lives from a vantage point of increasing self-esteem and self-acceptance. There is a tremendous relief as their tasks of parenting diminish and they begin to look forward to the years ahead of them.

As we, the baby boomers, evolve through our forties, we're unlikely to forgo our hard-won sexuality by default of a partner, marriage, societal expectations, or our hormones. We can and should expect a continuation of our sexuality in this decade and the many to come.

HORMONE FACTORS AND SEXUALITY IN OUR FORTIES

Let's get to the more concrete. We know that our hormones are "a-changing"; how does this affect our sexual response? We have a general decline in estrogen production years before we're menopausal, with a resulting decrease in vaginal blood flow and the quantity and quality of vaginal secretions. We may not get adequate lubrication with sexual arousal or may require a longer period of sexual stimulation before we have enough lubrication to allow for comfortable penetration. Lack of lubrication and accompanying discomfort eventually trigger a self-defensive tensing of our vaginal muscles, making penetration even more difficult. "Hurt" replaces pleasure. Our response and that of our partner are understandably negative. We feel that there is a decline in our sexual viability, and our partners feel that they are not performing adequately and can't excite us. Desire is a function of expectation and memory, and if we remember negative sexual experiences, we can lose our desire—and fail again.

The genital action of estrogen may not be the only one we have to consider in our forties. This hormone also affects our sensory perception. Estrogen can potentiate our capacity to develop muscle tension and acts on the central and local nerve functions that relate to our sexual response. As estrogen levels decline, some women develop nerve "apathy." They have more numbness, itching, and aversion to touch. Caresses may become unpleasant or even irritating. Finally, lower estrogen levels may increase our PMS. Depression, bloating, and breast tenderness certainly don't enhance our desire for sexual contact. If we develop hot flashes, we may not want any body contact, and if the hot flashes interrupt our REM sleep, we're just too tired!

Libido per se (if we can separate it from the memory of physical discomfort) is probably not affected by declining estrogen. But, alas, our sex drive is not "hormone-free." Our male hormones appear to be the facilitators of our sex drive. Higher androgen levels are associated with greater sexual desire, frequency of sexual fantasies, and sexual arousal. Theoretically, in our forties, these should not be diminishing at the same rate as our estrogen. Our male hormone production usually remains "up" until we're menopausal.

So hormonally, our desire and fantasies should be unaffected in our forties. Our only real hormonal complaint relates to lubrication and skin response. Both can easily be corrected. Lubricants can make all the difference, allowing us to glide our way into the sexual responses we expect. If lowered estrogen levels affect our psychologic well-being, and we don't smoke, we should consider low-dose birth control pills. These may alleviate some of our lubrication problems, help us maintain vaginal health, and prevent the continued natural decline of our estrogen. We also get contraception. One word of birth control pill caution: Rarely, women find that their sex drive diminishes while they are on the Pill. We know that oral contraception suppresses pituitary function and FSH and LH are not produced; as a result, there can be less stimulation of male hormone production by the ovary. For those women who develop this complaint, I prescribe a 2 percent testosterone cream to be applied to the labia and clitoris before sleep. Its sexual mode of action is not clear, but it helps thicken the labial skin and may increase blood flow to the clitoris. If this doesn't work, I suggest stopping the birth control pill and trying estrogen replacement therapy.

Sexual Function During and After Menopause

DOES THE FIRE BURN OUT?

We've dealt with turning 50 or older, but Hollywood and the media haven't; actually, they've given up on us! Sexuality in the next third of our lives is rarely portrayed or discussed. If it does come up, it's "put down"; witness the books written by older feminists who celebrate their newfound freedom from sexuality. They suggest that we should be relieved of our need to be sexual or submit to a continuation of a "male conspiracy." I disagree; most women who have had orgasmic, enjoyable sex do not want it withdrawn (literally or figuratively). If we accept a de facto sexual decline as a part of our inevitable hormonal decline, or if we let the media tell us we're not sexy, ergo we shouldn't have sex (or want it), we do become victims of a greater conspiracy—that of misinformation and ignorance of our human need for bonding, affection, and sexual pleasure.

FACTS AND FICTION ABOUT MENOPAUSE AND SEXUAL RESPONSE

Facts

1. *Diminished vaginal "health" affects our response to genital stimulation and intercourse.* Decrease in our vaginal blood supply as a result of estrogen loss can lead to thinning of pubic hair, loss of fat tissue around and in the labia (unfortunately, fat isn't lost in other parts of our bodies), and shrinking of the clitoris. Vaginal changes from lack of estrogen have already been described in detail. Whereas in our forties we simply had to contend with lubrication problems, we now have more general vaginal atrophy. If left untreated, this can lead to significant dryness and pain during intercourse; narrowing of the vaginal entrance and cavity, making penetration difficult; and less vaginal elasticity (so that the vaginal walls can't expand even if penetration is attained).

2. *Sexual desire decreases with loss of estrogen.* Yes, but the put-down of our desire with loss of estrogen is primarily due to the takedown of our vaginal health. Pain and impenetrability may cause us to avoid sexual contact. With the return of vaginal health, desire usually follows.

3. *Sexual desire decreases with loss of male hormone.* We lose nearly all of our ovarian estrogen with menopause and between 30 and 50 percent of our male hormone. This latter loss is more gradual and can continue for many years. Male hormones help mediate our desires, fantasies, and state of arousal. The levels of androgens have been found to be higher in women who continue to be sexually active in their later years. If male hormone is given (together with estrogen) to women who have undergone surgical menopause, their sex drive, fantasies, and rates of intercourse "better" those of similar women treated with estrogen only or who receive no hormonal therapy.

Fiction

1. *Orgasms decrease as a result of hormonal loss.* Studies have shown that orgasmic response is not impaired after menopause. Women who continue to be sexually active have little or no decrease in orgasms and, indeed, can continue to be multiorgasmic. The 1993 *Janus Report* found that 85 percent of the women interviewed between the ages of 27 and 38 had orgasms at least "sometimes during lovemaking." That number increased to 87 percent for women over the age of 51 and did not decline in women 65 or older. Fifty-one percent of women between 27 and 38 had orgasm "often," and this figure declined only slightly—to 44 and 42 percent for the older age groups. If we actually measure the intensity of orgasmic and rectal contractions, we "scientifically" find that they are somewhat reduced, but few of us notice this. In short, our psychological experience of sexual pleasure is considerable and will become diminished only if penetration and/or thrusting is painful.

2. *The reason most women stop having intercourse after menopause is menopause.* At least 35 percent of men over the age of 60 have erection problems; this is our major reason for lack of sexual activity! We don't want to confront the issue (they are too vulnerable), and rather than risk their performance failure, we often negate our own sexual needs or convince ourselves that these needs have been hormonally swept away.

PSYCHOLOGICAL FACTORS AND POSTMENOPAUSAL SEX

How we feel about ourselves as we outgrow the reproductive capacity that has so wrongly been associated with our sexual attractiveness will determine whether we pursue or abandon our sexuality. If we enjoyed sex in the past, we're more likely to be positive and even willing to become assertive in continuing our sexual activity in the future. If sex was never a "big deal," we tend to greet the waning sexual demands of our partner and society with relief. But not all women with poor sexual histories welcome asexual freedom after menopause. I recently saw a women in her late fifties; she had decided to begin estrogen replacement therapy for medical reasons. After several visits, she confided to me that she had never experienced an orgasm (10 percent of women don't) and wondered if hormone therapy would cure this problem. Hormones may enable her to be more comfortable during intercourse, but her lifelong sexual dysfunction will require intense psychological examination. I referred her to an excellent psychologist who specializes in sexual counseling. This patient wants to experience what she's missed, and her age should not be a factor. Few physicians would hesitate to refer a 30-year-old for sexual counseling. Why is it absurd to pursue this need in our fifties or sixties?

THE SOCIALIZATION OF OUR SEXUALITY

The major social factor affecting our sexual function is partner function. The "three Ds"—disinterest, divorce, and death—decimate partner participation. By our mid- to late adulthood, 65 percent of all first marriages and 55 percent of all second marriages will have ended in divorce. We outlive men by an average of ten years, and if our partners are older, we can expect to be widowed for as long as fifteen to twenty years. The majority of us will do something about this. Sixty-five percent of divorced women between 40 and 60 will remarry, 50 percent within three years of their divorce. Another encouraging statistic is that over 40 percent of widowed women resume sexual activity, most within a year of their spouse's death.

Disinterest can be mutual, but seems to occur more frequently in men after the age of 45. Sexual response in males in this age group does appear to diminish, although some studies show men peak sexually at age 18, when any stimulus causes an immediate erection. (It's probably just as well that they come down from this state of constant and rapid arousal. At some point, they need to function as social beings and, who knows?, they might want to go into politics!) Midlife sexual burnout occurs in 20 percent of men, but appears to be less common in women. Libido and erotic passion are not really burnt out, they are just lost. Men and women may try to recapture it by changing their sexual partners (some men try new cars first), but many couples have found that a change in their now boring sexual routines may "do the trick."

Medical Disease and Our Sexual Function: If We're Sick, Can We "Do It"?

At any age, medical problems can affect our physical ability to have intercourse in certain positions. Back problems affect many of us (some might even be caused by our own sexual acrobatics) and result in the need for special positioning of ourselves and our pillows. Our joints and bones can undergo a lot of degenerative changes as we age. Rheumatoid arthritis causes stiffness and pain. A hot, relaxing, sensual bath can do wonders for this condition and, if done with our partner, allows us to establish a warmth of intimacy. The pain caused by degenerative changes in our joints (osteoarthritis) may distract us from our ability to enjoy sexual activity. The doctor's traditional advice, "Take two aspirin and call me in the morning," applies in part: take an aspirin (or any anti-inflammatory medication), but there's no need to make that morning call.

Autoimmune disease can damage blood vessels and nerves anywhere in the body; if it occurs in the genital area, we may develop a decrease in lubrication, sensitivity, and orgasmic response. A friend and patient of mine who moved to Chicago spent years going from one specialist to another complaining of vaginal dryness and loss of vaginal sensitivity. She also had dry eyes, a dry mouth, and joint pain. A diagnosis of Sjögren's syndrome was finally made, but only after she was told that her sexual dysfunction had to do with mental dysfunction. Hypothyroidism, another autoimmune disease, may cause us to become fatigued and depressed, and gain weight. To add to the moroseness of this condition, our libido and ability to reach orgasm can also diminish. There is no question that the right hormone (in this case, thyroid) can "cure" this disease-specific form of sexual dysfunction.

Diabetes develops in 4 percent of our population. Its effect on male sexual dysfunction has been thoroughly addressed. Sexual problems in diabetic women, however, were not even mentioned in the medical literature until 1970. The unfortunate fact is that about one third of diabetic women lose orgasmic function four to six years after this disease is diagnosed.

Chronic heart disease, lung disease, and any other disorder that make us physically unfit can cause us to avoid sex if we are afraid that we'll exacerbate our condition (e.g., die of a heart attack) while having sex or be unable to muster our diminished reserves for intercourse. In these circumstances, we need to ask our doctors what we can and cannot do. If we undergo cardiac rehabilitation so that we can perform other physical activities, why can't we include intercourse? The amount of energy expended is equivalent to climbing about two flights of stairs (but *a lot* more fun!). If we're physically incapable of intercourse, mutual fondling and touching may give us the intimacy and pleasure we crave.

Surgery can radically alter our bodies, but with few exceptions (such as radical pelvic surgery that shortens or abolishes the vagina) it does not physically prevent us from continuing our sexual lives. The real question is what it does to us psychologically and how we and our partners react to a change in body image. We can't simply dismiss the disfigurement of procedures such as mastectomy or colostomy. Between 22 and 30 percent of women who undergo mastectomy report a decrease in their frequency of intercourse or ability to reach orgasm. Many of these women also have to deal with vaginal atrophy because they have stopped or never started estrogen replacement therapy. Breast reconstruction is probably the best way to adjust, but there are less invasive methods, such as wearing a bra with a prosthesis under an attractive nightgown when going to bed with a partner. Vaginal estrogen and lubricants can certainly eliminate physical discomfort while we deal with (and hopefully overcome) our psychological discomfort.

Hysterectomy is a surgical fact of life for one third of us by the time we've reached our sixties. It should not affect our sexual response unless we and our partners believe that the uterus is the source of our female competency. Our postoperative sexual function depends on whether our ovaries were removed (with no correction of subsequent hormonal loss), the medical necessity for the surgery, and our knowledge about the real physiology and function of the uterus. There is some evidence that suggests that the cervix has a role in triggering vaginal orgasm and that the uterus contracts during orgasmic response, yet most women who had good sex before their surgery continue to have it afterward. A New Zealand study found that 42 percent of women who had undergone hysterectomy reported improvement of their sexual lives, and 52 percent said there was no change in their sexual enjoyment after surgery.

Medications, Alcohol, and Drugs: How Do They Affect Our Sexual Response?

Have you ever noticed how pills multiply and clutter our medicine cabinets, kitchens, and purses as we get older? Both legitimate prescription medications and the over-the-counter stuff we're encouraged to take for our sniffles and coughs can be detrimental to our sexual health.

Heart disease and hypertension are often treated with beta blockers. Depending on the dosage, these medications can decrease libido and ability to achieve arousal and orgasm in up to 50 percent of women (and men) who use them. If this happens, changing the beta blocker or trying to lower the dose may help.

Tranquilizers and antidepressants may aid us in dealing with our life crises, but they can also inhibit our sexual response (another crisis).

Antihistamines dry us up, in both our upper airways and lower vagina. They are "at fault" for decreased lubrication and drowsiness. Chronic sinus problems and long-term use of antihistamines both hurt and diminish our sexual response. This association gives new meaning to the statement "Not tonight, honey, I have a headache."

Alcohol may allow some of us to imbibe away our stress and inhibitions so that we feel we can peak sexually. The contrary often occurs; sexual arousal is actually lowered for 40 percent of us who are under the influence and rarely meets our inebriated expectations.

Improving with Age: Managing Our Sexual Health

Aging is a biologic phenomenon. It does not preclude our emotional need for intimacy, arousal, and sexual pleasure. Many of the psychological and physiological changes that we have been told will reduce our sexual capacity are either nonexistent or treatable. We don't need to give up because we grew up. We can take charge of our sexual lives in the following ways.

THE RIGHT MENTAL ATTITUDE: WE'RE "TOO SEXY FOR OUR BODIES"

Our capacity for sexual giving or receiving will always belong to us. It's time for us to match the maturity of our cellular components with a maturity of attitude. If we have a partner, we may need to initiate sexual intimacy. If we don't, self-arousal will bring sexual pleasure and should not be thought of with shame or embarrassment. (I feel very comfortable offering this advice, since I am not seeking appointment to the post of Surgeon General!) Several recent studies have shown that more than 70 percent of American women masturbate and that 37 percent of women in their sixties continue (or begin) to do so. Masturbation, just like intercourse, will help us maintain our vulvar and vaginal health after menopause.

APPRECIATING FAMILY CHANGES

We've made it. The kids are out of the house, and we finally have the privacy and time to explore our relationship with our partner or perhaps explore relationships with new partners. The empty-nest syndrome is, for most of us, feathered with the gifts of peace and contentment. So let's forget about locking the bedroom door, put on soft music (or adult rock or adult videos), and slowly explore the forms of intimacy we've neglected while rushing through our midlife chores. We deserve this pleasure!

AIDING AND ABETTING VAGINAL AND SEXUAL HEALTH WITH HORMONES

Estrogen therapy will prevent and reverse the atrophic vaginal changes of menopause. Intercourse becomes comfortable and, more important, pleasurable as improved vaginal blood flow affects our sexual response. There is more swelling of the vulva, clitoris, and lower third of the vagina and more secretion of fluid into the vagina during sexual stimulation. Estrogen may also increase the pleasurable sensitivity of our skin and enhance our responses to fondling and caressing.

Estrogen vaginal cream has an excellent local effect. It can be used in addition to pills or patches (especially if we start hormonal therapy relatively late and the blood flow to this area is already diminished). This very low dose of estrogen cream can be used to maintain our vaginal health even when we can't or won't use "systemic" estrogen therapy.

For those of us who feel that menopause has suddenly (with surgery) or slowly (with advancing years) robbed us of our sexual desire, fantasies, and level of gratification, adding male hormone to estrogen therapy may help overcome these sexual woes. Studies have shown that when younger women who undergo surgical menopause are given estrogen and male hormone, they experience an increase in fantasies as compared with similar women given estrogen alone. They also live out these fantasies with increased coital activity. Older women given the same estrogen and testosterone therapy experience the fantasies and sensuality but don't match these feelings with more frequent intercourse. Their male hormone levels are only as good as the males around them, and it appears that they are less likely to initiate sex. Perhaps as the more aggressive baby boomers become menopausal boomers, their decision to add appropriate hormones will allow them to match their fantasies with coital activity (this is our form of virtual reality!).

MOISTURIZE, LUBRICATE, AND LUBRICATE

Even with estrogen therapy—and certainly without it—we may need additional lubrication. Our choices include Astroglide, Lubrin, Today Personal Lubricant, and K-Y Jelly (I prefer these water-based lubricants). If estrogen cream is not an option, we can still moisturize. We do it for the rest of our skin; why should we neglect our most sensitive area? Two excellent products are available: Replense and Gyne-Moistrin.

SEXUAL TIMING

Staying up late and fooling around was fun when we were younger, but now most of us prefer an earlier bedtime and fall asleep when our heads hit the pillows. If we're tired, have had a late or large meal, or have had alcohol, we and our partners are less likely to be sexually responsive and we're at risk for performance failure. Morning sex after a good night's sleep may be more au courant as we get older. Noon siestas or late-afternoon "Let's get into bed and cuddle" engagements will also allow us to deploy our sexual energies before we have exhausted all energy with our daily routines.

PRESEXUAL ACTIVITIES

Hot baths can soothe joint problems as well as get us into a warm, relaxed mood.

EXPLORING NEW OR NONCOITAL
MODES OF SEXUAL EXPRESSION

Couples often develop routines for coupling, and sexual boredom can set in. Exploring new positions (if your imagination runs out, books and videos are good references) and noncoital sex may ignite old or new sexual fires. Oral-genital stimulation is a common sexual activity for older couples. A recent study of Americans age 50 or older found that 56 percent of men said they gave oral stimulation and 49 percent of women said they received it. More important, 95 percent of the men and 82 percent of women who engaged in this behavior reported enjoying it.

SEEKING PHYSICAL AFFECTION AT ANY AGE IN ANY SETTING

We need to caress and hug at every age in our human development; yet elderly women and men are separated and discouraged from seeking physical contact in hospitals, institutions, and retirement homes. We'd better encourage a change of rules for our grandparents and parents or we will face the same contact deprivation in our later years.

CORRECTING PELVIC PATHOLOGY
THAT INTERFERES WITH OUR SEXUAL FUNCTION

Pelvic prolapse and urinary incontinence may require medical or surgical correction before we can comfortably have intercourse. The desire for coital activity should suffice as an indication for this needed gynecologic attention.

GETTING SEXUAL THERAPY IF WE NEED IT

Hormones, music, lubricants, and even the right partner may not work for all of us. It's never too late to get professional help for sexual problems.

Sexual activity and pleasure are lifelong human experiences. They express the core of our emotions and being. This music of life comes in so many melodies. We may not need orchestras or rock bands to play them, but we should be able to sing for as long as we want. . . .

17

PREVENTION
We Are Too Young To Get Sick

We live in an age of information glut—television, print media, and even our computer superhighways deluge us with so much material that we all think we know what we're supposed to do to keep healthy. I call it the EVES code of life—eat right, vitamins, exercise, and stop our excesses. Every public health agency has presented us with guidelines, charts, and tables. This hardly makes for exciting reading. More titillating are the "experts" who write best-sellers telling us these guidelines are wrong and that the real truth and wisdom allowing us to achieve weight loss, health, general perfection, and longevity can be obtained by following the ten easy guidelines presented *only* in their books or seminars. We also have the single-study approach, whereby one bit of research is presented as the absolute and final truth: Oat bran will protect us from heart attack; butter is bad, margarine is better—no, wait, it isn't; or a very-low-fat diet deprives us of essential fatty acids, which causes us to have an increase in our risk of heart disease; and so it goes. This information frenzy and our subsequent behavior are further fed by an excess of product pushers. One night of TV would have us believe that vitamins keep us young and fit (note the gray-haired couple riding their bicycles); that protein mixes added to our regular food will keep on "taking care of both of us"; that a large cheeseburger, fries, and Coke are inexpensive, easy, and delicious; that we can lose weight by eating diet chocolate bars, and, finally, that we can treat our constipation gently so we awaken in the morning feeling ready to go (and, of course, consume again!). The ad agencies' budgeting, marketing, and commercial skills are more than a match for the statistics and charts of our national health institutes.

Now comes the hard part: Who will we allow to define us? Hopefully, we've rejected media-portrayed ageism as we pass through our fifth decade. Let's also ignore their espoused belief that we "midlife consumers" are dumb enough to succumb to what they deem we will or should consume. This means we have to make life-pattern commitments to health in spite of the ever-present media-pattern commitments to sales. In this chapter, I hope to provide some incentive for this goal. Here are "just the facts, ma'am" to use as a general guide. What we do now while we're young can indeed have a major impact on whether we get sick in the future, and we're talking about major diseases here: diabetes, high blood pressure, heart disease, stroke, osteoporosis, and cancer. EVES—here we come!

Eating Right: How Much, What, and When

Food provides us with essential fuel, pleasure, socialization, and guilt. It also, to a large extent, determines our appearance and our health. There is no constant here. We have to make choices and commitments about food every few hours, every day, for our entire lives. We may regret some of these choices, but there is still plenty of time (the next half of our lives) to change them.

Quantity—The Ideal: What Goes In Gets Burned Up

Our body is wonderfully sensitive to our energy fuel (otherwise known as food) and adapts to maintain a set weight. So if we have been a certain weight for the past ten years or have gained weight after the age of 18, we might not be that happy with it, but the weight management center in our brain is, and it directs our body's utilization of energy so that it maintains this weight. That means if we're consuming too much, the body will tend to use up more energy to burn off the calories. On the

other hand, when we reduce fuel intake or diet, our body cruelly becomes more efficient and less wasteful in burning up whatever calories
we consume. Most of us know—at least roughly—what our body needs
to maintain our present weight. The estimated caloric intake that
women generally need ranges from 1,600 to 2,200 calories, depending on
our size, frame, amount of muscle (which burns more calories than fat),
activity level, and age. This last factor is important; apparently at age 65
we need only 1,600 calories to maintain our body weight. This is due to a
combination of factors: the lowering of our metabolism with age (estimated to be about 2 percent a decade), our gradual tendency to increase
fat over muscle, and diminished physical activity (remember, we're talking averages here).

If we want to figure out how many calories we use on an individual
basis, we have to figure out our basal metabolic rate—or calorie consumption while we're at rest—and add to that the calories we burn during physical activity. Machines can do the former (by measuring how
much oxygen we breathe in and CO_2 we breathe out while we're at rest
and before eating), or you can ask your doctor to calculate your appropriate caloric intake with the Harris-Benedict equation (the current standard) for your present weight or, for thinner circumstances, your ideal
weight.

Not all calories are created equal, nor do all food groups render the
same caloric energy (or price, depending on how we view calories). One
gram of protein or carbohydrate gives us 4 calories, while one gram of fat
gives us 9. So not only do we want to chose a combination that gives us
the right caloric intake, but we need to mix and match the factors of 4
and 9 in arriving at this final number. Thankfully, manufacturers must
now print the "Nutrition Facts" on all packaged goods. They tell us the
calories, caloric components, and what this constitutes in an "average"
diet. (I love the fact that this "average" is routinely set at 2,000 and
2,500 calories a day, nicely applicable to men, but a high norm for
women.)

Fats, Proteins, and Carbohydrates: How Little, How Much, and Why

Let's start with the diet component that has the worst nutritional and
health rap—fat. If we're going to make efforts to follow guidelines from

the American Heart Association, the American Cancer Society, the National Institutes of Health, and our mothers, we should understand why.

FATS: FROM THE NECESSARY TO THE (KNACK)WURST

Fats are a necessary component of our nutrition; gram for gram, they are our most concentrated energy source. Fats carry fat-soluble vitamins (A, D, E, and K), they help us absorb vitamin D, and they help convert carotene to vitamin A. Fats slow down our digestive process by reducing stomach acid secretion, giving food more time to be digested and absorbed. Fats make us feel full after a meal, and, most important, they taste good. A fat's flavor, texture, and melting point are influenced by its content of fatty acids. There are two main types: saturated and unsaturated.

SATURATED FATTY ACIDS

These are solid at room temperature and include fat from animals, dairy products made from whole milk, and certain plant foods: coconut oil and palm kernel oil (called tropical oils), and cocoa butter.

UNSATURATED FATTY ACIDS

These are usually liquid at room temperature and come from vegetable sources. They are divided into two types:

1. *Polyunsaturated fatty acids* include safflower, sesame, and sunflower seeds; corn; soybeans; many nuts and seeds; and their oils.

2. *Monounsaturated fatty acids* include olive oil, peanut oil, and avocados.

Many of these oils are converted to a more solid consistency through a process called hydrogenation. This creates new types of synthetic fats called *trans fats*. Hydrogenation turns liquid oils into creamy spreads or solid sticks. These man-made (or, to be more PC, person-made) fats can increase our LDLs to the same degree that saturated fats do. But, unlike "natural" saturated fats, they compound cholesterol damage by lowering our good protective HDLs. It's estimated that our intake of trans fats may account for 2 percent of our daily calories.

Our knowledge of trans fats has created a "political" dilemma: Whose side should we take in the great butter-versus-margarine debate? A tablespoon of margarine can have up to 2 grams of saturated fat and up to 2 grams of trans fatty acids, a total of 4 grams of "bad" fat. That's not good, but it's still better than butter's 7 grams of saturated fat per tablespoon. The diet or light margarines are probably still our best bet. Soft is better than hard, and in all cases, we should use it sparingly. We should also beware of the many sources of hidden trans fats in products made with hydrogenated or partially hydrogenated vegetable oils (deep-fried foods, packaged snack foods). Even as their labels are trumpeting claims of low or no cholesterol, many products have trans fats—which may be worse than cholesterol—lurking silently within. Always read the list of ingredients.

Some fatty acids are essential because our bodies don't make them. Fatty acids function in the transport and breakdown of another fat-related substance or lipid, *cholesterol*. This, too, is needed by our body. It's a component of most of our tissues and organs and is the starting point for synthesis of the hormones made by our ovaries and adrenals. Cholesterol forms vitamin D, which is needed for absorption of calcium, and it is the main component of bile, which help us digest fats. Our dietary sources of cholesterol are all in animal fats such as meat, fish, poultry, and dairy products (these are the same foods that are sources of saturated fat). Egg yolks and organ meats (liver and kidney) are especially high in cholesterol.

Unless we are starving or suffering from certain rare diseases, none of us has a fat deficiency. It just doesn't occur in adults, so I'm not going to devote any time explaining how we should get our essential fat. The majority of us are, however, in a chronic state of excessive fat intake, and the implications on our health are enormous.

In this country most of us derive 37 percent or more of our calories from fat. What happens if we continue to "grease" our way through our fifth decade? If we change our level of fat consumption, can we improve our health destiny? The answer is yes.

Fat and Cancer

Breast Cancer   We have significant data that show that women who have consumed large amounts of saturated fat have a 50 percent increase in their relative risk of breast cancer as compared with women who consumed low amounts. One study showed that for every 77 grams of fat we consume daily, we increase our risk by 35 percent!

These and other data seem to indicate that to appreciably lower our risk of breast cancer, we have to lower our fat intake to less than 20 percent of our total food. This could also help women who already have been treated for breast cancer. Analysis of diets of Western women who have estrogen receptor–positive breast cancer have shown that those who failed treatment had a higher level of total fat than those who were treated successfully. In analyzing the numbers, it was determined that for each 1 percent increase in total fat content, there was an 8 percent increase in the risk of treatment failure.

A high-fiber, low-fat diet based on the American Cancer Society Guidelines may improve the immune function of women treated for breast cancer. Women on this diet appear to increase their counts of certain fighter T cells that help prevent tumor recurrence. This immunity has also been shown in certain tissue studies to improve with the addition of omega-3 fatty acids, which are found in cold-water fish.

Having made these antifat reports with great assurance, I now have to self-edit. The very newest analysis (or metanalysis) in *The New England Journal of Medicine* purports to show no correlation between fat consumption and breast cancer. We're all looking at the same data, but drawing different conclusions. I, at least, will continue to espouse a "lower fat, lower breast cancer" dictum for myself and my patients.

OVARIAN CANCER

Several studies have shown a direct correlation between high levels of dietary fat and ovarian cancer. It's estimated that if we reduce our meat intake and/or we consume only lean meat, avoid egg yolks, and increase our consumption of high-fiber vegetables, we might cut our risk of ovarian cancer by as much as half.

COLON AND RECTAL CANCER

The correlation between dietary fat and cancer of our lower bowel is probably the most obvious. Certainly the mechanism seems the clearest, since we know that the process of digesting and processing fat creates cancer-promoting agents. We also have statistics and studies that have determined that lowering our fat consumption by half translates into a two-thirds reduction in our relative risk for colon cancer and a one-third reduction in relative risk for rectal cancer.

OTHER CANCERS

Fat consumption probably plays a role in at least seven types of cancer. In addition to the cancers I just discussed, there is an increased risk of endometrial, lung, gallbladder, and prostate cancer (that last, of course, doesn't strike women but should be cause for concern, as we share our meals and lives with men). When we total these cancers and consider the statistics of relative risk, we come up with the very real possibility that 35 percent of fatal cancers might be reduced by dietary modification. Future research may reveal that cancer reduction could be as great as 60 percent, but even if it's "only" 20 percent, that's substantial enough to warrant making changes in what we eat.

Fat and Atherosclerosis (and Ultimately Heart Attack and Stroke)

Let's face it: For most of us, the fat and cholesterol we consume become the fat and cholesterol we contain and store (in addition to what our bodies make). On average, we eat a diet containing three times as much saturated fat as polyunsaturated fat, and then we add insult to injury by consuming 320 to 400 milligrams of cholesterol. If we were to keep the same amount of fat but switched the ratio so that we ate equal proportions of saturated and polyunsaturated fats, and we kept our cholesterol intake to less than 300 milligrams a day, we would quickly achieve some amazing results. Our body's cholesterol concentration would drop, for the most part, by 10 to 15 percent within two weeks and remain that way as long as we kept to this diet.

Our average cholesterol level is related to our consumption of animal fats, egg yolks, and milk products. The good news is that we can often reverse atherosclerotic changes with a low-fat, low-cholesterol diet. A 1 percent reduction in our total cholesterol levels can cause a 2 percent reduction in our risk of heart attack. (See Table 9.1 for cholesterol guidelines.)

The American Heart Association strongly recommends we lower our fat and follow simple dietary guidelines to protect our hearts. To get a general idea of what we want to consume in grams of fat, we simply take

TABLE 17.1   DIETARY FAT GUIDELINES

Total Daily Calories	Total Fat Calories		Grams of Fat	
	20%	30%	20%	30%
1,400	280	420	27	42
1,600	320	480	35	53
1,800	360	540	41	60
2,000	400	600	46	66

our total calories, figure 30 percent, 20 percent, or below, and divide by 9. (See Table 17.1.)

ARE THERE FAT "EXCEPTIONS"?

Olive Oil   This is a monounsaturated fat; and monounsaturated fats (like all unsaturated fats) have no undesirable effects on our cholesterol. But let's not kid ourselves; they are still fattening (9 calories per gram), and if we gain weight, we tend to increase our cholesterol. There is no free "greasing." It would appear, however, that not all unsaturated oils are equal. Mediterranean populations whose diet contains 30 to 40 percent of their calories as fat, much of which is olive oil, have been shown to have a low incidence of heart disease. A recent study also documented a 50 percent lower risk of breast cancer in women in these regions, and olive oil was credited for this fact.

The problem with taking a purely Mediterranean approach to our diet is that most of us are very selective in our information retrieval. We hear that olive oil is good, so we add it to what we're already eating. We smugly enter Italian restaurants, pour the oil onto a plate, mop it up with bread, and go on to order large portions of meat, fish, or pasta Bolognese, followed by ice cream (now called gelato). I fear telling women to "up" their fat intake in any form unless they exercise, rigorously control their total calories, and significantly cut back on or cut out nearly all saturated fats. However, when I have a choice between butter and olive oil, or even margarine and olive oil, I choose the latter.

Fish and Fish Oils Cold-water fish, other seafood, and their oils contain a special form of polyunsaturated fatty acid called omega-3. These oils may prevent our platelets from sticking together and forming clots and in this way could protect us from heart attack and stroke. But this anticlotting benefit is very weak, especially when we compare it with aspirin. Large amounts of fish oil sometimes lower blood pressure but, once more, this is a weak and inconsistent response. Fish fatty acids also seem to reduce serum triglyceride levels, but don't lower our LDL cholesterol and may even increase it.

Recently, the effect of fish consumption *in men* was investigated by a Harvard study following the diets of over 51,000 health professionals (mostly dentists) for six years. Those who consumed six or more servings a week had only a 14 percent decrease in their relative risk of coronary heart disease as compared with those who ate one serving a month or less. The risk of death from coronary disease among men who ate any amount of fish, as compared with the non–fish eaters, was about 25 percent less, but didn't improve as they increased their consumption to six portions. The investigators concluded that any beneficial effect from fish fat is obtained with just one or two servings of fish per week, and that more is not better. This should extend to fish oil capsules, which provide much higher amounts of omega-3 fatty acids than fish. I would retitle this study "Real Men Don't Eat Too Much Fish." It could also be subtitled "Where Did the Female Dentists Go?"

A Word About Shellfish Shrimp, lobster, and crayfish are higher in cholesterol than most other types of fish and seafood, but they raise our cholesterol less than eggs and are still lower in total fat and saturated fatty acids than most meats and poultry. So if we have to decide between a shrimp salad and a chicken salad, we can go for the shrimp (and low-fat dressing) without too much guilt.

A Postscript on Low-Fat Diets

If we follow the advice of the American Heart Association and the National Institutes of Health, we'll restrict fat to less than 30 percent of our total caloric intake. But if we're at risk, maybe we shouldn't stop at 30 percent and should make the effort to get down to or below 20 percent; this is what the National Cancer Institute is recommending (and appears to be what we need for cancer prevention). However, a disturbing study from Rockefeller University showed that when fat content got below 20 percent in individuals who were on strict diets, they began making fat out of the carbohydrates they were eating, and the fat they made was saturated. So on one side of the scale we're told to cut out fats, especially the saturated ones, and then we are weighed down with the information that we may go on to produce our own!

CARBOHYDRATES

Carbohydrates are our chief source of energy. They keep us going and going—from the baseline processes of our body functions to the more voluntary efforts of our muscles (and hopefully outright exercise). Our food carbohydrates consist of sugars, starches, and fiber. Sugars can be simple—such as those in honey and fruits—or processed, such as table sugar. Starches need to be broken down into simple sugars by digestion. Our body converts all digested sugar and starches into glucose (our blood sugar) or fructose. The glucose is either immediately utilized by our body as fuel or converted to glycogen and stored in our liver and muscles. This will provide future energy and gives us a needed reserve. If we still have excess glucose (we're "carbing out"), it's converted to fat and stored. Theoretically, this is a long-term energy reserve, but for many of us, it is just excess lumpy poundage. Because our body can manufacture its own carbohydrates from some amino acids and components of fat, we don't have a list of "essential" carbohydrates—just those that are good for our nutrition and health.

When carbohydrates require enzymatic digestion to be absorbed and aren't just sugar, we call them complex carbohydrates. These are chiefly starches and include the worldwide staples—rice, potatoes, grains, beans, as well as fruits and vegetables. Fiber consists of the indigestable part of grains, vegetables, and fruits. There are two kinds: water-soluble fiber, which is mostly found in whole grains and the skin of fruit and vegetables; and water-insoluble fiber, found in oat and oat bran, certain fruits, and dried peas and beans. Each carbohydrate component has its ups (energy) and downs (fat production). We are told by most institutes and agencies that complex carbohydrates should be our major food component, accounting for more than 50 percent of our calories. If we're going to eat it, we should know why we need it.

Refinement: Sugars and Starches That Fail to Refine Our Bodies

Sugar gives us a quick surge of instant energy as it causes a rapid rise in our blood sugar levels, but like most good things that come quickly and effortlessly, our energy euphoria rapidly disappears. Blood sugar levels drop, and we feel tired and may experience dizziness, weakness, and headaches. This, in turn, causes us to want to re-elevate our blood sugar, and we crave more sweet or starchy food. Unfortunately, sugar and refined carbohydrates (foods made from white flour, white sugar, and white rice) are low in natural vitamins and minerals and, most important, fiber.

Some of us may overreact to the ingestion of sugar and simple starches, and we overproduce glucose. A call for help then goes out to our glucose mediator, the pancreas, and we end up overproducing insulin. This hormone determines how much glucose gets converted to energy and how much becomes fat. It appears that the higher our levels of insulin, the more glucose calories we convert to fat. This overproduction of insulin as a response to sugar and certain carbohydrates is termed *insulin resistance* and may occur in as much as 25 percent of the U.S. population.

Our Unrefined Starches: Complexity Is Good

Our complex carbohydrates have been given the dietary seal of approval as our best alternative to fat and excess protein. They contain no animal fat, give us necessary calories, and, when not refined and stripped, provide us with vitamins, minerals, phyto (plant) chemicals, and fiber. Let's make a "complex" subject simpler and examine the nutritional advantage of these components.

FIBER

Fiber is more than just something we have to eat so that we have regular bowel movements. Here are some fiber facts:

Heart Disease   Increased fiber intake appears to decrease our risk of coronary heart disease. Insoluble fiber can enhance the cholesterol-lowering effect of a low-fat diet, by decreasing LDL. (The "hype" about oat bran and a lot of other grains is probably true.)

Cancer   High fiber intake may decrease our risk for all forms of cancer, especially colon. A study in the Netherlands showed that overall cancer deaths were reduced by one-third in people with high-fiber diet compared to those with low-fiber diets.

Diabetes   High fiber intake offers protection from diabetes and may help control diabetes if we already have it (it improves blood sugar control and increases our body's sensitivity to insulin).

Weight Management   Fiber helps us keep our weight down. Foods high in fiber are low in fat and calories, and because our bodies work harder and longer to digest them, we feel full longer. Our blood insulin levels are not raised, which also helps curb our appetite. High-fiber foods decrease starch absorption, so ultimately we get fewer calories per mouthful of food.

Gastrointestinal Disorders   High fiber intake reduces our risk of gastrointestinal problems and diseases. We all know that fiber prevents or relieves constipation; that's what Metamucil and all those other powders we're told to mix with water and drink consist of. But this food component also helps stop disease, namely diverticulitis. A fiber-rich diet prevents the development of saclike protrusions through the weakened muscle layers of the colon wall. If we eat too little fiber, we have less fecal bulk; the colon narrows, and we need more pressure to move the stool through, which can cause the colon muscles to herniate or rupture. This can occur in 20 to 50 percent of men and women over the age of 50 (somewhat more in men) who consume "refined," nonfibrous diets. Once these sacs develop, they can get clogged and inflamed, especially if constipation develops. Diverticulitis can be a serious and very painful illness that may ultimately require removal of a portion of the bowel.

Unfortunately, most of us don't get enough fiber in our diet. Our average ranges from 10 to 23 grams daily. The experts now recommend we have 20 to 35 grams a day. We can increase fiber by leaving skins on our fruits and vegetables and consuming at least five servings a day. We should have six to eleven servings of whole bread, cereals, and rice a day. Product information panels tell us the amount of fiber in a portion of packaged food. Having a cup of cereal in the morning may give us as much as 20 grams of fiber (if we choose the right cereal). Two pieces of whole wheat bread can give us another 3 grams, and then we can add the rest with prunes, beans, and, yes, broccoli, or even fresh raspberries. Remember, 1 cup of fruits and vegetables counts as two servings, so the total number required is not overwhelming. We don't have to become grazers, constantly chomping on twigs and berries to get our fiber.

One word of caution: If we decide to go from our usual 10 grams of fiber to 35, we should do it gradually; otherwise we'll bloat, have gas, and feel fat. Fiber can also decrease our absorption of calcium and vitamins, so we shouldn't exceed the suggested 35 grams. If we take supplements, we should probably do so with our least fibrous meal.

A SPECIAL ODE TO FRUITS AND VEGETABLES: WHAT THE VITAMIN MANUFACTURERS DON'T TELL US

We expect a lot from scientists. If something is good for us, why can't it be isolated, compounded, and squeezed into a pill so we can just pop it and get on with our lives? Getting on with our lives usually means eating fast food on the run. For those of us who do sit down, the right vitamin pill could still excuse us from eating our minimum of five portions of fruits and vegetables a day. Just pass that high-potency vitamin C (and we'll forget the citrus fruit), the beta-carotene (carrots and other yellow vegetables have to be washed and prepared), and, if possible, give us a pill of sulforaphane (instead of broccoli, which even some Democrats dislike!). Our pack-it-in-a-pill expectations are not going to be met. Vitamins cannot fix what we break by not eating right. At most, they may give us some higher-potency "edges" in the prevention of certain body malfunctions.

A vegetable or fruit is not just a large container of vitamins; it has fiber, complex carbohydrates, and a myriad of chemicals and compounds that have amazing abilities to nourish and care for our cells, organs, and perhaps our souls. We are only just beginning to discover these plant compounds and their impact on our body functions. The compounds are called phytochemicals ("phyto" has no connection with canines; it's the Greek word for "plant"), and many of them evolved with the plants to protect them from sunlight. One day, we may succeed in isolating and taming these phytochemicals into pills. Indeed, the National Cancer Institute and many private pharmaceutical companies have started to invest millions of dollars to do this. But for now, better health through phytochemicals remains simple: eating fruits and vegetables. Table 17.2

TABLE 17.2   "CHEMICAL" PROTECTION FROM NATURE

Plant Source	Phytochemical
Broccoli (also cauliflower, brussels sprouts, turnips, and kale)	*Sulforaphane:* Increases production of anticancer enzymes and human cells that are grown in cultures. Not destroyed by cooking.
Tomatoes (also green peppers, pineapples, strawberries, and carrots)	*P-coumaric acid and chlorogenic acid:* Prevent formation of nitrosamines, which are cancer-causing substances. Not destroyed by cooking.
Cabbage and turnips	*PIETC (phenylethyl isothiocyanate):* Protects DNA of cells from a carcinogen in tobacco smoke.
Strawberries, grapes, and raspberries	*Ellagic acid:* Deactivates carcinogens
Soybeans	*Genistein:* Prevents small blood vessel growth that supplies malignant tumors. A lower incidence of breast cancer (and prostate cancer) in the Japanese population may be partly due to their soy-rich diet.
Cauliflower	*Indole-3-carbinol:* Promotes the breakdown of certain potent forms of estrogen and may decrease breast cancer.
Onion and garlic	*Allylic sulfide:* Increases enzymatic breakdown of certain carcinogens.
Hot peppers	*Capsaicin:* Prevents certain toxins from initiating DNA changes that lead to cancer.
Most fruits and vegetables	*Flavonoids:* Sit on hormone-binding sites in the cells and prevent overstimulation by hormones.

is a short list of just a few "new" chemicals and their "old" fruit and vegetable sources.

PROTEIN

Sugar and spice and everything nice are not what we're made of. We're primarily composed of water, followed by protein. This organic compound is the major building material for our muscles, bones, all of our internal organs, our blood, other body fluids, and our skin, nails, and hair.

Hormones and enzymes, as well as antibodies, are made from proteins. Protein is also an energy source, but we don't need to use it for this purpose if we ingest enough carbohydrates and, of course, fat. Excess protein, like excess anything we consume, is converted to fat and stored in our tissues.

Proteins are composed of amino acids. Our body requires twenty-two of these to make our human proteins. All but eight can be self-produced. These eight that we need to assimilate from an outside source (namely food) are thus termed *essential amino acids*. We need all of these essential amino acids present and in the right proportion to produce our human protein, and if one is low or missing, it shuts down our protein-building conveyer belt. A food that contains all of the essential amino acids is called a *complete protein*. Most meats and dairy products are complete; most vegetables and fruits are not. So if we cut out the former, we have to combine the latter in a way that completes our ingested amino acid profile. The recommendation is that we eat 0.42 gram of protein per pound of body weight a day. At 130 pounds, we would need only 55 grams of protein, which is much less than what most of us consume.

The Right Proteins: A Steak a Day Does Not Keep the Doctor Away

Converting between grams of protein, ounces of meat, and cups of fruits and vegetables can be confusing. Some of us want red meat; others figure we'll get our protein from fish and poultry. There are those of us who use dairy products, others who don't, and some of us are or will become complete vegetarians. In order to get our minimum protein requirements and not exceed the maximum, we have to know something about protein sources.

Protein from Meat, Fish, and Poultry

We don't need more than 6 ounces a day. This will provide us with 30 to 40 grams of protein.

RED MEAT

Make sure it's lean. A 3-ounce portion is the size of a deck of playing cards (in case you're wondering how to weigh your cooked meat without carrying a scale in your purse). A 3-ounce portion of lean roast beef would equal two thin slices measuring 3 by 3 inches and ¼ inch thick. Or, if you plan to get all of your meat protein in one meal, this would be a 6-inch-wide, one-half-inch-thick piece of meat, certainly not a microscopic portion. Apply the same measurements to other cooked meats, and make sure that all fat has been trimmed. If you make hamburgers, have the meat department grind up lean sirloin or loin.

CHICKEN

Three ounces would be half a chicken breast or one chicken leg with thigh (the skin should be off when we cook it to reduce the fat).

FISH

If it's flaked, it will fill three fourths of a cup. In solid form, it has the same-size dimensions as meat (see above).

Protein from Dairy Products

Skim milk products are fine. We don't need the fat of whole milk to make this a complete protein.

PRODUCT	PROTEIN
Milk	8-oz glass = 8.4 gr
1 cup nonfat yogurt	13 gr
Low-fat fruit yogurt	9 gr
1 cup ricotta cheese	28 gr
½ cup nonfat cottage cheese	15 gr
1 ounce cut cheeses (Monterey jack, Gouda, Muenster, provolone)	7 gr
Eggs	
1 large egg	6 gr
1 egg white	3.35 gr

Protein from Nuts and Seeds

These are one of the important sources of protein if we're complete vegetarians.

TYPE OF NUT *(people are not listed here!)*	PROTEIN
1 cup almonds, cashews, or pistachio nuts	25 gr
1 cup pecans	10 gr
1 cup walnuts	15 gr
1 cup peanuts	37 gr

Protein from Fruits

These are not high in protein, but some fruits give enough to count. Here are some of the protein-worthy.

TYPE OF FRUIT	PROTEIN
¹/₂ cantaloupe	2.3 gr
1 papaya	1.8 gr
10 dried peach halves	4.7 gr
10 dried pear halves	3.28 gr
1 cup packed raisins	4 gr
10 prunes	2.2 gr
1 banana	1.2 gr
1 cup grapefruit juice	1.2 gr
1 cup orange juice	1.7 gr

Protein from Vegetables

If we think (or better yet, eat) legumes, we'll get lots of terrific low-fat, high-fiber vegetable protein.

TYPE OF VEGETABLE	PROTEIN
1 cup dried black beans	14 gr
1 cup cooked kidney beans	14 gr
1 cup cooked lentils	14 gr
1 cup cooked navy beans	14 gr
1 cup cooked lima beans	14 gr
1 cup cooked soy beans	12 gr

Note: 1 cup of these can replace
   3 oz of meat, poultry, or fish

1 cup peas	7.9 gr
1 cup broccoli or cauliflower	3 gr
1 cup corn	5 gr
1 cup asparagus	4.1 gr
1 large baked potato with skin	4 gr

Note: For those of us who are total vegetarians (and consequently need to complete our incomplete proteins), it would probably be worthwhile to consult nutritional guides for vegetarians or talk to a licensed nutritionist.

The "Right" Healthy Diet: Plans, Pyramids, and Reality

Health institutes, dieticians, and weight control centers love to give us plans. They may formulate these as pyramids: the fats on top, because we should limit them; and the complex carbohydrates on the broad-based bottom, because this should be our largest food group and, theoretically, will not cause *us* to develop broad-based bottoms. The plan put out by the American Heart Institute is our "classic." It consists of the following:

> *Total fat:* Less than 30 percent of total calories
>
> *Saturated fat:* Less than 10 percent of total calories
>
> *Unsaturated fat:* Less than 10 percent of total calories
>
> *Cholesterol:* Less than 300 milligrams a day
>
> *Carbohydrates* (emphasis on complex): More than 50 percent of total calories
>
> *Protein:* The remainder
>
> *Sodium:* Less than 3 grams a day

The above requires some degree of translation to actual servings of food groups. This serving plan is also recommended by the National Academy of Sciences:

FATS

Less than 5 to 8 servings of fats and oil, where a serving size equals:

1 teaspoon vegetable oil or regular margarine

2 teaspoons diet margarine

1 tablespoon salad dressing

2 teaspoons mayonnaise or peanut butter

1 teaspoon seeds or nuts

$^1/_8$ avocado

10 small or 5 large olives

This sounds like a lot of fat and oil, but we have to allow for what's in our bakery goods and what we use for cooking.

CARBOHYDRATES

A minimum of five servings of fruits and vegetables a day; a serving equals:

1 medium fruit

$^1/_2$ cup chopped, cooked, or canned fruit

$^3/_4$ cup fruit juice

$^1/_2$ cup vegetables

Six or more servings of breads, cereal, and starchy vegetables; a serving equals:

1 slice of bread

$^1/_4$ cup nugget or bud-type cereal

$^1/_2$ cup hot cereal (low-fat)

1 cup flake cereal

1 cup cooked rice or pasta (not made with egg yolks)

$^1/_2$ cup of starchy vegetables (potatoes, corn, yams, sweet potatoes, lima beans, or peas)

1 cup low-fat soup

PROTEIN

Meat, poultry, or fish: No more than two servings a day
(3 ounces cooked, four ounces raw) = 1 serving

Vegetable: 1 cup cooked beans, peas, or lentils

3 ounces tofu

We can follow this plan and not feel hungry or deprived. It necessitates cutting down our huge American portions of fatty meat (the meat industry doesn't like this) and whole milk products. High-fat desserts are out, but we can substitute fruit, low-fat frozen yogurt, sorbets, and special low-fat cakes. We can snack, but it should be on fruits, raw vegetables, low-fat crackers and cookies, air-popped popcorn, or unsalted pretzels. We'll need to substitute jams and jellies or mustard for butter on our breads and low-fat muffins.

The question is, Is this plan enough? For cancer prevention, it appears that we have to go below 20 percent in fat calories. That means reducing our five to eight servings of fats and oils to three to five servings. If we steam, poach, or broil without oil; substitute mustard for mayonnaise; avoid nuts, avocados, and olives; and use nonfat salad dressings (or

TABLE 17.3   VERY-LOW-FAT DIET GUIDELINES

	Ornish Reversal Diet (to reverse atherosclerotic changes)	Pritikin Diet
Total fat	10% of total calories	5 to 10% of total calories
Saturated fatty acids	Exclude as much as possible	Exclude as much as possible
Polyunsaturated fatty acids	Total fat composed primarily of polyunsaturated and monosaturated fats	Only fat found naturally in food
Cholesterol	5 mg a day	100 mg a day
Carbohydrates	70 to 75% of total calories (mostly complex)	Up to 80%
Protein	15 to 20% of total calories	10 to 15% of total calories

just vinegar and spices), we can probably do this without living on a diet of sushi, steamed fish, seaweed, and tofu (although that would be a pretty healthy diet). Restricting fat to less than 20 percent is an effort and requires our reading every packaged food label and becoming real pests in restaurants.

Finally, we can restrict our diet to what I call ground zero. The two best-known "super-low-fat" diets were designed primarily for people with severe cardiovascular disease. Their basic guidelines are shown in Table 17.3.

We have to decide how far we want to commit ourselves to health through diet. There will be times when we just can't eat the way we want or should, but if these are the exceptions rather then the rule, we've come a long way from hot dogs and apple pie!

VITAMINS: HOW VITAL ARE THEY?

We've assigned vitamins a maternal role. They're supposed to be the "vitameres" of our nutrition; condensed encapsulated mommies that will make everything right. Proponents of vitamins boast that they will help prevent cancer, heart attack, cataracts, and, in general, aging, while the vitamin reactionaries respond that the health claims for vitamins are, at best, not valid and, at worse, lies. So what do we do about vitamins?

FROM D (DEFICIENCIES) TO M (MEGADOSES): THE VITAMIN CONTROVERSIES

The Antioxidants

Oxygen is the essence of our lives, but it also destroys our tissues. We use oxygen for the most basic chemical reactions that keep our bodies going. Unfortunately, as these reactions occur, oxidants and free radicals are formed. Their unsolicited creation is accelerated by adverse external influences such as air pollution and tobacco smoke. These *free radicals* have no political affiliation; they are just unstable molecules in search of an electron they "lost" during the oxidation process. They bombard the intact borders of billions of cells in our bodies, attempting to pair up with their missing electrons. These collisions can damage the cells and their DNA so that they can't reproduce or, if they do, they're genetically altered and can become cancerous. When the bombardment strikes our collagen molecules, we develop liver spots and wrinkles. When our cholesterol is attacked and LDL cholesterol is oxidized, it forms artery-clogging plaque. If our joint tissues undergo an electron "search and seizure," we may develop arthritis.

The antioxidants are supposed to act like a sponge and sop up and neutralize these harmful radicals. Sounds great, but do they become the quellers of disturbances through simple ingestion in our food, or do we need to amass larger protective forces in the form of vitamin pill "radical" deactivation?

VITAMIN A AND BETA-CAROTENE

Vitamin A is a fat-soluble vitamin. Our bodies produce this vitamin from preformed vitamin A or carotenoids, the most "famous" of which is beta-carotene. The only way we can naturally consume ready-made vitamin A is through animal tissues; our best source is fish, and the most concentrated form is found in fish liver oil. We can also get it through cream and butter (a small asset amid the liabilities of these saturated fats). Vitamin A aids in the growth and repair of our tissues and is believed to protect the mucous membranes of our airways (mouth, nose, throat, and lungs), as well as the lining of our gastrointestinal tract. It promotes gastric secretion of acid that we need for digestion. Additionally, vitamin A is used in the formation of our teeth, bones, and blood, and it gives us "visual purple," a substance in our eyes that we need for night vision.

Carotenoids come from the pigments in vegetables. We know we get them from carrots (hence, the name), but they are also concentrated in leafy green vegetables, spinach, broccoli, sweet potatoes, peaches, apricots, cantaloupe, and yellow vegetables. In general, the greener or yellower the vegetable or fruit, the more carotenoids it contains. About one fourth to one third of the carotenoids we consume are converted into vitamin A. The rest is either stored in our fat tissues or excreted in our stool.

What can vitamin A do for us? When we add vitamin A to cancer-causing agents in cell cultures, it seems to prevent growth of human breast cancer cells. Researchers have looked at the effects of antioxidants and vitamin A on our development of breast cancer. They followed over 89,000 American women between the ages of 35 and 59 for nine years. Those with very low intakes of vitamin A had a 25 percent higher risk for breast cancer than women who had what was considered normal or high vitamin A or carotene intake. Vegetables themselves seemed to account for much of this correlation. If the women consumed less than 0.9 serving a day, their breast-cancer risk was almost 30 percent higher than that of women who had just two servings a day. The only women who benefited breast cancer–wise from vitamin A supplements were those with very-low-vitamin-A diets. If they took 10,000 units of vitamin A per day, they decreased their risk to about half that of the "low-A nonsupplemented women."

Vitamin A and beta-carotene have disappointingly "struck out" in three other studies. A Finnish study of over 29,000 *men* who were smokers found a slight increase in the death rates of those who took beta-carotene for five to eight years. They took only 20 milligrams a day, and possibly this wasn't enough to afford protection. Larger doses of beta-carotene (50 milligrams) were taken by half of the 22,000 doctors (again all male) in the Physician's Health Study. Twelve years later, no protection against cancer or heart disease was found with use of this supplement. The third investigation, called the Beta Carotene and Retinol Efficacy Trial (CARET), followed 18,000 smokers and asbestos workers (obviously at a high risk for lung cancer). The study group took 30 milligrams of beta-carotene or 25,000 international units of vitamin A, or both. Those taking these vitamins had a 28 percent higher death rate from lung cancer and a 17 percent increased mortality from heart disease compared with the control group who took placebos. When these results came in, the researchers "de-vitaminized" the test group and halted the study almost two years ahead of schedule.

An ongoing study of *women* (40,000 female health professionals) who were taking beta-carotene, vitamin E, and aspirin was altered after similar findings. Beta-carotene was declared null and void, and its testing was eliminated.

Vitamin A in supplement form may not only be of little health value, but in megadoses it can be health harming. It is chemically classified as a retinoid. We know that a synthetic member of this retinoid family, isotretinoin or Accutane, which is used to treat acne, is extremely teratogenic, increasing fetal malformations 25-fold. The results of a recent study published in *The New England Journal of Medicine* confirmed that high doses of vitamin A were likewise harmful to fetal development. Twenty-two thousand pregnant women were followed, and those who took more than 10,000 international units of vitamin A per day, especially before the seventh week of gestation, had a 1 in 57 chance of delivering an infant with malformations of the head, face, central nervous system, thymus gland, and heart. These findings did not relate to the vitamin A precursor, beta-carotene. Strict warnings have now been issued for women of reproductive age (and that obviously includes those of us in our forties who might conceive) to limit vitamin A supplementation.

Whatever protection we do get from vitamin A or beta-carotene seems to be through their natural providers—fruits and vegetables—and that's what we should supplement.

VITAMIN C (ASCORBIC ACID)

This is a water-soluble vitamin found in most of our fresh fruits and vegetables. It's our "collagen vitamin": it helps maintain this essential component of our skin, bones, and connective tissue. We need vitamin C to form our red blood cells. It helps our wounds and "boo-boo"s heal. Vitamin C appears to help us fight bacterial infection and the effects of allergy-causing substances. We need vitamin C to absorb iron and utilize folic acid; it also helps form adrenaline, which is our stress-reacting hormone.

Because it's water-soluble, vitamin C doesn't stay in our bodies for long. We usually excrete it in our urine just three to four hours after we ingest it. The more C we take, the less we absorb (our GI tract seems to be protecting us and our kidneys from vitamin C overload). We absorb even less if we smoke, have a high fever, experience high stress, or take aspirin, antibiotics, or steroids.

Aside from the controversy over vitamin C's ability to fight colds, there is a larger (and ultimately more interesting) debate over its other antioxidant properties. Does C protect us from C-diseases (cardiovascular and cancer)? A recent epidemiologic and nutrition survey of over 11,000 adults followed for ten years says yes, resoundingly for men and less emphatically for women. Men with the highest vitamin C intake had what is termed a standardized mortality ratio of 0.65 for all causes, 0.78 for all cancers, and 0.58 for all cardiovascular diseases (this is a terrible phrase, but 1 is the expected mortality for their age group, and their deaths were compared to this standard of 1). We women rated only a "high-C" mortality ratio of 0.90 for all causes, 0.86 for all cancers, and 0.75 for all cardiovascular diseases. The average user of vitamin C pills consumed about 800 milligrams a day. We have to assume that many individuals in the study who regularly used supplements of C were also taking vitamins E, A, and other nutrients. But when C was analyzed on its own, it appeared to have its own anti–C disease effect.

Since cooking, storage, and long-term exposure to air can destroy C in fruits and vegetables, we need to make sure we're getting the fresh stuff. If not, it seems reasonable to supplement.

VITAMIN E

This is a fat-soluble vitamin made of compounds called *tocopherols*, which are given Greek alphabetic designations from alpha to zeta. Thankfully, we don't have to remember the entire Greek alphabet. The first one, alpha, is the most potent and the one we look for in our foods and vitamins. *Alpha-tocopherol* is found in raw seeds, nuts, and soybeans and is concentrated in cold-pressed vegetable oils.

Vitamin E protects vitamins A, B-complex, and C from oxidation and destruction. As an antioxidant, it has been shown to prevent the oxidation of LDL cholesterol and, therefore, should protect us from deposits of fatty plaque. As a fat-soluble vitamin, it does this more effectively than C, since the plaque is formed in a fatty, not watery, environment in the lining of our vessels. Vitamin E (together with beta-carotene) has been shown to protect cell membranes from oxidation by acting as a decoy, attracting the free radicals that would otherwise attack the fatty acids in the membranes. It has been shown to stimulate our immune system and enhance its response to mutations and cancers. Together with vitamin C it reduces nitrite and prevents production of compounds called nitrosamines and nitrosamides that induce tumors in animals and probably do the same in humans. Vitamins E and C also reduce chromosomal damage produced by radiation and chemicals that cause cancer. The tocopherols help our muscles to better utilize oxygen, decrease the stickiness of platelets and, hence, the formation of clots, and have a protective effect on blood cells. We use vitamin E to help prevent abnormal scarring and to reduce pain and swelling associated with fibrocystic breast changes.

This is a pretty impressive list of vitamin qualities, but it's mostly laboratory data. What about us? The Nurses' Study, which followed over 87,000 *female* nurses, ages 34 to 59, for eight years, showed that those women who took separate vitamin E supplements of at least 100 international units for more than two years lowered their risk of major coronary disease by 40 percent compared to women who did not take these supplements. One hundred international units seemed to do the trick, and higher doses made no difference. Those nurses who took "standard" multivitamins, which usually contain less than 30 international units of E, reduced their risk by less than 25 percent. What's impressive is that separate supplementation of vitamin E bestowed its 40 percent cardiac benefit even if the nurses were "graded" for other factors like age, weight, smoking, hormone use, exercise, hypertension, diabetes, and regular use of aspirin.

A recent study of 162 men who had had coronary bypass surgery showed that those who took 100 units a day of vitamin E had significantly less reblockage of their arteries as seen in two-year follow-up X rays than men who did not (I know this is a male study, but it's still fairly impressive).

We can't naturally consume 100 international units of E in our diets (we'd have to drown ourselves in vegetable oils), so if we want this cardiovascular protection, we'll have to be dedicated E supplementers.

Now on to cancer: Another study conducted on women—over 35,000 in Iowa between the ages of 55 and 69 who were followed for four years—showed that those who took high doses of vitamin E in the form of supplements decreased their risk for colon cancer by nearly 70 percent as compared with women whose intake of vitamin E was low. This benefit was even more pronounced (more than 80 percent) in the younger women between the ages of 55 and 59. This protection was not found for other vitamins they tested: namely A, beta-carotene, and C.

Researchers have looked at breast cancer to see if vitamin E might work some magic there. Sadly, a Harvard study of 90,000 women failed to demonstrate any protective effect. Conflicting conclusions from several recent studies have left the lung cancer protection by vitamin E more debatable than ever. Some previous studies showed that higher intakes of E and beta-carotene were associated with a reduced risk of lung cancer. An initial finding of E protection was recently reversed: Finnish men who smoked had no decrease in their rate of cancer after five to eight years of vitamin E and beta-carotene supplementation.

There's no question that we should be consuming as many fruits and vegetables as we can to get our antioxidant vitamin naturally, but even this won't give us enough E. Until we've got all the right studies to satisfy the medical purists (or pessimists), taking C (500 to 1,000 milligrams a day) and vitamin E (100 to 400 international units a day) won't hurt (or at least we don't have data to show it hurts) and it may be, or probably is, beneficial. How's that for couching terms?

VITAMIN D

This is another fat-soluble vitamin. We can either ingest it, produce it (in small amounts) in our kidneys, or soak it in through our skin's exposure to the sun's ultraviolet rays. UV light activate a process that converts a cholesterol compound in our skin to vitamin D. The darker we are with protective pigment, the less ray-sensitive we are (to both skin cancers and vitamin D production).

The natural form of vitamin D is D_3, and it's found in fish liver oils. D_3 can also be made synthetically, as can another form of vitamin D, called D_2 or calciferol. Milk and milk products are "fortified" with D, so we no longer have to count on fish oil to get our D during sunless days or months. Even if we consume the fish oil or fortified milk products, we need fat, bile, and vitamin A to absorb vitamin D through our intestines. We can then store it in our liver or other organs.

This vitamin is our "calcium vitamin." It helps us absorb this essential mineral from our intestine and incorporate it into our bone. If we eat an adequate diet with dairy products or get some sunlight exposure (10 to 15 minutes of UV exposure a day will suffice), we are most likely vitamin D "sufficient." But if we're homebound, live in sunless climates, and eat few or no dairy products, we should supplement 400 units a day. If we're over 70, this dose should be doubled to adequately protect our bones. Obviously, high doses of vitamin D will have no effect if we don't also ingest calcium.

B Vitamins

This group of vitamins is water-soluble and is created by bacteria in our own intestines as well as yeasts, fungi, and molds. The B-complex vitamins are our energy source creators. They convert the carbohydrates we eat into glucose. We also need the Bs to metabolize fat and protein. They are essential for the functioning of our nervous system and the muscles that propel our food in our gastrointestinal tract. We get B vitamins in brewer's yeast, liver, whole grain cereals, and green vegetables. The intestinal bacteria that produce our "in-house" Bs grow best if we supply them with milk, sugar, and small amounts of fat.

Because these are water-soluble vitamins, we don't store them, so we have to ensure a daily supply. The B vitamins are created and work together in vitamin harmony, so if we choose to supplement, we usually do so in a "B-grouped" fashion.

Two of the B-complex vitamins—B_6 and folic acid—have been shown to provide women with special benefits.

VITAMIN B_6

This aids the function of a fatty acid called linoleic acid. It is converted into prostacyclins, which may alter some of our PMS symptoms. B_6 also helps release glycogen from the liver and muscles, another possible PMS-altering phenomena. Specifically formulated PMS vitamins have fairly high amounts of B_6.

FOLIC ACID

This is also included in the vitamin B complex. It helps form *heme*, the iron-containing protein found in hemoglobin, which is needed to form our red blood cells. Folic acid is concentrated in our spinal fluid, and it's necessary for proper brain development and function. It's especially crucial for any fetus we're carrying, since a lack of folic acid in our diet has been shown to be a factor in neural tube defects (see chapter 4). Folic acid also decreases the amino acid homocysteine, which may cause damage to our coronary vessels. Four hundred micrograms may help protect us from heart attack. It is one of the nutrients most often lacking in our diets when we don't consume leafy green vegetables, whole grains, liver, or brewer's yeast; so supplementation is reasonable.

MINERAL SUPPLEMENTS OF SPECIAL INTEREST TO WOMEN

Calcium

"Calcium" and "bones" are practically synonymous. Indeed, more than 99 percent of our total body calcium is found in our bones. This mineral is also essential to maintaining many of our vital functions: the pH of our blood, our electrolyte balance, and the contraction of all of our muscles, including our heart. When calcium is supplemented above and beyond our usual inadequate intake, it can help prevent a number of "nonbone" diseases such as high blood pressure and preeclampsia (or toxemia of pregnancy).

Unfortunately, calcium is not allowed to just sit in our bones, where it belongs. Our skeletal system acts as a huge reservoir, and if a call for calcium is made by other parts of our body, this reservoir can become depleted and we develop osteoporosis. As women, we are especially vulnerable to this devastating cause of disability and death.

We need 1,000 to 1,500 milligrams of calcium a day, and this can easily be obtained through diet and calcium supplements. For the full story on calcium and the crucial role it plays in our present and future health, see chapter 11.

OUR CALCIUM "BIND"

Excess of any nutrient can cause a loss of balance in the complex interdependent absorption that is taking place in our GI tract. If we eat too much protein, we excrete or lose more calcium. Too much dietary fiber may bind calcium and other minerals so they don't get absorbed (this is not a problem for most of us who are "underfibered"; 25 to 30 milligrams a day should not harm our calcium balance). There are other healthy foods that contain oxalates, which interfere with calcium absorption. These include rhubarb, dark leafy vegetables (such as spinach and Swiss chard), as well as beets, parsley, legumes, peanuts, tea, and cocoa. So if we're having spinach as a vegetable and rhubarb pie with a cup of tea as dessert, we might consider waiting and taking our calcium with a different meal.

Magnesium

This is a relatively small element of our body's composition, accounting for only 0.05 percent of our total body weight. Seventy percent of it is in our bones. Magnesium is necessary for the activation of enzymes that metabolize our carbohydrates and amino acids; it counteracts calcium stimulation of muscle contractions; it helps us utilize important vitamins; and we need it for the functioning of our nerves, muscles, and heart and the regulation of our body temperature. It also helps form the hard enamel on our teeth. Magnesium has one more important function: We need it to help us absorb other minerals, especially calcium.

Certain foods may decrease our absorption of magnesium. These include protein, foods with oxalic acid (like spinach) and alcohol. Cooking can also destroy or remove some of the magnesium in our foods.

If we eat a healthy diet and have two portions of milk products a day (each containing about 30 milligrams of magnesium), two portions of green vegetables (each with 20 to 60 milligrams), and a cup of wheat bran (279 milligrams), bran flakes (102 milligrams), oat flakes (58 milligrams), or brown rice (172 milligrams), and have six ounces of poultry (average 30 to 40 grams) or fish (50 to 100 grams), we can get our needed magnesium and protect our calcium. But if our diet has little fish, no milk products, and is not green- or grain-rich, we might want to add the magnesium when we add our calcium. Women with diabetes seem to be especially prone to magnesium deficiency and might want to discuss special supplementation with their doctors.

EXERCISE: BODY OVER MIND

We're no longer planting fields, gathering firewood, or carrying water from the well, nor does fleetness of foot or physical prowess affect our ability to feed ourselves and protect our families. We're so "developed" that many of us have gotten to the point where we don't even walk. We drive everywhere (and sometimes don't even get out of the car to get or eat our food), use people movers, elevators, and escalators to "advance" in public places, and use our fingers to access the world—through our TVs, computers, and telephones. Our minds have shown us how to abandon the large muscle groups in our bodies. I often wonder if thousands of years of future disuse won't cause us to evolve into heads and hands supported by rudimentary legs (I guess our rears will be our main support; we have to sit on something!). We're told to exercise our minds to succeed. But if we don't exercise our bodies, we'll succeed in putting our minds to rest much too soon through premature illness and mortality.

It's estimated that physical inactivity accounts for 25 percent of all deaths from chronic disease in this country. Add to this the fact that 70 percent of adult women are sedentary or only irregularly active, and we have to conclude that better living through ease is killing us. Since sound advice should be supported with facts, here are some exercise facts that should move us . . .

Cardiovascular Disease

We know what contributes to the failure of our coronary vessels to function in their designated role of cardiac nutrition and maintenance. Most of these factors, except for our declining estrogen, can be positively affected by exercise.

Our Lipid Profile   Exercise lowers our total cholesterol, triglycerides, and "bad" low-density lipoproteins; it raises our "good" high-density lipoproteins.

Hypertension   Exercise lowers our blood pressure.

Obesity   Exercise helps us burn calories. To lose 1 pound, we need to use up 3,500 more calories than we take in. The arithmatic is simple; we need to increase exercise, decrease our intake, or combine the two. This can be done slowly, without even changing our diet. An example given by the American Heart Association is that of a 200-pound person who keeps on eating the same amount of calories, but walks briskly 1.5 miles every day. After one year, she or he will lose about 14 pounds. This may be too slow for those of us who feel weight-challenged. If we want to get more vigorous, we'll be able to burn more calories. Table 17.4 shows the average calories spent per hour by a 150-pound person. Our weight determines the number of calories expended in each activity. For example, a 100-pound person would reduce the listed calories by one third; a 200-pound person would need to multiply them by $1^1/_3$.

Muscles   Aside from keeping us leaner, exercise builds our muscles. The more muscle we have, the higher our metabolic rate. We don't enter the vicious cycle of fat, with its poor use of calories, leading to production of more fat.

Insulin Levels and Diabetes   Exercise lowers our insulin levels. Remember, a high level of insulin promotes the deposition of fatty plaque in our coronary vessels and "encourages" fat to accumulate in our bodies

TABLE 17.4
CALORIES EXPENDED
PER HOUR OF EXERCISE

Bicycling, 6 mph	240
Bicycling, 12 mph	410
Cross-country skiing	700
Jogging, 5½ mph	740
Jogging, 7 mph	920
Jumping rope	750
Running in place	650
Running, 10 mph	1,280
Swimming, 25 yds/min	275
Swimming, 50 yds/min	500
Tennis (singles)	400
Walking, 2 mph	240
Walking, 3 mph	320
Walking, 4½ mph	440

Reproduced from the American Heart
Association Guide.

in the "apple" pattern. High insulin levels can also raise our blood pressure by preventing us from excreting salt through our kidneys. The more we retain salt, the more we retain fluid in our vascular system, and the more our vessels are "under pressure."

Clotting Factors   Exercise increases our fibrinolytic activity, which is our "in-body" clot-buster system that helps dissolve small, but potentially dangerous, clots. Exercise also decreases the adhesiveness of our platelets so they won't stick together and form these clots.

Heart Muscle Tone and Quality   Exercise improves the mechanical performance of our hearts. A "well-conditioned" heart beating 45 to 50 times a minute will circulate the same amount of blood as the average person's heart beating 70 to 75 times a minute. The "average" heart has to pump up to 36,000 more times per day than the "conditioned" heart and 13.1 million more times per year.

Building our cardiac muscles should diminish our risk of heart attack, but it also gives us one more safeguard. If, for some reason, we should have a "coronary accident" and a vessel is blocked, the better the muscle is conditioned, the more likely it will be able to keep pumping. We've reduced the chances that this "accident" will be fatal.

Fitness   A 1989 study of physical fitness (the obvious end result of physical exercise) followed 10,000 men and 3,000 women for eight years. Those whose exercise programs enabled them to perform best on tread-mill exercise tests had an 8-fold decreased risk of death from heart attacks as compared with those who were "unfit." This mortality-to-fitness ratio was the same for both the men and the women. What was also encouraging in this study is that becoming fit occurred without marathon training. A decrease in death rates plateaued with regular moderate exercise—as little as a brisk walk for thirty to sixty minutes a day.

Cancer

Exercise has been found to decrease the incidence of several types of cancer, including colon and breast, possibly by increasing substances that help our cellular immunity, decreasing production of cancer-potentiating substances, and lowering obesity. The same study that related physical fitness to cardiovascular disease showed that women who were fit had an age-adjusted death rate that was six to nine times lower for all cancers than that of unfit women.

Osteoporosis and Muscle Strength

(See chapter 11.)

Menopausal Symptoms

Exercise releases endorphins (our self-made, feel-better "drug"), which may help decrease hot flashes. A Swedish study found that only 6 percent of menopausal women who were physically active had severe hot flashes, whereas 25 percent of women who were inactive sat and suffered.

Does Exercise Keep Us from Aging?

If we consider aging a loss of heart and lung function, frailty from loss of muscle tone and mass, and deformity from osteoporosis, the answer is an emphatic yes. If we're physically fit, we also have a central nervous system edge. Exercise increases blood flow to our brains, improves our reaction times, and in some cases allows us to perform better on mental ability tests. It improves our balance so that we're less likely to fall, break something, and become bedridden. It helps us fall asleep more readily and sleep longer (aging does not have to equate with sleep deprivation and zombie status).

A reactive, alert, and active mind in an active, vital body defies much of what we consider to be aging. Exercise will help keep us young enough to achieve this goal.

How Much and How Hard?

Since science has entered the field of fitness, we expect, or even demand, an "exercise formula." How many hours a week do we need to exercise, and how hard do we need to do it to maintain quality of life and longevity? As busy women, we would like the answer to fit into our time schedule, and as middle-aged or later-aged women, we would prefer not to have to wear skimpy leotards and prance to rap music with 20-year-olds.

Exercise recommendations seem to be changing (and challenging us to keep up) as quickly as our progeny. We used to be told that the "how much" we needed to improve the condition of our hearts and lungs was defined by three factors: raising our heartbeat and breathing rate, maintaining the exercise for thirty to sixty minutes without interruption, and repeating this at least three or four times a week. The "how hard" was calculated as a percentage of the fastest rate our hearts could beat. The ideal activity level would raise our heartbeats to between 50 and 75 percent of this maximum rate. This is called our target heart rate zone (see Table 17.5). We can also get "zoned in" on our maximum heart rate by subtracting our age from 220. If we exercise according to this schedule, we should warm up for five minutes beforehand, with either stretching or a slower-paced exercise, and take five minutes at the end to cool down with the same technique.

This seemed enough to stave off morbidity, at least in men, through

TABLE 17.5   TARGET HEART RATE ZONE

Age	Target Heart Rate 50 to 75% (in beats per minute)	Average Maximum Heart Rate 100%
20	100–150	200
25	98–146	195
30	95–142	190
35	93–138	185
40	90–135	180
45	88–131	175
50	85–127	170
55	83–123	165
60	80–120	160
65	78–116	155
70	75–113	150

1986. A Harvard study published that year reported that *moderate* physical exercise in adult life increased life expectancy. Men who walked, climbed stairs, and participated in sports that caused them to burn 2,000 or more calories a week had death rates one quarter to one third lower than those who were not active. So about 30 percent of us (women) continued our moderate exercise routines with the blessing of the American Heart Association and Harvard. Studies from the Institute of Aerobics Research in Dallas upheld this blessing. Women who went from being unfit to moderately fit had a 50 percent decline in deaths from all causes.

Life was made even easier for those of us who wanted to "move forward" in the world of exercise when, in February 1995, the Centers for Disease Control and Prevention and the American College of Sports Medicine formed a committee (an entity necessary to get consensus between medical experts). It came out with new recommendations: Every U.S. adult should accumulate thirty minutes or more of moderate-intensity physical activity on most, preferably all, days of the week. Unlike the previous American Heart Association recommendations, this committee felt that it was okay to get our exercise in spurts, eight to ten minutes at a time, as long as the spurts added up to thirty minutes and we expended about 200 calories a day. They excused us from formal exercise programs and suggested instead that we walk up stairs (rather than taking an elevator), walk short distances (instead of driving), do calisthenics, garden, do housework (I guess vacuuming is in; sitting and watching the Cuisinart is out), rake leaves, dance, and play actively with children. As long as these activities contributed to our daily thirty-minute total and we performed them at an intensity corresponding to a brisk walk, the committee stated, the program would substantially decrease the 250,000 U.S. deaths per year that are attributable to a lack of regular physical activity.

This program is very "do-able" and is really designed to get the 70 percent of us who don't "actively" exercise to become more fit. The greatest drop in disease and death (50 percent) is with that initial start-up as we go from being unfit to moderately fit. If we choose to do more and become highly fit, we probably improve on that number. How much is not clear, since "maximum" exercise was much more likely to have been evaluated in men than in women.

The male-dominated world of fitness and sports was quite upset by the latest Harvard study published in April 1995. Questionnaires were sent to over 21,000 alumni (men—no Radcliffe graduates were included), who provided self-evaluations of their exercise habits. *Only* those men who spent years performing three or more hours a week of vigorous exercise (which caused them to sweat) had a decreased risk of dying that was 0.75 to 0.87 that of men who did nonvigorous or no exercise. The authors were somewhat at a loss to explain this, but went on to say that they believe that "even nonvigorous exercise is preferable to sedentariness."

So which study, statistics, and recommendations do we consider to be most valid for our fitness and health? What is our feminine "exercise-ique"? The answer is similar to that given by the beleaguered authors of this latest Harvard exercise and longevity study. Some is better than none; more is probably best. Minimally, we should fit ourselves into an exercise routine that gives us a total of thirty minutes of moderate exercise (see Table 17.6) most every day. While we're doing this, we increase our consumption of oxygen to three to six times that which we use at rest, and we burn 4 to 7 calories a minute. This should be manageable for all of us and promotes us to the CDC category of moderately fit. Statistically (and, more important, individually), this should decrease our future chance of disease and mortality by as much as 50 percent. Since calisthenics and conditioning exercise are listed in this moderate category, they should account for at least two sessions a week for a minimum of fifteen minutes; that's half of our "allotted" exercise for the day. That means using weight-resisting machines or free weights. It's recommended that if we're novices, we start with weights that we can comfortably lift or move for fifteen repetitions (and two to three sets of these repetitions should be performed). With time, weight is added in 5 percent increments until it's too hard to complete ten repetitions. At that point, the weight is too heavy and should be decreased. Most gyms will give one or two free training sessions to entice us to join. At some point, we should be comfortable on our own or may find we can duplicate these exercises with free weights at home. If we want to go for "more fit," we can build up to the previous program suggested by the American Heart Association and the Academy of Sports Medicine. This involves twenty to sixty

TABLE 17.6 SUGGESTED EXERCISE

Moderate (4 to 7 calories per minute)	Hard/Vigorous (more than 7 calories per minute)
Walking, briskly (3 to 4 mph)	Walking, briskly uphill or with a load
Cycling for pleasure or transportation (less than 10 mph)	Cycling, fast or racing (more than 10 mph)
Swimming, moderate effort	Swimming, fast treading or crawl
Conditioning exercise, general calisthenics	Conditioning exercise, stair ergometer, ski machine
Racket sports, table tennis	Racket sports, singles tennis, racketball
Golf, pulling cart or carrying clubs	
Fishing, standing/casting	Fishing in stream
Canoeing, leisurely (2.0 to 3.9 mph)	Canoeing, rapidly (3 to 4 mph)
Home care, general cleaning	Moving furniture
Mowing lawn, power mower	Mowing lawn, hand mower
Home repair, painting	

Data from Ainsworth *et al.*; Leon and McCardie, *et al.*

minutes of moderate- to high-intensity endurance exercise performed three or more times a week (see Table 17.6). These activities raise our oxygen consumption to more than six times what we burn at rest, use more than 7 calories a minute, and raise our heart rate to 60 to 90 percent of its maximum (at our age, we probably should be trained athletes before we go over 75 percent). We should spend at least five minutes warming up and cooling down, and always stretch. Again, adding weight-resistance exercise twice a week will give us a break from this strenuous regimen and also build the muscles and bones we don't stress, even if we're aerobically superior.

Despite the many controversies, it's clear that fitness can be achieved by many measures, great and small. As long as we're aware of our choices, we can "fit" the program that allows consistency and enjoyment into our lives and our ongoing woman care.

Stop! In the Name of Life

Admittedly, this title is presumptuous, but what we stop doing in our midlife may ultimately be more important than what we do. Stopping is not just an absence of action. For most of us, it's a tremendous effort in self-discipline and habit reversal, especially when applied to obesity, smoking, and excessive consumption of alcohol and caffeine. Here are some facts that can motivate us to stop in our (bad habit) tracks.

OBESITY: IS THIS A SIN OF OVEREATING?

Thin women obviously eat right, and those of us with weight problems don't. We bear the ultimate responsibility for our poundage; we're gluttons, give in to our cravings, and we're lazy. Buying clothes that are size 16 or larger is the price we pay for these psychologic weaknesses. This has been the weight message that has been "pounded" into our psyches for decades. Consequently, we feel that if we just eat the right foods and get onto the right program (and about $50 million are spent yearly by those of us in search of these foods and programs), we could express the thin souls trapped in our overweight bodies. But if this is just a situation of mental turpitude and "all" we have to do is overcome bad eating habits, why do 90 to 95 percent of us fail to maintain our weight loss for five years? Most cancers have a far better five-year cure rate!

Medical studies have provided us with some fascinating information that indicates that weight excess is not necessary indulgent excess. Our appetite, cravings, choice of foods, and body build are a complex mix of genetic, neurologic, physiologic, and psychologic factors. We can work on some of these, but there is no single "fixable" factor or solution. We certainly can't moralize obesity away. More than 37 percent of us are overweight, and this number rises with age until we're 80 (see Table 17.7). Does a preponderance of "weighty" women make obesity our midage norm? Not if it's a cause of significant abnormal diseases such as diabetes, high blood pressure, coronary heart disease, stroke, arthritis, and some forms of cancer. We spend over $39 billion a year in health-care costs because of obesity. That's a financial norm that is far too heavy.

WEIGHT FACTS

In medical terms, we're obese if we're 20 percent over our desirable weight. (Desirable here means average; it's defined as the midpoint in the range of weights of a woman with a medium frame based on the 1983

TABLE 17.7
PERCENTAGE OF WOMEN
WHO ARE OVERWEIGHT

Age	Percentage of Overweight Women
30–39	34.3
40–49	37.6
50–59	52.0
60–69	42.5
70–79	37.2
80 and over	26.2

Journal of the American Medical Association, The National Health and Nutrition Examination Surveys.

TABLE 17.8 AVERAGE DESIRABLE WEIGHTS FOR WOMEN

Height	Small Frame	Medium Frame	Large Frame
4'10"	102–111	109–121	118–130
4'11"	103–113	111–123	120–134
5'0"	104–115	113–126	122–137
5'1"	106–118	115–129	125–140
5'2"	108–121	118–132	128–143
5'3"	111–124	121–135	131–147
5'4"	114–127	124–138	134–151
5'5"	117–130	127–141	137–155
5'6"	120–133	130–144	140–159
5'7"	123–136	133–147	143–163
5'8"	126–139	136–150	146–167
5'9"	129–142	139–153	149–170
5'10"	132–145	142–156	152–173
5'11"	135–148	145–159	155–176
6'0"	139–151	148–162	158–179

Source: Metropolitan Life Insurance Company.
These are "dressed" figures—women wearing indoor clothing and one-inch heels. (I guess it wasn't proper to take off our shoes and clothes to get weighed in 1983.)

Metropolitan Life Insurance Company Height and Weight tables; see Table 17.8.)

We deviate from these Metropolitan weight norms as we decrease our exercise, have our babies, follow our genetic patterns, and, yes, overeat. Our weight at 18 seems to set standards for problems to come. According to the data from the Harvard Nurses' Study, we double our risk of diabetes and increase our risk of coronary heart disease by 50 percent by simply gaining 11 to 17 pounds from the age of 18. Diabetes increases 2.5-fold if we gain 17 to 24 pounds. If we go up 45 pounds or more by our fifties, we increase our risk of hypertension and heart disease by a factor of 3, diabetes by a factor of 10, and gallstones by a factor of 4, compared to women who gain only 10 pounds. (As bad as it sounds, the magnitude of these risks is still less than that associated with smoking!) Further analysis of the Nurses' Study showed that one-third of cancer deaths and more than half of cardiovascular deaths in these women (who were followed for sixteen years) were due to obesity. The lowest mortality rate was found in women who weighed less than the U.S. "average" for women of similar age, or whose weight had not changed from early adulthood. Our averages may be "overages."

As we go through adulthood and our pregnancies, we set our fat levels through our *adipose*-stat (adipose is a medical term for fat). This is the central fat setting that is present in the hypothalamus of our brains. If we lower our calories once this fat monitor is set, it "sets" about correcting the situation by ordering the body to recalibrate itself and expend less energy to "save" what it "thinks" is the right fat content. Genetically, some of us may have a predetermined "high" fat setting or an obesity gene that issues the "wrong" orders to our fat monitor. There appears to be a protein or satiety factor that signals our brain with information about our bodies' store of fat tissue. One such substance is a hormone that has been identified in mice; it's called leptin, and scientists have found the mouse gene that controls leptin production. They're certain that mice and men (and, of course, women) are alike in possessing this gene and gene product. If the gene is defective, resulting in inadequate production of leptin, or if there is a genetic insensitivity to this satiety hormone so that leptin is not "read" by the brain's fat center, we lose our internal weight control.

Pharmaceutical companies are aggressively working to develop medications that could work like leptin or improve our brain's sensitivity to leptin. Their leap into leptin is obviously propelled by expectations of enormous profit.

CAN WE RESET OUR FAT SETTINGS?

Yes, if we're willing to do it slowly and don't expect an immediate "skinny fix" from our diet experts or ourselves. If we go on a very-low-calorie diet, we might lose weight quickly, but we can't continue a state of nutritional deprivation for prolonged periods. Our body won't let us; it just readjusts to lower our caloric needs. Hence, our 90 to 95 percent five-year failure rate (and the term "yo-yo diets"). But if we're willing to attempt to change our eating patterns, increase exercise, and go for the realistic goal of 5 to 10 percent decrease in our body weight, most of us can do it. This loss might not put us into a size 8 dress, but it will give us a healthier body composition.

TAKING IT OFF ON OUR OWN

If we're not clinically obese, but want to take off the 11 to 17 pounds we've gained over the last few decades, we can do the usual: cut our calories to 1,000 to 1,200 a day and increase our exercise. The composition of what we should eat for this weight loss is still under debate. The American Diabetes Association recommends a diet rich in fiber (up to 25 grams per 1,000 calories a day) composed of 60 percent carbohydrates, 20 percent fat, and 20 percent protein. This may not always accomplish our goal of losing fat without losing muscle. Studies have shown that a higher-protein diet with 45 percent protein, 35 percent carbohydrates, and 20 percent fat will do this, especially if we belong to the 25 percent of the population that has developed some degree of insulin resistance. For those of us who don't lose weight despite caloric deprivation on our high-carbohydrate, low-fat, low-protein diet, this is a very reasonable "new" approach. Our ideal weight loss should be 1 to 2 pounds a week. We'll probably reach an impasse where this weight loss decreases as our bodies readjust to this lower energy input. If we want to keep the weight off, we'll have to maintain our exercise program and a caloric balance that may be lower than that calculated for naturally thinner women who are not attempting to reset their adipose stats (this is an unfair burden, but so is our weight).

TAKING IT OFF WITH HELP

If we're clinically obese or need to lose more than 25 pounds, we should consult a physician for proper monitoring during our more heroic attempts. Very-low-calorie diets (800 calories or less) can result in a lack of essential nutrients, dehydration, electrolyte imbalance, and even death. Trying on our own to use commercial drinks and powders without adding the meal they advise on the label might make us drop pounds faster, but could result in us simply dropping. The problem with these diets is that we cannot continue them indefinitely, and as we reintroduce real food (and this should be done with medical supervision), our literally starved bodies go into a state of constant craving. This translates into a need to overeat and the body's tendency to store reaccumulated fat (after all, our adipose-stats never know when our poor bodies will once more be put in such a terrible state of deprivation).

DIET PILLS: IS THIS THE HELP WE NEED?

If an antibiotic can cure a bacterial infection, why can't we take a pill to reset our adipose stats (or at least block the instructions of that "dumb" fat controller so we can curb our appetite and increase our metabolism)? The issue is that we are not dealing with a temporary disorder akin to strep throat, which we cure with a short course of penicillin. The problem is chronic, so if we're looking to use medications, we'll have to use them for the long run (and, hopefully, while we're running as exercise).

In the past, our diet pills were the "classic" amphetamines, which would temporarily suppress our appetite and speed up our metabolism (and everything else). We couldn't sleep, our hands trembled, and we chanced addiction. New research on old, preexisting drugs has given us insight into long-term appetite suppression that doesn't wreak havoc on our nervous system. Two of these anorectic (appetite suppressant) drugs have been tested for over three and a half years. One is phentermine, which increases the neurotransmitters dopamine and norepinephrine (these give signals that are necessary for many of the essential functions of our bodies, including our heartbeat, blood flow, and reaction to stress). This drug has been tested in combination with fenfluramine, which acts on another neurotransmitter, serotonin. Increased levels of serotonin reduce our feelings of deprivation and hunger and improve our mood. One reason we're obese may be that we're serotonin-deficient. If we increase our serotonin levels, we feel satiated, but we may also feel sleepy and slow. Phentermine is a stimulant and can counteract this effect. In turn, the fenfluramine prevents this stimulant from causing anxiety and sleeplessness. When we combine the two, we get a yin-and-yang effect on our nervous system that permits appetite control and little else.

A major four-year study on these medications was carried out by Dr. Michael Weintraub at the University of Rochester School of Medicine and Dentistry. He took a group of 121 obese people (two thirds of them women) who were 50 percent or more over their ideal body weight. They were all put on the typical caloric restriction of 1,000 to 1,200 calories a day and exercise programs three times a week where they expended 300 calories. He then divided them into two groups, medicated and nonmedicated, and followed them for thirty-four weeks. Those who received fenfluramine and phentermine lost an average of nearly 15.9 percent of their initial weight (more than 25 pounds), and those who took a placebo lost only 4.9 percent (or less than 10 pounds). The most common side effect was dry mouth. Some medicated dieters complained of fatigue, sleep disturbances, nightmares, dizziness, nervousness, sadness, and decreased libido. Most of these complaints stopped after four to six weeks of treatment (other patients outside the study have also complained of mental "fogginess," decreased motivation, and loss of short-term memory).

After thirty-four weeks, all of the participants in Dr. Weintraub's study were given the active drugs, some continuously and others starting and then stopping them. Meanwhile, they also continued their diet and exercise. He found that the intermittent group would start to gain weight as soon as they stopped "fen" and "phen," but that they could catch up with the weight loss of the continuous users if they restarted these drugs. The problem was that each time they restarted, they had some of the side effects listed above. It became evident that if the drugs are to be used for continued weight loss, they should be used continuously. The participants were allowed to stay on "fen" and "phen" for three and a half years. They were then followed for another five months, during which time these patient dieters continued their caloric restrictions, behavior modification, and exercise. They gained back most of their weight. After four years of dieting, they were only 3 to 5 pounds below the weights with which they had begun the study (many had also dropped out; only 48 remained out of the original 110). Only 13 were still 5 percent below their initial weights, and just 7 dieters had achieved a 10 percent or greater weight loss. This means that even after three and a half years, most of these initially obese individuals did not reset their weight control mechanisms. Dr. Weintraub believed that at least their new behavior modifications helped prevent these men and women from gaining more weight during this period and that they diminished their risk factors while they were losing weight. Ultimately, they also improved their health with diet and exercise.

Those of us who decide to use these anorectics won't be on a strict four-year study. We can start, lose weight, and possibly adjust the dosage of the medication as needed (increase it if we start to gain weight, decrease it if we're at a desired level or have side effects). We can also taper doses, continue our healthy dietary and exercise routines, and restart treatments months or years later at times of unacceptable weight gain. We probably need to consider this a chronic, ongoing therapy and, like our thyroid medication, we'll need to use it forever. This type of use has not been approved by the FDA, whose literature states that the medication should be given for twelve weeks at a time. So physicians who prescribe this will be doing so "off-label," which is acceptable as long as we are under their close supervision. None of us should cavalierly enter this world of improved thinness through chemistry. Three and a half years of follow-up without serious complications is encouraging but no match for decades of experience with tens of thousands of women. Our only experience is decades of uncured obesity, and we know what a medical calamity that can be . . .

Dexfenfluramine

An additional serotonin-affecting, appetite-suppressing, weight-loss-enhancing, and hence news-promoting drug has just been approved by the FDA. Its generic name is dexfenfluramine, and it is a chemical variant of fenfluramine (technically, it's an active isomer). This drug inhibits reuptake of serotonin and creates a higher "serotonin milieu" for the synapses or communication links of the brain. This improved central world of serotonin helps reduce our appetite and, in turn, our body weight.

Studies have shown that dexfenfluramine can be effective when other weight reduction strategies have failed. It can help maintain weight loss as well as "correct" disturbed eating patterns (such as snacking on carbohydrates) that are associated with PMS, seasonal affective disorder, and nicotine withdrawal (translation: some of us could use it after ovulation; others, after the fall [season]).

Dexfenfluramine may do more than "just" diminish hunger; it appears to improve lipid profiles and glucose metabolism and has been used to help some insulin-dependent diabetic patients control their blood sugars. There are, of course, side effects, and these are similar to those of its cousin fenfluramine: sleepiness, dry mouth, headache, nausea, and diarrhea. Most symptoms are reported to diminish with time. Like other anorectics, this drug works as long as we continue to take it (although it may peak in its effectiveness after six months). Once we stop medicating our weight control we tend to lose control and the pounds creep back. We have not been cured but may have been helped in our ongoing struggle to achieve a more ideal weight, figure, and health.

We're too young to become obese, and it would appear that our model of STOP has to begin from early adulthood. Our forties and future decades have to be a continuation of this battle of the bulge. If we don't add fat, we won't let it settle into our bodies as a standard for our internal fat controls.

Smoking: Converting Our Bodies to Toxic Waste

This chapter (indeed, the entire book) has been devoted to woman care, yet nearly a quarter of us (23.5 percent, to be exact) don't care enough to stop inhaling 4,000 chemicals that waste our bodies. If we've heard it once, we should hear it four thousand times: Smoking is the number-one cause of preventable death in this country. Just to put us into the right mortality perspective, illicit drug use accounts for less than 1 percent of deaths in this country; motor vehicle accidents 1 percent; firearms 2 percent; alcohol 5 percent; and tobacco 19 percent. Another horrifying way of putting it: smoking accounts for nearly 1 in 5 deaths among those of us between the ages of 35 and 64. If we smoke, our average life expectancy at 30 is 17.9 years shorter than that of our contemporaries who have never smoked (we certainly won't be contemporaries in our old age).

These are some of the diseases we and our daughters (most adults begin to smoke before the age of 20) can look forward to as the tobacco companies help us to come a long way—in our self-destruction.

Cardiovascular Disease   We estimate that one fifth of all deaths from cardiovascular disease are due to smoking. The chemicals of cigarette smoke "waste" our blood vessels and heart muscles in a number of interacting ways (one chemical may help another, and with 4,000, that's a lot of combinations and permutations).

The Nurses' Health Study has shown that smoking "just" one to four cigarettes a day was associated with a 2-fold increase in the risk of coronary artery disease. Five to fourteen cigarettes a day increased that risk 2- to 3-fold, and 25 cigarettes a day was associated with a 5.5 relative risk of fatal heart attack, 5.8 risk for nonfatal heart attack, and 2.6 risk for angina (versus 1 for nonsmokers).

Stroke   Most of what smoking does to the vessels of our heart is also occurring to the blood vessels supplying our brains. In the Nurses' Study, current smokers of just one to fourteen cigarettes a day have more than a

2.5 times increased risk of stroke compared with nonsmokers. This risk increases to 3.7 for those who smoke twenty-four or more cigarettes a day.

Cancer   Smoking damages our cellular DNA and causes the cells that line our airways to become atypical. Ninety-three percent of smokers versus 6.0 percent of ex-smokers, and 1.2 percent of people who never smoked, have these damaged airway cells. When this atypia goes "all the way," the cells become cancerous. Smoking is responsible for over 85 percent of lung cancers. This disease is now the number-one cause of cancer death in women, killing 62,000 of us in 1995.

The carcinogenic affect of inhaled chemicals doesn't stop with our lungs. As we smoke, we swallow many of these chemicals, which increase our risk of cancers of the mouth (by 2 to 18 times), pharynx and larynx (82 percent of these cancers are due to smoking), esophagus (80 percent are due to smoking), and stomach. From our gastrointestinal tract, the chemicals get to our pancreas, and we have an increase in pancreatic cancer. Excretion of these toxins occurs through our kidneys, ureter, and bladder. All of these "exposed" urological organs are made more susceptible to cancer. The chemicals that are not excreted in our urine are absorbed in our blood and some, like benzene, are associated with leukemias. Breast cancer rates may be 60 percent higher in long-term smokers. A Danish study showed that the median age of smokers with breast cancer was eight years younger than that of nonsmokers. Thirty percent of cervical cancers are probably due to by-products of cigarettes that are concentrated in our cervical mucus (decreasing our local immunity so that we're more susceptible to HPV infections). When we add these up, smoking accounts for about 30 percent of all our deaths from cancer! If we smoke, we're twice as likely to develop cancer as nonsmokers, and if we smoke heavily, that factor increases to four. Stopping is the most effective "treatment" we have to prevent our most feared disease.

Lung Disease   Coroners can look at the lungs of a smoker and figure out how many years and how many packs it took to tar and destroy them. We suffer from chronic inflammations of our airways that decrease our ability to breathe long before our lungs end up as pathology specimens. In clinical terms, we're developing recurrent pneumonias, bronchitis, and emphysema. Seventy-nine percent of chronic lung disease in women is caused by cigarette smoking. A constant oxygen "hookup" may be the only way many of us can continue to survive. Even this won't help the 84,000 men and women who die yearly from their nonventilating lungs.

Early Menopause   Those of us who smoke experience menopause one to two years earlier than nonsmokers, perhaps because tobacco smoke has a toxic affect on our ovaries.

Osteoporosis   Smokers not only enter menopause earlier but also lose bone mass at a faster rate in the first years after this transition (see chapter 11).

Pregnancy Loss and Complications   Smoking reduces our fertility (and the number of years we remain fertile) and increases our rate of miscarriage and other complications of pregnancy (see chapter 4).

Cataracts   If the smoke we exhale doesn't cloud our vision, cataracts will. Studies suggest that about 20 percent of cataracts are due to smoking.

Thyroid Disease   Cyanide is a component of tobacco smoke (we really are talking poisons here!) It diminishes our thyroid's ability to take up iodide and synthesize thyroid hormone. Those of us who already have low thyroid hormone levels may have a worsening of this condition. Smokers seem to be more prevalent among women suffering from Graves' disease and they are more likely to have the bulging eyes associated with this disease.

Aging   Smoking can age our skin by ten years or more. The toxins in cigarette smoke damage the small vessels that nourish our skin (especially around our lips and eyes). These chemicals also lower our estrogen level, which, in turn, causes a loss of our skin's collagen content and the resulting "pruniness." We not only look old before our time, but as time passes and we're over the age of 65, those of us who smoke lose our balance and have weakened physical performance. Essentially, we're cosmetically ten years older and physically five years older than our chronological age if we smoke. We're also more likely to be dead; the rate of mortality for smokers over 65 is twice that of nonsmokers.

Passive Smoking   Smoking has become an environmental issue. It's not enough that we individually decide to stop as part of our woman care, but if we don't get cigarette smoke out of the air we breathe, we are all, by default, at fault for significant health abuse. Here are some facts about environmental tobacco smoke that the tobacco companies don't want us to know.

There are two kinds of environmental tobacco smoke: mainstream smoke, which is exhaled by the smoker, and sidestream smoke, which is emitted from the burning tobacco between puffs. It's the sidestream smoke that does most of the polluting of our air, since it hasn't been "cleared" by the unfortunate lungs of the smoker. It contains more small particles, which are likely to be deposited in our "nonsmoking" lungs. This sidestream smoke may actually have a higher concentration of some toxins and carcinogens than the smoke inhaled by a smoker. What's most worrisome is that we nonsmokers have not adapted to what these toxins can do, and when we're exposed to them, they "do it" out of proportion to their absolute quantity. Sidestream smoke generates the most carbon monoxide, which, when the rest of us breathe it, reduces our blood's ability to carry oxygen. Our heart's energy potential is also diminished. The enzyme that converts oxygen to cardiac energy is reduced (or smoked out) by 25 percent in animals exposed to just thirty minutes of secondhand smoke. If this exposure is repeated daily for eight weeks, the enzyme activity is reduced by half!

Secondhand smoke is responsible for 30,000 to 60,000 heart disease deaths a year and three times as many nonfatal heart attacks and strokes. It causes us, the nonsmokers, to have most of the problems and complications that occur to smokers (without even trying). The tobacco companies often tell us that secondhand smoke will be no more harmful than smoking "just" one cigarette. If we already have heart disease, this one cigarette increases our risk of heart attack by 30 percent and our risk of dying from it by 70 percent. "A little goes a long way" also applies to our risk of cancer. Environmental tobacco smoke has been classified as a known human carcinogen.

Children do very poorly when we expose their developing lungs to tobacco smoke. Between 150,000 and 300,000 infants and young children who breathe smoke develop bronchitis and pneumonia. They also have an increase in middle-ear problems and colds. Smoking parents cause an estimated 26,000 new cases of asthma in their children each year, and the 1 million children in this country who have asthma suffer more frequent and severe attacks due to their environmental exposure to tobacco smoke.

Passive smoking is our third leading preventable cause of death. The fight to eliminate it has become dirty, but while we fight for freedom (the smokers want the freedom to light up; the nonsmokers want tobacco-free air), let's remember where the real dirt lies—in the smoke given off by burning tobacco.

STOPPING: THE GAINS JUSTIFY ALL EFFORTS

When used "as directed," this product lays waste to our bodies. When we stop, our bodies miraculously repair most of these ravages. Our risk of heart attack is rapidly reduced after just one year of quitting, and after ten years, that risk is essentially the same as a nonsmoker's. Our risk of lung cancer is reduced, but this takes a longer time (probably because we are already dealing with the early cancers that are developing from the carcinogens we inhaled ten to fifteen years ago). After fifteen years, our "retained" risk is reduced 80 to 90 percent. Our risk of other cancers is reduced even more, approaching that of those who have never smoked. If we stop smoking, our 2.5 increased risk of stroke is reduced and almost equals that of nonsmokers after four years.

It's never too early or too late to stop smoking. If we quit before the age of 50, we decrease our risk of dying of smoke-related illnesses by 50 percent over the next fifteen years. If we're already over the age of 65, cessation of smoking reverses our doubled mortality rates.

Ways to Stop: How to Succeed by Really Trying

The nicotine in cigarettes has been declared by the Surgeon General to be as addictive as heroin! Many of the symptoms of nicotine withdrawal are similar to those experienced by illicit drug withdrawal—anxiety, awakening during sleep, depression, difficulty concentrating, impatience, irritability, anger, and restlessness. These symptoms peak after two days and diminish after two weeks. It appears that we're far more nicotine-vulnerable (or addictable, if there is such a word) than men. We metabolize this substance more slowly and need fewer cigarettes than men to reach the same nicotine blood levels. Not surprisingly, it may be harder for us to stop.

It's as difficult for a smoker to listen to advice from a nonsmoker as it is for the obese to be counseled by the thin. This reference to weight is not accidental. Many of us started smoking to control our weight, and now the fear of weight gain keeps us puffing. About two thirds of smokers who quit will gain weight, but the average weight gain is less than 5 pounds. It appears that smoking decreases our bodies' weight set point and that once we stop, this goes up. Putting food into our mouths to make up for cigarette cravings will also contribute to this weight gain. As nasty as it sounds, our increased weight has less adverse impact on our health than our state of smoking toxification. We would have to gain 75 pounds to equal the harm we do to our bodies by smoking!

There are numerous programs that have been devised to help us in our quest to stop smoking. They share some common guidelines:

Motivation   That's what this preceding section is all about. The facts are convincing enough that 75 percent of all smokers report they want to stop (the other 25 percent must think they're invincible!).

Access to Available Treatments   There's a lot out there to help us—group therapy, behavior modification plans, hypnosis, acupuncture, and relaxation techniques. The American Cancer Society will provide lists of local programs, as well as written information which they will mail at the "drop" of a toll-free phone call (1-800-ACS-2345).

A Quit Date   Once we've set this, we should let everyone we know, know.

Coping with Nicotine Withdrawal   The world of better living through pharmacology has entered our nicotine war by supplying us with prescribed doses of this substance. We no longer have to go "cold turkey" (I'm not quite sure what a chilled fowl has to do with withdrawal symptoms!). Nicotine can be provided through chewing gum, which has just become available "over the counter" (but probably not on the gum and Life Savers counter). If this type of nicotine substitution isn't palatable, prescription patches can be used. These maintain our nicotine levels without the tar, carbon monoxide, and the other 3,998 chemicals found in cigarettes. This form of nicotine substitution is expensive (the patches cost $30 to $35 a week). Nicotine patches can be worn for either sixteen or twenty-four hours and are recommended for daily use up to twenty weeks. The twenty-four-hour patch may cause vivid dreams (most of us are not used to smoking in our sleep). This problem is lessened with the sixteen-hour patch. But a continuous twenty-four-hour nicotine supply will minimize the early-morning craving for that first cigarette (which seems to be the most satisfying for many smokers). The larger-size patches (21 milligrams) provide a steady replacement of approximately 50 percent of the average nicotine level that would be present if we smoked one to one and a half packs of cigarettes a day. After four to six weeks the dose can be reduced. Both cigarettes and the patch share the same adverse nicotine effects: They raise our heart rate about 10 beats per minute and our blood pressure by 5 points. So we shouldn't kid ourselves that because it is prescribed and not available from vending machines that long-term use of the patch is "okay." What is okay is that we're twice as likely to be successful in our efforts to stop smoking if we temporarily use these nicotine systems.

Coping with Initial Failure   If, by four weeks, we're still smoking and using the patch, we're in trouble, for two reasons. First, we're increasing our blood nicotine levels through two sources, and this can potentially increase our risk of heart attack and stroke. Second, we are doomed to failure for this treatment schedule. There is no sense in continuing the patch this time.

Try Again   It may take two or three attempts before we succeed in making such a drastic reversal of "miss"-fortune. But once we do, we have taken the most important step we can ever make to improve our health and increase our life span.

Alcohol: Do We Drink for Our Hearts or Abstain for Our Breasts?

We can look at alcohol in so many ways: As an adjunct to roses and romance, as a fattening source of "empty" calories (at 7 calories a gram), as a nutrient that has a positive effect on our stress, as a medicinal substance that may decrease our incidence of heart attack, as a potentiator of breast cancer and bone degeneration, or as a cause of inebriation, auto accidents, and death.

BACCHUS WAS A MAN

We're much more susceptible to the wrath of fermented grapes and grains than men. We produce fewer enzymes to break down alcohol in our stomachs, so when we drink alcohol, we're more likely to absorb a higher percentage in its raw potent form (as ethanol). This goes straight into our bloodstream, whence it quickly reaches our brain, and since our blood–brain perfusion also seems to be more rapid (or better) than men's, we get a central nervous system "bang" faster. Add to this the fact that we're generally smaller than men and have less blood to dilute the ethanol, and one drink can "do" for us what two do for the opposite sex.

No matter who's drinking it, one shot of hard liquor in a standard drink equals a glass of wine or a can of beer. These each contain about 14.8 milliliters of ethanol. Two of these drinks equal 25 grams. If we have two drinks in two hours and weigh 150 pounds, our blood alcohol level will be at least 0.05, which, in many states, is above the legal limit for driving. If we weigh less, we'll "get there" (and may be arrested for drunk driving if we don't kill or get killed on the road) with less!

There may be times when we all go above our personal or legal limits, but that doesn't mean that this places us into one of two chronic categories: alcohol abuse (when drinking impairs our life function) or alcohol dependence (when the same impairment continues together with an unremitting compulsion to continue to use alcohol). Biologic and genetic factors affect our tolerance of alcohol and our susceptibility to dependence. If a parent or sibling is an alcoholic, we're four times more likely to be at risk for this disease. But despite the similar genetic propensities to our brothers, we're one fourth as likely to be heavy drinkers as men. This, however, should not be heralded as a female triumph over alcoholism. Because of our decreased alcohol tolerance, we're unfairly destined to suffer the health consequences more quickly and completely than men. These include high blood pressure, stroke, heart disease, anemia, malnutrition, gastrointestinal hemorrhage, early menopause (obviously not a male worry), and finally, cirrhosis and liver failure. The mortality rate for alcoholic women is increased by a factor of 4.5, and life expectancy is cut short by an average of fifteen years (being too young to get old becomes a moot point; we don't get old if we're alcoholics).

LIGHT TO MODERATE DRINKING: "L'CHAIM" ("TO LIFE")

The question for most of us is not whether or not we should abuse alcohol, but whether light to moderate consumption is good or bad for our health. Since so much of this section on STOP has been negative, let's look at some of the positive health benefits that have made the wine and liquor industry very happy.

The Nurses' Study showed that moderate consumption of alcohol can be good for our hearts. One to three drinks a week was associated with a decrease in deaths from heart attack by 17 percent compared to that of nondrinkers, and one-half to two drinks a day afforded a 12 percent benefit. More than two drinks a day canceled this cardiac advantage, and the nurses had a 19 percent increase in their death rate, usually from nonvascular diseases such as breast cancer and cirrhosis. When the study looked at those women who were 50 or older, the light to moderate drinkers had a very pronounced 41 percent decrease in their risk of fatal heart attack, but only if they had one or more risk factors for coronary artery disease (such factors included high cholesterol, diabetes, high blood pressure, smoking, and heart attack of a parent before age 60). There was, however, no appreciable reduction in total mortality among women without these coronary risk factors. Other studies using coronary heart disease and not death as the end point found that women who consumed one-half to two drinks a day had a 20 to 40 percent decrease in their risk of heart disease, compared with nondrinkers, but again risk seems to play a part in alcohol's "protection." For example, smokers had a 30 percent reduction in risk while nonsmokers had a 10 percent reduction. A drink a day "to save our hearts" may work only if our hearts are at risk.

How imbibed alcohol imbues this cardiac protection is under scientific investigation (a grant to do research on this topic in the South of France would be a delightful "grapefall" for interested researchers). Alcohol appears to raise two of the components of high-density lipoproteins, and this may account for about 50 percent of the reduction of our risk in heart attack. The other 50 percent may be due to alcohol's relaxing effect on the smooth muscles of our cardiac vessels. Alcohol also reduces clot formation, an attribute that is good for heart attacks, but bad for hemorrhagic strokes. Indeed, there is an increase in these strokes in women who are moderate to heavy drinkers. Red wine may have a special cardiac effect; it seems to have nutrients that diminish low-density lipoprotein adherence to plaque in our vessels. Scientists have used this to explain the relative low incidence of heart disease and heart attack among Europeans (especially the French, who drink large amounts of red wine and may have diets that are quite high in cholesterol—the proverbial red wine and cheese).

A DRINK OR TWO WON'T KEEP
OTHER DISEASES (AND PROBLEMS) AWAY

Cancer   In 1987 two major studies demonstrating a link between women's alcohol consumption and increased rates of breast cancer grabbed headlines everywhere (see page 258).

Osteoporosis   Alcohol affects the health of our bones in many ways, from inhibiting our absorption of calcium to increasing our risk for falls. (see chapter 11).

Alcohol and Pregnancy: This Is Never a Mix   Mild to moderate drinking increases our risk of miscarriage, fetal growth retardation, and fetal malformation (see chapter 4).

AA: Alcohol and Accidents   While we're listing the adverse effects of alcohol on our health, it's imperative that we consider the issue of drinking and driving. Motor vehicle accidents are the leading cause of death in this country for children and young adults (this includes ages 1 to 34), and half of these traffic accidents are alcohol-related. Forty percent of us will be involved in a car crash involving an intoxicated driver during our lives.

Caffeine: Espresso, Cappuccino, Osteoporoso?

Caffeine is our most commonly used legal psychoactive substance. It stimulates our central nervous system, temporarily raising our blood pressure and increasing our heart rate. Many of us "need it" to get up, become alert, and keep going. We get 80 percent of our caffeine through coffee, and over 80 percent of us consume doses that qualify as behavioral stimulants. Our average daily consumption of caffeine is about 280 milligrams, which translates into about two and a half 6-ounce cups of brewed coffee (but maybe less if it's strong espresso or cappuccino). Our sources of caffeine are numerous and ubiquitous (see Table 17.9). Does this natural alkaloid, which provides us with the pleasures of taste and aroma, stimulation, and socialization (in short, what they promise us in the coffee commercials minus the donkey), have to be categorized as medically "incorrect"? Will Seattle's economy and fame have to rely on software, grunge rock, and Boeing?

Let's sip our coffee and peruse the medical areas of caffeine concern . . .

Osteoporosis   Caffeine increases our urinary loss of calcium. It may also directly affect our bones, reducing bone remodeling and calcium turnover. If we get enough calcium, we may negate these caffeine effects.

Heart Disease   Caffeine temporarily raises our blood pressure and increases our heart rate. Fortunately, however, coffee consumption doesn't seem to be associated with the development of high blood pressure, probably because our bodies quickly develop a tolerance to its blood pressure effects. Some studies have implicated coffee in elevating our cholesterol levels, but it turns out that only boiled coffee has this potential, and it doesn't occur if the coffee is dripped through a filter.

Coffee may be associated with palpitations and abnormal changes in our cardiac rhythm. Eliminating coffee helps controls these arrhythmias, but that seems to be the only heart-related problem we can blame on "normal" consumption of caffeine.

For those of us who like the taste of coffee, but want to avoid caffeine, there were some "disheartening" decaf data coming from a Harvard study. Decaffeinated coffee was the only type of coffee correlating with some increased risk for heart attack and stroke. A Stanford study showed that drinking more than three cups of decaffeinated coffee a day raised LDL cholesterol levels. (I have to report that I'm actually drinking a cup of decaf coffee as I write this.)

Breast Disease   Caffeine is a harmless-sounding term, but the minute we give it a more chemical description as a methylxanthine compound, its tenor becomes more sinister. Whatever we call it, it has been found to inhibit certain enzyme activity in our breast tissue. When the substances that are supposed to be broken down by these enzymes accumulate, they

TABLE 17.9 SOURCES OF CAFFEINE

Item	Portion	Caffeine (mg)
Coffee		
Brewed	6 oz	103–164
Instant	1 tsp	57
Brewed decaf	6 oz	2–5
Instant decaf	1 tsp	2
Tea		
Brewed	6 oz	40–60
Iced	12 oz	70
Caffeinated soft drinks	1 can	30–45
Baking chocolate	1 oz	58
Milk chocolate	1.6 oz	11
Cocoa		
Hot cocoa mix	1 oz	5
Cocoa powder (unsweetened)	1 tbsp	12
Prescription drugs		
Cafergot (for migraine headaches)		100
Fiorinol (for tension headaches)		40
Darvon Compound (pain reliever)		32.4
Over-the-counter drugs		
Anacin and Anacin Maximum Strength		32
Excedrin Extra-Strength		65
Midol		32.4

There are over 100 nonprescription drugs that contain caffeine. These include cold remedies (in which the caffeine counteracts the soporific effect of antihistamines), diet pills, pills to keep us alert, and diuretics. The caffeine content is listed on each medication.

stimulate fibrocystic changes. Studies have shown that daily intake of 30 to 250 milligrams of caffeine (less than our average national dose) increases our risk of fibrocystic breasts (they become lumpy and tender) by

50 percent. With ingestion of more than 500 milligrams, this risk was found to increase 230 percent. Fibrocystic changes scare us; we don't know if we're feeling good or bad lumps. We may undergo more diagnostic tests such as ultrasound, mammography, and even biopsies. No study has equated caffeine consumption with an increased incidence of breast cancer, yet we shouldn't dismiss the caffeine-breast factor because it stimulates "only" benign disease.

Cancer   Good news: We have no credible evidence that implicates caffeine as a cause of cancer.

Fertility and Pregnancy   It may be that coffee decreases our fertility. Two studies have shown that two to three cups of coffee may be enough to more than double our infertility rates. Trying to get pregnant over 40 is hard enough.

Adverse Caffeine Stimulation   Caffeine stimulates more than our general sense of well-being. It affects our temperature control center in our brain and increases hot flashes. It can trigger anxiety and panic attacks by increasing our brain's level of neurotransmitters, raising our pulse and breathing rates, and stimulating release of stress hormones from our adrenal glands. It certainly disturbs our sleep, both our ability to fall asleep and the quality of our sleep. Since caffeine remains in our system for four to seven hours, even a 4:00 P.M. coffee break can affect our 11:00 P.M. bedtime.

Caffeine also "stimulates" our kidneys and bladders in ways that range from annoying (having to void more frequently because of its diuretic effect) to embarrassing (urge incontinence where we don't make it to the toilet).

One more system can be adversely stimulated by caffeine: our GI tract. Caffeine causes an increase in the secretion of acid from the stomach and can cause heartburn and reflux. It also has a laxative effect by increasing intestinal peristalsis and may cause frequent bowel movements or even diarrhea.

Premenstrual Syndrome (PMS)   PMS symptoms have been shown to increase more than 3-fold when we drink three to four cups of coffee a day, and if we go higher (four and a half to eight cups), we're more than eight times as likely to suffer.

ARE WE ADDICTED TO THIS BEVERAGE?

If we're dependent on a substance that affects our psychologic well-being, and if stopping that substance is difficult and causes withdrawal symptoms, then it would be medically reasonable to use the term "addictive" to describe the substance. We may feel that our energy levels are mildly enhanced with small doses of caffeine (20 to 200 milligrams), but higher doses of 200 to 800 milligrams can, like other drug dependencies, cause negative effects such as nervousness and anxiety. Yet, even if we're aware of this problem and want to stop, studies have shown that over 90 percent of us will experience withdrawal and find it difficult to stop. If we consume as little as 100 milligrams per day (one cup of coffee, two cups of tea, or three cans of caffeinated soft drinks), withdrawal symptoms occur if we suddenly quit. These symptoms include moderate to severe headaches, depression, anxiety, drowsiness, and an inability to concentrate. Yes, we're addicted.

SHOULD WE STOP?

Some of us should, if we suffer from palpitations, rapid heartbeat, fibrocystic breast problems, anxiety, panic attacks, PMS, or heartburn. If we have inadequate calcium intake (something we can obviously fix), or are at significant risk for osteoporosis, we probably should consider caffeine abstinence. None of us should be drinking more than three cups of coffee a day.

If we decide to "withdraw" from caffeine, we should do so gradually, mixing caffeinated and decaffeinated coffee, and slowly reduce the amount we drink until we decaffeinate. Or, better yet, eventually substitute water, juices, or even skim milk as our beverage of choice.

18

A WOMAN-CARE CHECKLIST AND HEALTH PLAN

Knowing Our Risks

Living is our ultimate risk for getting sick and dying. But before we get too philosophical about our inevitable mortality (something we're less likely to do when we're healthy and death is theoretical), let's look at the hard-won medical facts. Many of our life-threatening or life-affecting diseases are preventable or curable with early detection.

Like it or not, we are a genetic composite of our ancestors. Superficial similarities such as wispy, fine hair may come from our mother, a dark complexion from our father, and more involved attributes, such as our intelligence, might have come from both of them. But did Aunt Jean's diabetes, Grandma Sarah's stroke, or the heart attacks that killed Grandpa Sam and Uncle Jack contribute to more than our monetary inheritance? The answer is yes.

At the same time, we are more than the macrocosmic expression of our genes. With awareness, information, and the right behavior, we can suppress some genetic predispositions and expose and/or manage others. Much of what happens to us biologically may have no inherited basis. For example, 90 percent of women who develop breast cancer have no family history of this disease. The absence of known "bad" genetic factors does not make us risk-free. How we treated our bodies—those excesses and deficiencies that we ignored the first forty years of our lives and may unfortunately continue to ignore now—represent some of our most important risks.

It is never too late to start taking charge of your health. Below are listed the known major genetic and behavioral risk factors for a number of diseases, as well as lists of other diseases that can lead to them.

TABLE 18.1   DETERMINING YOUR RISK FACTORS

Disease	Inherited Risk Factors	Behavioral Risk Factor	Disease Risk Factor
Heart disease (See chapter 9.)	Family history of premature coronary heart disease (heart attack or sudden death before age 55 years in a father or brother, or before age 65 in a mother or sister)	Smoking Obesity High-fat diet Sedentary lifestyle Lack of estrogen therapy after menopause	Diabetes High blood pressure Hyperlipidemia
	History of a parent or sibling with blood cholesterol greater than 249 mg/dl		
Stroke (See chapter 10.)	Developmental malformations of the vessels	Smoking Obesity High-fat diet Sedentary lifestyle	High blood pressure Hyperlipidemia Atrial fibrillation Atherosclerosis
Cancer (See chapter 12.)			
Lung cancer		Smoking (primary and secondary exposure) Asbestos exposure	Chronic lung diseases

(table continues)

TABLE 18.1 *continued*

Disease	Inherited Risk Factor	Behavioral Risk Factor	Disease Risk Factor
Breast cancer	A first-degree relative (mother or sister) who had premenopausal breast cancer Cancer family syndrome (several family members with cancers of the colon, rectum, ovary, and/or breast) Ethnicity (Ashkenazi Jewish heritage)	Delayed or absent childbearing High-fat diet Obesity Smoking Sedentary lifestyle Alcohol consumption	Previous breast cancer Previous colon or ovarian cancer
Colon or rectal cancer	A first- or second-degree relative with colorectal cancer A family history of familial polyposis (multiple polyps) of the colon Cancer family syndrome (see above)	High-fat diet Sedentary lifestyle	Previous colon polyps or cancer Previous breast or ovarian cancer
Ovarian cancer	One or two first-degree relatives with ovarian cancer Family history of first- and second-degree relatives with breast and ovarian cancers Family history of several cancers, including colorectal, endometrial, and cancer of the upper gastrointestinal tract (gallbladder, pancreas, small bowel)	Absence of childbearing Use of asbestos-containing talcum powder in the vulvar area Long-term use of fertility drugs Smoking High-fat diet	Previous breast or colon cancer

(table continues)

TABLE **18.1** *continued*

Disease	Inherited Risk Factor	Behavioral Risk Factor	Disease Risk Factor
Cervical cancer		High-risk sexual behavior at an early age Exposure to sexually transmitted diseases Smoking DES exposure	Previous cervical dysplasia or cancer Human papillomavirus or herpes infection
Uterine cancer		Obesity Use of unopposed estrogen Use of tamoxifen	History of polycystic ovarian syndrome
Skin cancer	A first-degree relative with melanoma	Sun exposure Smoking	History of precursor lesions (dysplastic nevi or certain congenital nevi) Previous skin cancer
Thyroid cancer	More than one relative (first- or second-degree) with thyroid cancer and/or parathyroid, pituitary, or pancreatic tumors	Radiation of thyroid, neck, or face	History of autoimmune disease
Osteoporosis (See chapter 11.)	A first-degree relative with significant osteoporosis Ethnicity (light-skinned Caucasian or Asian)	Lack of adequate calcium intake Lack of weight-bearing exercise Smoking Excessive alcohol consumption Excessive caffeine consumption Excessive weight loss or exercise with prolonged absence of menstrual periods	Hyperparathyroidism

(table continues)

TABLE 18.1 *continued*

Disease	Inherited Risk Factor	Behavioral Risk Factor	Disease Risk Factor
		Long-term or excessive use of thyroid medications	
		Use of steroids	
Sexually transmitted diseases (See chapter 2.)		Sexual activity; the risk increases with multiple sexual partners or sexual partner with multiple contacts	
		Sexual contacts with culture-proven STDs	
Diabetes	First- or second-degree relative with diabetes	Obesity	Gestational diabetes
	Ethnicity (Native American, Hispanic, or African American)		High blood pressure
			Hyperlipidemia
Thyroid disease (See page 318.) (see also thyroid cancer, above)	First- and second-degree relatives with thyroid disease and autoimmune diseases	Radiation of thyroid, neck, or face	History of autoimmune disease
Alzheimer's disease	One or more relatives who developed Alzheimer's before the age of 65		
Obesity (See chapter 17).	One or more first- and second-degree relatives who have lifelong obesity	High-fat diet	Diabetes
		Sedentary lifestyle	Insulin resistance
			Hypothyroidism
			Polycystic ovarian syndrome
Trauma injuries		Driving without a seat belt	
		Alcohol	
		Using any illicit drugs	
		Abusing prescribed drugs	

The Woman-Care Health Plan

Once we've truthfully compiled our individual list of genetic, behavioral, and disease-associated risks, we can formulate a program of woman-care screening after the age of 40. The general program applies to all of us, but we need to have special tests or increase the frequency of regular tests in the categories in which we have been labeled (not branded, since we can do something about this) "at risk." The following chart is a compilation of recommendations by the American College of Obstetricians and Gynecologists, the American Heart Association, the American Medical Association, and the American Cancer Society, as well as my own recommendations. The institutions looked at large populations and factored in cost-benefit ratios. My ratio to my patients is one-to-one, and I tend to err on the side of maximum rather than minimal testing.

This schedule is our "ideal" basis for screening and early detection of health problems and diseases. We may need more (depending on our development of symptoms and illnesses), but we shouldn't look for excuses to do less. A note from home or an "A" in behavior is not going to "get us off." The ultimate medical authority figure is not our physician; she or he can only advise. The one in charge of making decisions and taking action is you, me, and every woman who wants to become more than a passive being in the human life cycle.

TABLE 18.2 WOMAN CARE OVER 40: SCHEDULE OF EXAMINATIONS AND TESTS

Examination/ Test/Procedure	All ages over 40	40 to 49	50 to 64	65 and over	High Risk at Any Age
Full Physical Examination	Every year				Every year, or at patient and physican discretion
Height; weight; blood pressure; mouth, throat, neck glands; thyroid and large vessels; breasts, axillae; abdomen; pelvic and rectal exam; skin; extremities; pulses; neurological					
Blood					
Cholesterol lipid panel	Every 3 to 5 years if first reading is normal			Every 1 to 3 years	Every 1 to 3 years
CBC (complete blood count)				Every year	Every year if history or symptoms of anemia
Fasting blood glucose					Every year if at risk for diabetes
Cardiovascular					
ECG (electrocardiogram)	Baseline at 40	Every 5 years if at low risk			Every year if at high risk
Stress ECG	Baseline at 40				Every 3 years if at high risk and/or Immediately after onset of angina

(table continues)

TABLE 18.2 continued

Examination/Test/Procedure	All ages over 40	40 to 49	50 to 64	65 and over	High Risk at Any Age
Chest X ray					Every year for smokers
					At physician and patient discretion for nonsmokers
Colorectal					
Fecal occult blood test	Every year				
Sigmoidoscopy			Every 3 to 5 years after 50		
Colonoscopy					Every 3 years if high risk for colon cancer; begin at 35 if 1st- or 2nd-degree relative had colon cancer before age 55
					After positive fecal occult blood test
Gynecological					
Pap test	Every 3 years if 3 consecutive tests are normal More frequently at physician and patient discretion				Every year if at risk for cervical cancer

(table continues)

TABLE 18.2 continued

Examination/ Test/Procedure	All ages over 40	40 to 49	50 to 64	65 and over	High Risk at Any Age
STD (sexually transmitted disease) testing					Cervical cultures (GC, chlamydia) and blood VDRL and HIV if at risk
					Couple HIV testing before and 6 months after starting new relationship
Pelvic ultrasound					Post menopausal bleeding if not on HRT
					Pelvic mass of unknown origin
					At physician and patient discretion after menopause if on HRT and/or at risk for ovarian cancer
Breast					
Mammogram		Every 1 to 2 years	Every year	Every year	
Breast ultrasound					Palpable mass or questionable finding on mammogram
Breast MRI (magnetic resonance imaging)					As possible adjunct to mammogram if very high risk
					As possible adjunct to suspicious mammogram prior to surgery

(table continues)

TABLE 18.2 continued

Examination/ Test/Procedure	All ages over 40	40 to 49	50 to 64	65 and over	High Risk at Any Age
Bone					
Bone-density scan					Baseline during perimenopause or menopause if high risk for osteoporosis, or if question use of HRT
					Every 2 to 3 years after menopause if not on HRT or high risk
					Every 2 years if on therapy for significant osteoporosis
Thyroid					
TSH (thyroid-stimulating hormone) (indicator of thyroid function)				Every 3 to 5 years	Begin testing after 40 if high risk, have symptoms, or at physician and patient discretion
Other Tests					
Urinalysis (dipstick) (check for blood, white cells, protein, and sugar)			Every year	Every year	Every year if high risk for diabetes, infections, kidney stones
CA-125					At physician and patient discretion after menopause
					Every year after menopause if high risk for ovarian cancer

19

WEAR, NOT TEAR
A Personal Odyssey

I've spent the last year and a half writing this book. During that time, I completed more than the book; I ended my personal odyssey through the fifth decade and started my sixth. At my fiftieth birthday party, a friend of mine declared that we had now entered the age of stuttering (not doddering), and when asked our age, the understandable response was "fif-fif-fif" (*-ty* being a very difficult syllable to roll off of our tongues). Well, my birthday has not left me tongue-tied, I'm 50 (one word) and feel much too young to get old.

Obviously, I can't stop the clock, but I can do the '90s thing and become "pro-active." I love that term; the antonym must be "anti-active," which, of course, has not gained wide usage. I thought I had good health habits before I began my book, but in doing the research, especially for chapter 17, I discovered that I was due for some woman-care reevaluation.

I grew up in the 1950s and 1960s and was fed what was then considered a healthy, nutritious diet: red meat nearly every day, egg sandwiches for lunch, and lots of whole milk. In the summers we went to the North Jersey beaches, where I baked in the sun. There's a lot wrong with this picture of my youth, but I remember it (especially the beach) with tremendous nostalgia. I wonder if I would have such fond memories of a fish-and-vegetable diet and constraint under a sun umbrella. It's astounding how our health values have changed in just three decades. We thought we knew it all then and, of course, we're sure we know it all now.

On the positive side of my medical past, I initially trained to be a ballet dancer. That meant up to three hours of strenuous exercise daily, lack of breast development (my daughters overtook my bra size when they purchased their first training bras), and low body fat. We now know that this helps protect against future breast cancer and obesity. I didn't become a professional ballet dancer. The choice was made for me, not by me—my second toe projects beyond my first (a "no-no" for point shoes), my torso is too long, I grew to be too tall, and, most disappointingly, Balanchine didn't notice me. At 16, my body had failed me, so I decided to develop my mind.

I attended Barnard College, where I promptly discovered starches and fat in the cafeteria and put on 10 pounds. I tried to smoke, but thankfully, like Clinton, could never master the art of inhalation. I tried to drink and even proclaimed a fondness for scotch and soda (I'm sure I never liked it; I certainly don't now). I didn't know that binge drinking can cause a sudden elevation of blood pressure and stroke, or that a state of semiconscious inebriation can lead to aspiration of one's own vomit. After attempting to gulp down a bottle of ouzo (a strong licorice alcoholic beverage) in a Greek club on my way to my junior year abroad, I passed out and had to be carried back to our ship. My body was smarter than I, and the resultant hangover convinced me that drinking to get drunk was sickening. I and my friends didn't know about our special female susceptibility to alcohol.

The only things I exercised after my second year of college were my mind and my mouth. My skeletal muscles were never taxed; it seemed much more important to sit with my dorm mates (on our ever-expanding rears) and discuss the problems of life and death. Health was always evaluated in global terms—the health of the universe, civilization, and the Western world. Our own was too "micro" and, anyway, we took it for granted. Even though health care did not interest me, biology did, and I loftily proclaimed that if I was going to study about life, I would "go for" the most complex and interesting form of life: human beings. I would study medicine. Being a progressive women's college, Barnard had something to do with this choice. My advisors pushed me to apply to medical school; women were not being admitted in large numbers, and my generation, or at least my class, was expected to redress this imbalance.

I got married several months before I started medical school, to a dashing Israeli law student whom I had met during my junior year abroad. When I first saw him, he was wearing a paratrooper uniform and a red beret, and carried an Uzi submachine gun, a far cry from the college students I had dated. It was awe at first sight. Once we were married and "nesting," the cleaning and cooking fell under my jurisdiction (this was the '60s). We ate the fastest food I could make—a lot of fried eggs and meat—and fresh fruit and vegetables were rarely included. The milk in the refrigerator was used to lighten our coffee. The minute we visited his family, we were plied with cakes and cookies, a sign of love, and a need to stuff some home-cooked food into us—the "poor" students (I'm not sure if poor had to do with our financial status or the status of my cooking). I was far too busy in medical school learning about diseases to consider health. My diet was high in fat and protein, and my calcium sources were scarce. I never looked at a vitamin pill; they were for the "malnourished" (I considered only diseases such as rickets and scurvy worthy of vitamin and calcium supplementation). My only exercise was walking through the corridors of medical school and an occasional attempt at housework.

When I was 24, my husband and I decided to have a child. It took me six months to get pregnant, and I began to worry that my fertility was impaired. Once pregnant, I vomited for three months, lost considerable weight, and got pneumonia. Even this did not convince me that I and my body couldn't do it all, though I did make an effort to eat better, drink milk, and take prenatal vitamins. I marveled at the miracle of the life within me and anticipated my newborn child with a maternal love that was overwhelming. I was also overwhelmed with studies and exams. I delivered my daughter several days after I took my pathology test. Labor was far more difficult than any medical school exam! But I achieved the most important "grade" of my life—a healthy baby. Once she was born, I reverted to inconsistent nutrition, except where my daughter was concerned. I refused to give her prepared baby food and cooked and blended everything she ate from scratch. At least one of us was eating well!

Trying to raise a child and finish medical school (and, later, my internship and residency) was a strength-sapping effort for all of us. My daughter is now 27 and has become a wonderful, beautiful, and sensitive woman, despite some very inconsistent past "mommying" on my part. She writes, produces, and directs television shows, video magazines, and commercials. She works twelve to fourteen hours a day and thinks her body is invincible. It's ironic that I've become a woman-care advocate, but have little influence on her health habits! My mother, however, seems more receptive to my proffered advice!

Once I finished my internship, we moved to Chicago, where I did my residency in obstetrics and gynecology. Medical training offers an extraordinary opportunity to abuse one's health. As residents we worked thirteen-hour days and were on duty twenty-four hours every three days. Believe me, being on call interrupts REM sleep more violently than any hot flashes. At night, the hospital (a major *health* facility) gave us free vouchers so we could descend to its bowels, find a huge woman sweating over a grill, and order one of two choices: a cheeseburger swimming in fat or hot dogs, plus the ubiquitous fries. While I was on my obstetric rotation, I worked from 7:00 P.M. to 7:00 A.M., and this became my nightly fare. I drank coffee and Coke to keep going, saw no sun (well, it was Chicago in the winter), and, when I did have meals with my family, grabbed fried chicken on the way home. I was too tired to cook. But, oh, the babies I delivered, the diseases I helped cure, and the surgeries I learned to perform. It was a glorious three years!

The one pill I took religiously during my residency was my birth control pill. I was the only female resident in my year and was certainly the only one with a child. Another pregnancy was out of the question. After one and a half years of training, I "scrubbed in" (meaning I assisted) on a five-hour case, which had me standing immobile while my senior attending took forever to perform a hysterectomy. I limped out of the OR and soon discovered I had a clot in my leg. Within hours, I was a patient, in a bed in my own hospital, having heparin (a blood thinner) run through my veins. Everyone blamed the Pill and declared I could never take estrogen again. So, I dutifully had an IUD inserted and continued my training.

We returned to Israel in 1975. I was now a grown-up doctor, supposedly well versed in medical practice. But my personal health care was far from exemplary. The quality of the food we ate improved; we had regular dinners replete with vegetables or salad. I was on call just once a week and could actually complete a dream most nights. I wanted to wear a bathing suit in the summer, so I made sure I didn't gain weight. We did bask in the Mediterranean sun. My exercise was standing in the OR and making rounds with the residents. I was in my thirties and still oblivious to my personal health.

At 32, after having my IUD removed to relieve heavy crampy periods, I got pregnant again. I didn't want my colleagues to know, but I think they suspected something when I demanded that they stop smoking during our morning conferences. We still didn't have much data on secondary smoke, but it made me feel queasy. I planned to publicly reveal my pregnancy (or it would reveal itself) when I returned from an upcoming European vacation, so I smugly followed my own pregnancy with self-administered ultrasounds at 8 and 16 weeks. The second ultrasound showed my fetus and her heartbeat, but to my horror, I also discovered a large tumor adjacent to my uterus. After undergoing a more complete ultrasound and a pelvic exam, the large tumor was verified. A diagnosis of possible ovarian cancer was made. After years of loftily being the expert treating other women's diseases, I became a fearful patient who realized that health (even in our thirties) cannot be taken for granted. I didn't want the department chief and my residents performing surgery on me; our relationship was too close. So I flew back to the University of Chicago and assembled a team of cancer surgeons and obstetricians. I was put to sleep, not knowing if I would awaken to learn that I had cancer or would still be carrying my baby. I've never been more scared or more aware of the power of physicians. I awoke with my pregnancy intact and the wonderful news that the tumor was a benign fibroid, which was removed. But I had to make a postoperative recovery amid premature contractions. I hated my vulnerability as a patient, lying in a hospital bed, dependent on others for my care.

After four months of bed rest and prolonged use of new drugs to prevent premature labor, I gave birth to my second daughter. Her delivery was a miracle, and I felt blessed and humbled for years. Now 17 and a teenager, she's combating the world and trying to establish her identity. Being around her continues to be humbling in other ways as I ask myself, "Who is this beguiling, awesome young person that I brought into the world and love so much?" Like her older sister, she is oblivious to any connection between health habits and physical well-being. I cajole her to take vitamins and calcium, and she reluctantly does so (when at home) to humor me. Vegetables became unnecessary when she passed puberty, and diet cola is her beverage of choice. She has to spend the next six to eight years getting an education, avoiding the rites of excess and abuse offered to our youth (smoking, alcohol, and drugs), staying slim, establishing sexual relationships, protecting herself from sexually transmitted diseases, and learning how to be a responsible citizen in cyberspace. Oh, and yes, hopefully she will establish better health-care habits. As she pointed out to me, it's easier to stay young than to be young.

We came to Los Angeles when I was 35, ostensibly to spend two years on sabbatical. The academic job I had been promised had been incorrectly described, and funding was not available. I decided to rent space in another doctor's office and see patients privately for the next two years. I, who had run departments and supervised residents, began to treat women on a one-to-one basis. I loved it! For the first time, I had an opportunity to talk to them, find out about their lives, and see how other women managed their professional and personal problems. All of this while taking care of their obstetrical and gynecologic health. In developing long-term relationships with my patients, I learned about health care with an emphasis on "care."

Meanwhile, my marriage was stagnating; we grew away from each other. We had married when we were too young to contemplate being old as a married couple. After a year of intense self-examination and questioning (with the help of a trained psychoanalyst), I ended my fifteen-year marriage. I was a single mother with two children, a solo practice, and a large mortgage (to prove my independence, I bought a house). I had made a wrenching move to obtain mental health; I now began to care about my physical health. I took multivitamins, and I started exercising two to three times a week. First, I tried jogging and ran up to three miles a day. But after I fell in the street, scraping huge amounts of skin off my knees and elbows, I decided that outdoor running was dangerous. I biked and took tennis lessons. I changed our eating habits and made sure we ate fresh fruit and salad daily. I also started to dye the gray out of my hair.

At thirty-nine, I met a wonderful man who in many ways is my antithesis. I, a surgeon, found happiness with a highly creative man who is a movie director and producer. He's also an educator and, as a dean at UCLA, he is helping to mold our next generation of filmmakers. He's been the best thing for my health. There is no question that love and good sex help keep us young. I remarried at the age of 41.

A new impetus in my personal odyssey of woman care was the writing of this book. Researching the latest information on contraception, infertility, menopause, hormones, and diseases was easy; that's what I've been doing for the last twenty years. But I also read articles on nutrition, searched for scientific evidence about vitamins, sought information on fitness and exercise, and read everything I could on aging. The results of this quest will, hopefully, be evident in what I've written. They have most assuredly affected my personal health habits. So here's what I currently do . . .

I have valid concerns about my genetic propensity for cancer. My mother was diagnosed with early breast cancer (by mammogram) at the age of 46. She had radical surgery and, twenty-five years later, is fine. My grandfather had stomach cancer, my grandmother bladder cancer, and a great-uncle colon cancer. I stopped eating red meat seven years ago in hopes that this would reduce my chances for cancer, especially colon cancer. This also allowed me to easily lose eight pounds. I try to restrict my fat intake to less than 20 percent; that means no fried foods, cream sauces, or butter. If I want something sweet, I eat nonfat frozen yogurt. Dessert is fresh fruit; I snack on dried fruit. I've luckily developed a real liking for vegetables (which I hated as a growing child), and we have fresh steamed vegetables and salad with every dinner. When I learned how important fiber was, I went out and purchased All-Bran and started eating a cupful every morning. I then spent an inordinate amount of time running to the bathroom. I cut down, but try to get my 25-gram daily fiber allotment through cereal or fiber-rich breads in the morning, a daily portion of beans, and lots of fruits and vegetables.

I've stopped drinking wine. I'm concerned about the possible connection between alcohol intake and the risk of breast cancer. When I learned about the connection between soy and breast cancer protection, I ran to my health food store and bought everything that had soy in it. I admit I'm not crazy about soy milk, and can't always add tofu to my food, but I do boil soybeans and snack on them.

I take a multivitamin supplement, 600 milligrams of calcium, 400 units of vitamin E, and 1,000 milligrams of slow-release C. I'm sure I need the calcium and D. My attitude about the antioxidants is a cross between hoping they will work and being certain they won't hurt. I don't want to look back with vitamin regret when we know more (I hope) in twenty years.

During stressful periods in my life (divorce, moving, child rearing, and changing medical associates), I developed heart palpitations. They felt like inner hiccups as the steady pulse I had always taken for granted began to skip beats. Being a physician, I assumed I had a rare form of cardiac disease and, after a complete workup with ultrasound, EKG, treadmill, and a twenty-four-hour heart monitor, was told it was nothing (and probably due to stress). I diminished my caffeine consumption and noticed two things: My breasts became less lumpy and my heart rate regular. Over the past two years, I have virtually stopped caffeine. If I have a cup of something, it's always decaf, and I don't drink more than one a day.

I had my bone density checked two years ago. I already had an 11 percent bone loss in my hip (all these years of low calcium intake probably did it). My mother also has moderate osteoporosis. So I have attempted to increase my dairy consumption with nonfat yogurt and cottage cheese, and supplement 600 milligrams of calcium carbonate a day. I'm also diligent in doing weight-bearing and weight-resistance exercise.

The evidence that exercise and fitness prevent many of the consequences of aging is overwhelming. Once I discovered that we need at least thirty minutes of daily exercise to keep fit, I changed my exercise program. I now go to a gym twice a week after work. I get onto the treadmill and run two minutes and walk a minute, increasing the pace until I get to seven miles an hour. I do this for twenty or thirty minutes, and then spend an additional thirty minutes using the gym's weight-resistance machines for upper and lower body. Most other days of the week (if we don't have to go out to an early dinner), I get onto our treadmill at home and do a cardiovascular program for thirty minutes while I watch the evening news. Twice a week, I spend an additional twenty minutes pushing and pulling on my seven-pound dumbbells and my two-and-a-half-pound leg weights. I hate it; it's boring, I don't like to sweat, and my muscles ache. But I've found that over the last year, I have felt better and healthier than ever (and very virtuous). If I stop for a week, I begin to lose this sense of well-being; I don't sleep as well and feel tired. I then go through a mental effort to get myself to resume "the program"; guilt helps. I have achieved a small degree of what the trainers call muscle definition (in certain flexed positions, you can see the outline of my muscles). It's great to be 50 and see muscles I lost in my thirties. More important, I'm convinced that one of the reasons we gain weight is that we lose muscle and replace it with fat. I'm doing my best not to lose this muscle. A total of four to five hours a week doesn't seem too great a sacrifice to make for this goal.

These last few paragraphs make me sound like an intolerable "Ms. Goody Two-Shoes." I'm not; I cheat. At the first sign of a sniffle, swollen gland, or sore throat, I stop exercising, excusing myself from my routine of health because I might be getting sick. If we're going out, I'm delighted to cancel my before-dinner workout. Even if I have the time, I don't want to sweat and have to deal with my curly hair.

If I'm a guest and dinner includes foods that are not low-fat, I eat them, telling myself that it would be impolite not to do so (although I draw the line with red meat, which I politely refuse). In restaurants, I try to order wisely and can drive waiters crazy. I also drive my companions crazy; I have what I call a long-fork syndrome and will eagerly try all the "improper" foods and desserts they, especially my husband, have ordered. I have a basic belief that the calories and fat I eat from someone else's plate don't count! One last confession: There are days when I just don't get down my allotted fiber; I get tired of chewing the stuff!

The topics of nutrition, exercise, and vitamins now enter all of my conversations with patients. Some ask what I do, and I'm happy to tell them (I usually don't admit to the cheating part). But the aspect of my personal health care that interests them the most is whether I take hormones.

When I turned 47, I began to have irregular, heavy, and crampy periods. My PMS got worse. It was then that I pulled out my IUD (actually, I had a colleague do it), tried every PMS product around, and continued to suffer. My hormone levels "tested" normal, but I felt far from normal. I decided to go on a low-dose birth control pill, despite previous admonitions not to take estrogen. I've never felt better. My cycles are regular, my cramps are gone, and my PMS has practically disappeared. I also feel I'm protecting my bones, skin, and vaginal health from the consequences of lowered estrogen in my perimenopause. I've already gone through an ovarian cancer scare; the thought that I'm decreasing the risk of this disease with the Pill cheers me as I pop it. Although I'm at risk for breast cancer, there are no data that taking the Pill in our forties or fifties increases our risk. I check my FSH levels every six months (on my Pill-free week); the level is still below 20, so I'm not yet menopausal. I'll continue these pills as long as my readings "hold." My only complaint is the night sweats I develop on my week off the birth control pill. If they're any indication of how I'll perspire or flush when I'm truly menopausal, I know I'm in for a wet time.

This, however, is not the chief factor that will affect my personal decision about hormone replacement in the menopause. My review of the literature and my experience in treating thousands of women during and after this hormonal transition have made me decide that the positives outweigh the negatives. I've looked at osteoporosis, heart disease, stroke, Alzheimer's, poor vaginal health, and diminished quality of life with respect to my being, and have decided that I will do what I can to "be" without them. I plan to use hormone replacement therapy, cyclically at first, and then continuously after a few years (periods are not something I need to make me feel young). I am concerned about breast cancer, but I have (perhaps incorrectly) rationalized that my risk is not too great: I am thin, exercise, eat a low-fat diet, don't drink or smoke, and take after my father. So I'm willing to monitor my breasts while I maintain my hormone levels.

I am no longer a sandler in need of shoes. I go through all of the tests I recommend for my patients. I have yearly mammograms and have done so since age 40. I've even had a breast MRI to see what it's like and also to ascertain if a better picture can be achieved of my small, dense breasts. I do yearly tests for occult blood in my stool; I've had a sigmoid-oscopy (it wasn't bad at all) and plan to do it every three years. A dermatologist looks at my skin. I check my cholesterol, blood count, urine, and thyroid function. I've had EKGs, treadmill stress tests, and chest X rays. I grab one of the other doctors in my office to do a Pap smear and monitor my fibroids. I go to the dentist twice a year.

As I write all of this, it seems like a lot, but as I go about my day-to-day living, it doesn't feel that way. Finally becoming involved in my health in a pro-active fashion (there's that word again) has given me a sense of personal fulfillment; I have taken charge. Whatever my genetic destiny, I'll always know that at least after 40, I worked to get the most I could out of it. I will not go passively (or silently) through middle and late age. I will burst through the decades to come with a sense of excitement, adventure, and control over my well-being. You and I and the women of our generation are too young to get old.

The Middle
(never The End)

Suggested Reading and Resources

Books

Alternative Therapy

Lockie, Dr. Andrew. *The Family Guide to Homeopathy* (New York: Fireside, 1989).

Nowry, Daniel B. *The Scientific Validation of Herbal Medicine* (New Canaan, CT: Keats Publishing, 1986).

Cancer

Love, Susan, M.D., with Karen Lindsey. *Dr. Susan Love's Breast Book*, rev. ed. (New York: Addison-Wesley, 1995).

Nixon, Daniel W., M.D. *The Cancer Recovery Eating Plan* (New York: Times Books, 1996).

Runowicz, Carolyn D., M.D., and Donna Haupt. *To Be Alive: A Woman's Guide to a Full Life After Cancer* (New York: Henry Holt and Company, 1995).

Siegel, Bernie. *Love, Medicine, and Miracles* (New York: HarperCollins, 1990).

Spiegel, David, M.D. *Living Beyond Limits* (New York: Times Books, 1993).

Contraception

Harlap, S., K. Kost, and J. D. Forrest. *Preventing Pregnancy, Protecting Health* (New York: Alan Guttmacher Institute, 1991).

Fertility

Berger, Gary S., M.D., Mark Goldstein, M.D., and Mark Fuerst. *The Couples' Guide to Infertility* (New York: Doubleday, 1995).

Corson, Stephen L., M.D. *Conquering Infertility: A Guide for Couples*, rev. ed. (Englewood Cliffs, NJ: Prentice-Hall/Simon and Schuster, 1991).

Silber, Sherman J., M.D. *How to Get Pregnant* (New York: Warner Books, 1990).

General Interest

American Heart Association and American Cancer Society. *Living Well, Staying Well* (New York: Times Books, 1996).

American Medical Association; Charles B. Clayman, medical ed. *American Medical Association Family Medical Guide, 3d ed.* (New York: Random House, 1994).

American Medical Association. *American Medical Association Guide to Your Family's Symptoms* (New York: Random House, 1993).

The American Medical Women's Association. *The Women's Complete Health Book* (New York: Delacorte Press, 1995).

Larson, David E., ed. *Mayo Clinic Family Health Book* (New York: William Morrow, 1990).

Heart Disease

Diethrich, Edward, and Carol Cohan. *Women and Heart Disease* (New York: Times Books, 1992).

Ornish, Dean, M.D. *Dr. Dean Ornish's Program for Reversing Heart Disease* (New York: Ballantine Books, 1992).

Williams, Redford, M.D., and Virginia Williams. *Anger Kills* (New York: Times Books, 1993).

Williams, Redford, M.D. *The Trusting Heart* (New York: Times Books, 1989).

Menopause

Schiff, Isaac, M.D., with Ann Parson. *Menopause: The Massachusetts General Hospital Guide* (New York: Times Books, 1996).

Sheehy, Gail. *The Silent Passage* (New York: Random House, 1992).

Mental Health

Kass, Frederick T., M.D., John M. Oldman, M.D., Herbert Pardes, M.D., editorial director, and Lois B. Morris, eds. *The Columbia University College of Physicians and Surgeons Complete Home Guide to Mental Health* (New York: Henry Holt and Company, 1992).

Kramer, Peter D., M.D. *Listening to Prozac* (New York: Viking, 1993).

Nutrition

American Heart Association. *American Heart Association Brand Name Fat & Cholesterol Counter, 2d ed.* (New York: Times Books, 1995).

American Heart Association. *American Heart Association Cookbook, 5th ed.*, new and revised (New York: Times Books, 1991).

American Heart Association. *American Heart Association Low-Fat, Low-Cholesterol Cookbook* (New York: Times Books, 1995).

American Heart Association. *American Heart Association Low-Salt Cookbook* (New York: Times Books, 1995).

American Heart Association. *American Heart Association Quick and Easy Cookbook* (New York: Times Books, 1995).

Brody, Jane. *Jane Brody's Nutrition Book* (New York: Bantam Books, 1987).

Dunne, Lavon J. *Nutrition Almanac*, 3d ed. (New York: McGraw-Hill, 1990).

Wotecki, Catherine E., and P. T. Thomas, eds. *Eat for Life: The Food and Nutrition Board's Guide to Reducing Your Risk of Chronic Disease* (New York: HarperPerennial, 1993).

Osteoporosis

American Medical Association. *American Medical Association Pocket Guide to Calcium* (New York: Random House, 1995).

Pregnancy

Cherry, Sheldon, M.D. *Understanding Pregnancy and Childbirth* (New York: Maxwell Macmillan International, 1992).

Eisenberg, Arlene, Heidi E. Murkoff, and Sandee E. Hathaway. *What to Expect When You're Expecting* (New York: Workman Publishing, 1991).

Luke, Barbara. *Every Pregnant Woman's Guide to Preventing Premature Birth* (New York: Times Books, 1995).

Stroke

American Heart Association. *American Heart Association Family Guide to Stroke* (New York: Times Books, 1994).

Ancowitz, Arthur, M.D. *The Stroke Book: One-on-One Advice About Stroke Prevention, Management and Rehabilitation* (New York: William Morrow and Company, 1993).

Sexuality

Janus, Samuel S., and Cynthia L. Janus, M.D. *The Janus Report on Sexual Behavior* (New York: John Wiley and Sons, 1993).

Masters, William H., Virginia E. Johnson, and Robert Kolondy. *Masters and Johnson on Sex and Human Loving* (New York: Little, Brown and Company, 1986).

Michael, Robert T., John H. Gagnon, Edward O. Laumann, and Gina Kolata. *Sex in America: A Definitive Survey* (Boston: Little, Brown and Company, 1994).

Rosenthal, Saul H., M.D. *Sex over 40* (New York: Tarcher, Putnam, 1987).

Surgery

Harris, Dena E., M.D., and Helene MacLean. *Recovering from a Hysterectomy* (New York: HarperCollins, 1992).

Resources for Additional Information

Aging

Alzheimer's Association
919 North Michigan Avenue,
    Suite 1000
Chicago, IL 60611
(312)355-8700 or (800)272-3900

**American Association for Retired
    Persons**
601 E Street, NW
Washington, DC 20024
(202)434-2277

National Council on the Aging
409 Third Street, SW, 2nd Floor
Washington, DC 20024
(800)424-9046

**National Institutes of Health
    National Institute of Aging**
900 Rockville Pike
Bethesda, MD 20892
(800)222-2225

Autoimmune ("Our") Diseases

American Diabetes Association
1660 Duke Street
Alexandria, VA 22314
(703)232-3472 or (800)ADA-DISC

American Lupus Society
3914 Del Amo Boulevard, #922
Torrance, CA 90503
(310)542-8891

Arthritis Foundation
P.O. Box 19000
Atlanta, GA 30326
(404)872-7100 or (800)283-7800

**National Institutes of Health
National Institute of Diabetes and
    Digestive and Kidney Diseases**
900 Rockville Pike
Bethesda, MD 20892
(301)496-5877

Cancer

American Academy of Dermatology
P.O. Box 4014
Schaumberg, IL 60168
(708)330-0230

American Cancer Society
1599 Clifton Road NE
Atlanta, GA 30329
(404)325-2217 or (800)ACS-2345

**American Gastroenterological
    Association**
7910 Woodmont Avenue
Bethesda, MD 20814
(301)654-2055

American Lung Association
1740 Broadway
New York, NY 10019
(212)315-8700

National Cancer Institute
Bethesda, MD 20205
(301)496-5583 or (800)4-CANCER

Society of Gynecologic Oncologists
401 North Michigan Avenue
Chicago, IL 60611
(312) 644-6610

Diet and Nutrition

American Dietetic Association
216 West Jackson Boulevard, Suite 800
Chicago, IL 60606
(312)899-0040

Food and Drug Administration
5600 Fishers Lane
Rockville, MD 20857
(301)443-2410

**Human Nutrition Information Service
U.S. Department of Agriculture**
Hyattsville, MD 20782
(301)436-7725

Exercise

American College of Sports Medicine
P.O. Box 1440
Indianapolis, IN 46202
(317)637-9200

Fertility and Pregnancy

The Alan Guttmacher Institute
111 Fifth Avenue
New York, NY 10003
(212)254-5656

American College of Obstetrics and Gynecology
409 12th Street, NW
Washington, DC 20024
(800)673-8444 or (202)638-5577

American Fertility Society
1209 Montgomery Highway
Birmingham, AL 35216
(205)978-5000

National Center for Education in Maternal and Child Health
2000 15th Street North, Suite 701
Arlington, VA 22201
(703)524-7802

General

American Medical Association
515 North State Street
Chicago, IL 60610
(800)262-3211 or (312)464-5000

National Health Information Center
(800)336-4797

**National Institutes of Health
National Institute of Child Health and Human Development**
Building 31, Room 2A03
9000 Rockville Pike
Bethesda, MD 20892
(301)496-5133

**National Institutes of Health
Office of Alternative Medicine (OAM)**
6120 Executive Boulevard
Executive Plaza South, Suite 450
Rockville, MD 20892
(301)402-2466

**National Institutes of Health
Office of Research on Women's Health**
Building 1, Room 201
9000 Rockville Pike
Bethesda, MD 20892
(301)402-1770

**National Institutes of Health
Women's Health Initiative**
Federal Building, Room 6A09
9000 Rockville Pike
Bethesda, MD 20892
(800)54-WOMEN

National Medical Association
1012 12th Street, NW
Washington, DC 20001
(202)347-1895

Heart Disease

American College of Cardiology
9111 Old Georgetown Road
Bethesda, MD 20814
(301)897-5400

American Heart Association
7320 Greenville Avenue
Dallas, TX 75231
(214)373-6300 or (800)AHA-USA1

**National Institutes of Health
National Heart, Lung and Blood Institute**
4733 Bethesda Avenue, Suite 530
Bethesda, MD 20814
(301)951-3260

Medication

American Pharmaceutical Association
2215 Constitution Avenue, NW
Washington, DC 20037
(202)628-4410 or (800)237-APHA

Food and Drug Administration
8800 Rockville Pike
Bethesda, MD 20852
(301)295-8228

Menopause

North American Menopause Society
4074 Abington Road
Cleveland, OH 44106
(216)844-3334

Mental Health

American Psychiatric Association
1400 K Street, NW
Washington, DC 20005
(202)682-6000

American Psychological Association
750 First Street, NW
Washington, DC 20002
(202)336-5500

National Institute of Mental Health
5600 Fishers Lane, Room 15C-05
Rockville, MD 20857
(301)443-4513

Osteoporosis

National Institute on Aging Information Center
P.O. Box 8057
Gaithersburg, MD 20898
(301)496-1752

National Osteoporosis Foundation
2100 M Street, NW
Washington, DC 20037
(202)223-3336

Sexuality

American Association of Sex Educators, Counselors and Therapists
435 Michigan Avenue, Suite 1717
Chicago, IL 60611
(312)644-0828

Council for Sex Information and Education
2272 Colorado Boulevard, No. 1228
Los Angeles, CA 90041

Sexually Transmitted Diseases

Centers for Disease Control and Prevention (CDC)
Division of STD Prevention
1600 Clifton Road, NE
Atlanta, GA 30333
(404)639-3311

CDC National AIDS Hotline
(800)342-AIDS

CDC National Sexually Transmitted Disease Hotline
(800)227-8922

Stroke (see also Heart Disease Resources)

American Physical Therapy Association
1111 N. Fairfax Street
Alexandria, VA 22314
(703)684-2782

National Institutes of Health
National Institute of Neurological Disorders and Stroke (NINDS)
Building 31, Room 8A54
9000 Rockville Pike
Bethesda, MD 20892
(800)352-9424 or (301)496-5751

National Stroke Association
300 East Hampden Avenue
Englewood, CO 80110
(800)367-1990 or (303)771-1700

Urinary Incontinence

American Urological Association
1120 North Charles Street
Baltimore, MD 21201
(410)727-1100

Help for Incontinent People (HIP)
P.O. Box 544
Union, SC 29379
(803)579-7900 or (800)BLADDER

The Simon Foundation for Continence
P.O. Box 835
Wilmette, IL 60091
(800)23-SIMON

Index

····················

ABOUT THE AUTHOR

JUDITH REICHMAN, M.D., is a gynecologist in private practice at Cedars-Sinai Medical Center in Los Angeles and an associate clinical professor at UCLA. Dr. Reichman has been actively involved in the health education of women. She has appeared as medical consultant on the television programs *Woman to Woman* and *Group One Medical*, as well as *The Home Show*, *Hour Magazine*, and network news. Dr. Reichman recently wrote and hosted the two-part series on PBS titled *Straight Talk on Menopause*.